Formulation, Characterization and Systems of Drug Delivery

Formulation, Characterization and Systems of Drug Delivery

Editor: Joy Bartlett

AMERICAN
MEDICAL PUBLISHERS
www.americanmedicalpublishers.com

AMERICAN
MEDICAL PUBLISHERS
www.americanmedicalpublishers.com

Cataloging-in-Publication Data

Formulation, characterization and systems of drug delivery / edited by Joy Bartlett.
p. cm.
Includes bibliographical references and index.
ISBN 979-8-88740-072-3
1. Drug delivery systems. 2. Drugs--Administration. 3. Drugs--Dosage forms. 4. Pharmaceutical technology.
5. Biomedical engineering. 6. Pharmaceutical chemistry. I. Bartlett, Joy.
RS199.5 .F67 2023
615.6--dc23

American Medical Publishers,
41 Flatbush Avenue,
1st Floor, New York,
NY 11217, USA

ISBN 979-8-88740-072-3 (Hardback)

Contents

Preface

Drug delivery is the method of administering a pharmaceutical compound to achieve a desired therapeutic effect in humans or animals. The principles associated with the route of administration, drug preparation, metabolism, site-specific targeting, and toxicity are used in the process of drug delivery. The primary focus of these principles is to optimize safety and efficacy in order to improve a patient's convenience and compliance. The systems of drug delivery are characterized by the transportation of drug directly to the site, while avoiding non-diseased tissue. The recent developments in drug delivery systems include several topics such as controlled-release formulations, targeted delivery, nanomedicine, drug carriers, 3D printing, and the delivery of biologic drugs. Controlled or modified-release formulations have the potential to alter the timing and rate at which a drug is liberated. This further helps to produce adequate or sustained drug concentrations. This book provides significant information to help develop a good understanding of drug delivery. It aims to shed light on some of the unexplored aspects and the recent researches on the formulation, characterization and systems of drug delivery. The extensive content of this book provides the readers with a thorough understanding of the subject.

This book unites the global concepts and researches in an organized manner for a comprehensive understanding of the subject. It is a ripe text for all researchers, students, scientists or anyone else who is interested in acquiring a better knowledge of this dynamic field.

I extend my sincere thanks to the contributors for such eloquent research chapters. Finally, I thank my family for being a source of support and help.

Editor

1

Safety of Nanoclay/Spring Water Hydrogels: Assessment and Mobility of Hazardous Elements

Fátima García-Villén [1], Rita Sánchez-Espejo [2], Ana Borrego-Sánchez [2], Pilar Cerezo [1], Luana Perioli [3] and César Viseras [1,2,*]

[1] Department of Pharmacy and Pharmaceutical Technology, Faculty of Pharmacy, University of Granada, Campus of Cartuja, 18071 Granada, Spain; fgarvillen@ugr.es (F.G.-V.); mcerezo@ugr.es (P.C.)

[2] Andalusian Institute of Earth Sciences, CSIC-UGR, Avenida de las Palmeras 4, 18100 Armilla, Granada, Spain; ritase@correo.ugr.es (R.S.-E.); anaborrego@iact.ugr-csic.es (A.B.-S.)

[3] Department of Pharmaceutical Sciences, University of Perugia, via del Liceo 1, 06123 Perugia, Italy; luana.perioli@unipg.it

* Correspondence: cviseras@ugr.es

Abstract: The presence of impurities in medicinal products have to be controlled within safety limits from a pharmaceutical quality perspective. This matter is of special significance for those countries and regions where the directives, guidelines, or legislations, which prescribe the rules for the application of some products is quite selective or incomplete. Clay-based hydrogels are quite an example of this matter since they are topically administered, but, in some regions, they are not subjected to well-defined legal regulations. Since hydrogels establish an intimate contact with the skin, hazardous elements present in the ingredients could potentially be bioavailable and compromise their safety. The elemental composition and mobility of elements present in two hydrogels have been assessed. Sepiolite, palygorskite, and natural spring water were used as ingredients. The release of a particular element mainly depends on its position in the structure of the hydrogels, not only on its concentration in each ingredient. As a general trend, elements' mobility reduced with time. Among the most dangerous elements, whose presence in cosmetics is strictly forbidden by European legal regulations, As and Cd were mobile, although in very low amounts (0.1 and 0.2 μg/100 g of hydrogel, respectively). That is, assuming 100% bioavailability, the studied hydrogels would be completely safe at normal doses. Although there is no sufficient evidence to confirm that their presence is detrimental to hydrogels safety, legally speaking, their mobility could hinder the authorization of these hydrogels as medicines or cosmetics. In conclusion, the present study demonstrates that hydrogels prepared with sepiolite, palygorskite, and Alicún spring water could be topically applied without major intoxication risks.

Keywords: heavy metal; hazardous element; element mobility; clay minerals; spring water; hydrogel; toxicity; sepiolite; palygorskite

---

1. Introduction

The concentration and bioavailability of impurities such as hazardous elements in both health products and medicines is a main preformulation concern during their development. Different health care products must comply with specific normatives and guidelines, depending on the administration route, and most of the times, on the region or country in which they are written and applied. It is generally accepted that levels of elemental impurities below toxicity thresholds could be considered as safe, with diverse limits depending on the consulted normative. In Canada, natural health products that do not require a medical prescription, are included in a guide in which heavy metals (Pb, As, Cd, Hg, and Sb, among others) are banned or limited to a maximum amount, in accordance with the administration route [1]. In the USA, similar health products fail into FDA legislation, which only considers Hg as a forbidden element and limits the Pb concentration [2]. On the other hand, European cosmetic legislation is much more detailed and restrictive regarding the presence of elemental impurities [3].

Similar health products may also be considered into different categories depending on the country. The boundaries between medicinal products, natural health care products, cosmetics, and others, are not internationally normalized, even if generally accepted definitions have been achieved. In fact, the absence of clear boundaries made it necessary to address some products on a case-by-case basis. Particularly interesting is the cosmetic category, in which the presence of some ingredients, their origin, the administration route, and the scope of the product could raise doubts about their classification. A manual on the scope of the application of the cosmetics regulation EC 1223/2009 has been published by the working group on cosmetic products in order to shed some light on this matter [4]. The global cosmetics market have grown by an estimated 5.25% in 2019 [5], and, due to this continuous growth, the attention is being increasingly focused on the quality and safety of these products. Cosmetics are, according to the European Council Directive 2003/15/EC and the US Food Drug and Cosmetic Act, those products or mixtures of substances prepared and destined to be applied in different parts of the human body in order to clean, protect, maintain them in good conditions, improve their aspect, or relieve/eliminate body odors [6,7]. It has been recognized and demonstrated that, although cosmetics are intended to be applied on the surface of the body or mucous membranes, they may not remain there exclusively, since some topically applied substances may penetrate through the skin [8–10]. This fact is more pronounced for those cosmetics which are intended to remain at their application site for several hours or days, without subsequent rinse or wash. The European Union established a Regulation on Cosmetic Products (1223/2009) where it states that "cosmetic products should be safe under normal or reasonably foreseeable conditions of use. In particular, a risk-benefit reasoning should not justify a risk to human health" [3]. According to the European legislation, all cosmetic products should be subjected to safety assessments, taking into consideration the toxicology of all the ingredients used, as well as their chemical structure and their potential to produce local and systemic side effects.

The use of clay minerals in health care comes from prehistoric times, as reviewed in various paperwork and databases [11–15]. Some properties of these minerals have made them one of the most frequently used materials in pharmaceutical formulations and cosmetics, due to both their potential therapeutic activities and their useful properties as excipients. These features depend on colloidal dimensions and high surface areas of clay minerals, which give rise to optimal rheological and sorption capacities [13,16,17]. Kaolin, talc, smectites (montmorillonite and saponite), and fibrous clays (palygorskite and sepiolite) are some of the clay minerals most used in pharmacy. Hydrotherapy, and more particularly, balneotherapy, is one of the most frequent uses of clay minerals from a traditional and natural point of view. Clay minerals are used to prepare semisolid suspensions (frequently known as thermal muds or peloids) after the interposition of clays with spring waters, thus forming a nanoclay/spring water hydrogel. That is, thermal muds are semisolid, topical, natural medicinal hydrogels prepared by the interposition of organic and inorganic solids in mineral–medicinal water [11].

On the view of the uses and properties of these clay-based hydrogels, they could be considered as cosmetics with skin-care functions such as cleansing, degreasing, exfoliating, hydrating, invigorating, and firming activities [18–20]. These clay-based products could also be considered as medicinal products, as they have demonstrated activities against dermatological affections such as psoriasis [21–23], atopic dermatitis, vitiligo, eczemas, seborrhoeic dermatitis, fungal infections, or acne have also been treated by clay/spring water hydrogels [24–28]. Moreover, in view of the current Covid-19 worldwide state of emergency, Masiero et al. [29] have pointed out the already demonstrated positive effects of balneotherapy and thermal muds over the human immune system. Therefore, according to the guidelines of the borderline products manual [4], these formulations could fall either in the cosmetic or in the medicine category. Nonetheless, they are usually prepared in thermal stations, without a deep characterization of their therapeutical functions, activities, safety, or quality control. This unclear boundary between cosmetic and medical products showed by thermal muds, justifies the necessity of a harmonized regulation that compel for a full characterization of these products. Either way, since clay-based hydrogel formulations are intended to be applied over the skin (either health, ill, or injured skin), safety assessments should be one of the main milestones to be accomplished.

A remarkable feature of materials such as clays is the wide spectrum of mineralogical and chemical composition they have, something that is inevitable when it comes to natural products, most of the time accompanied by other naturally-associated mineral phases. Even if nanoclay/spring water hydrogels (thermal muds) are not legally considered as cosmetics or medicines and, therefore, they are not subjected to any kind of compulsory regulation; their accomplishment would highlight their quality constancy attributes and safety. The use of pharmaceutical-grade minerals in the preparation of thermal muds would guarantee the compositional safety of the gel-like system. In this regard, the chemical composition of the substances present in the formulation is crucial, since hazardous elements such as heavy metals and other elements are prohibited or limited in cosmetic products by different regulations. For instance, the ICH Harmonized Guideline for elemental impurities Q3D(R1) [30] published by the European Medicines Agency and Regulation No 1223/2009, European Parliament [3] are some of the regulations in which the discussion of this paperwork will be based. The safety assessment of the elements, such as heavy metals in cosmetics should start from the knowledge of the type and concentration of ingredients contained in the product in order to evaluate their potential intrinsic hazard [31]. The next step would include the analysis and studies of the mobility of those elements, either beneficial or harmful, in order to understand the potential biological and therapeutical effects of the formulation. This is especially important when it comes to "technically unavoidable" elements.

Recently, sepiolite and palygorskite (two inorganic excipients mainly composed of clay minerals) were mixed with natural spring water to prepare hydrogels intended for topical application. In previous studies, these excipients have demonstrated remarkable purity in terms of mineralogical composition (> 92% and > 58% of sepiolite and palygorksite richness, respectively) and quality performance [32]. Moreover, these very same hydrogels have also proved to possess wound healing effects.

The aim of this paper was to prepare, characterize, and address the elemental composition of nanoclay/spring water hydrogels made of sepiolite and palygorskite clay minerals and natural spring water. Since the present hydrogels are intended to be applied over potentially damaged or wounded skin, the mobility of their elements was also characterized. The final objective of this study was to assess the safety attributes of these formulations on the basis of the content and bioavailability of the elemental impurities.

2. Materials and Methods

2.1. Materials

Pangel S9 (PS9) and Cimsil G30 (G30) were kindly gifted by the TOLSA Group (Madrid, Spain). PS9 (d_{90} 23.9 μm) and G30 (d_{90} 49.3 μm) were mainly composed by sepiolite and palygorskite, respectively. According to their composition and properties, previously characterized by García-Villén et al. [32], they could be classified as "pharmaceutical-grade" excipients. Their corresponding pharmacopoeial denominations are "magnesium trisilicate" (PS9) and "Attapulgite" (G30) [33–35]. Sepiolite was present in PS9 in >92%, muscovite being the main mineralogical impurity detected. Palygorskite was present in G30 in 58%, accompanied by quartz (26%), fluorapatite (7%), smectites, and sepiolite (6%) and carbonates (3%) as associated minerals. Both PS9 and G30 excipients were dried in an oven at 40 °C for at least 48 h prior to being used in the preparation of the hydrogels. Spring water from Alicún thermal station (ALI), located in Granada (Spain) was used. ALI water is classified as hypothermal with strong mineralization [36,37].

Nanoclay/spring water hydrogels were prepared according to a process previously studied and optimized [32]. Briefly, clay minerals were mixed with ALI by means of a turbine high-speed agitator (Silverson LT, Chesham, UK), equipped with a high-traction stirrer head of square mesh, at 8000 rpm for 5 min. Samples were preserved in closed polyethylene containers, from which aliquots were sampled in order to monitor further analysis. Nanoclay/spring water hydrogels prepared had a 10% w/w of PS9 nanoclay concentration (ALIPS9) and 20% *w/w* of G30 nanoclay (ALIG30). Both of them were preserved and characterized in the same way.

2.2. Methods

2.2.1. Elemental Composition of Pristine Ingredients

Elements present in PS9 and G30 as well as ALI water has been addressed by Inductively Coupled Plasma mass spectrometry (ICP-MS) measurements. Solid samples were prepared by acid digestion in strong acids (HNO_3 and HF at a 3:5 ratio) inside a Teflon reactor, thus the samples were subjected to high pressure and temperature by heating in a microwave oven (Milestone ETHOS ONE, Sorisole, Italy). The quantification of the elements was done by a NexION-300 ICP-MS spectrometer (Perkin Elmer, Waltham, MA, USA) equipped with a triple cone interface and a quadrupole ion deflector using argon for plasma formation. Standard solutions of 100 and 1000 ppb were prepared for each element (Multi-Element standards, Perkin Elmer, Waltham, MA, USA), and Rh was employed as an internal standard. All standards were prepared from ICP single-element standard solutions (Merck, Darmstadt, Germany) after dilution with 10% HNO_3. Ultrapurified water (Milli-Q® grade, 18 MΩ·cm) was used during the whole experiment. The accuracy of the ICP-MS equipment used ranges between ±2 and ±5% for analyte concentrations between 50 and 5 ppm, respectively. The detection limits were <0.1 ppt for Ir and Ta; <1 ppt for Ba, Li, Cu, Mo, Sb, Sn, Ag, Au, Co, Ni, V, As, Cd, Pb, Zr, Be and Nd; <10 ppt for Cr, Hg and Te; < 1 ppb for P.

2.2.2. In Vitro Release of Elemental Impurities from Hydrogels

The element mobility from nanoclay/spring water hydrogels (ALIPS9, ALIG30) was assessed by in vitro cation release studies performed in a Franz diffusion cell system FDC40020FF (BioScientific Inc., Phoenix, AZ, USA) [38]. This system is designed to recreate conditions of formulations placed over the skin and mucosa membranes. Particularly, the selected Franz diffusion cells possessed a contact area of 0.64 cm^2 and an approximate total volume of 6.4 mL in the receptor chamber. In this study, the aim is to explore the potential number of elements that would be released by the formulation and that are potentially able to establish contact with the skin. To do so, dialysis membranes (cut-off 12–14 kDa (31.7 mm), Medicell International, London, UK) were placed and used to separate the donor and receptor chambers, just acting as physical support for the hydrogel and not as a permeation barrier. The membranes were boiled in ultra-purified water (Milli-Q® water) for 10 min in order to hydrate them. Over the membrane, in the donator chamber, 0.025 g of each hydrogel was placed. The receptor chamber of the Franz diffusion cells was filled with degassed, ultra-purified water, which was maintained at a constant temperature of 32 ± 0.5 °C (to reproduce human skin temperature) through a thermostatic bath circulation. The experiment lasted for 30 min, this being the typical time of topical nanoclay/spring water hydrogels application. At the end of the experiments, the receptor aqueous phase was withdrawn and filtered through 0.45 μm single-use, sterile filters. Then, the elemental composition on each sample was assessed by ICP-MS, following the same protocol previously described for the pristine materials. All samples (six replicates) were subjected to in vitro release experiments 48 h after the preparation and after one month. During the experiment, the manipulation of different materials and instruments could contaminate the ultra-purified water of the Franz cell receptor chamber. To eliminate this error, blanks were also analyzed in order to monitor the elements coming from the materials and the ultra-purified water itself. Briefly, it consisted of analyzing the ultra-purified water that was placed in the receptor chamber of the Franz cell device. The concentration of the elements detected in the Milli-Q water (which was considered the blank, data not shown) were subtracted from the concentration detected in the receptor chamber. This way, it will be possible to discern the real number of elements exchanged/released from the semisolid formulation and, thus, able to establish contact with the patient skin.

2.3. Result Discussion and Interpretation Bases and Criteria

Different regulations could be used for the interpretation of the obtained results. In this paperwork, the discussion and interpretation of the results will be centered on the documents summarized in Table 1.

Table 1. Documents used during the interpretation and discussion of the obtained results.

Type of Document	Region	Year	Ref
Regulation of the European Parliament and Council of the European Union on cosmetic products (EC 1223/2009)	EU	2009	[3]
Guidance on Heavy Metal Impurities in Cosmetics (HC-SC)	Canada	2012	[1]
Quality of Natural Health Products Guide - Natural and Non-prescription Health Products Directorate (NNPHD)	Canada	2015	[39]
Guideline for Elemental Impurities Q3D(R1)	EU	2019	[30]

The HC-SC guideline is focused on heavy metals (As, Pb, Cd, Hg, and Sb). Other metal elements such as Se, Ba, and Cr are considered less significant in terms of toxicity; therefore, no impurity limits are found for these elements in this document [1]. The Natural and Non-prescription Health Products Directorate (NNPHD) [39] is a guidance document intended to give support to stakeholders "in assuring that natural health products are produced in a high-quality manner". NNPHD is focused on natural and non-prescription health products, which is the case of PS9, G30, and ALI ingredients and resultant hydrogels. Acceptable limits for As, Cd, Pb, Hg, Cr, and Sb elemental impurities are defined in this guide, including the limits for topical administration (Figure 1).

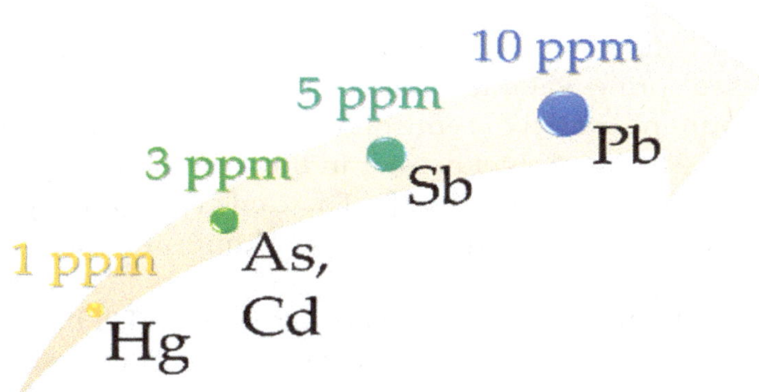

Figure 1. Acceptable limits for heavy metals in topical products [39].

The ICH guideline for Elemental Impurities Q3D(R1) refers to medicinal products and classifies elements into four groups based on their toxicity and likelihood of occurrence in these products (Figure 2). The fourth group called "other elements" includes elements for which Permitted Daily Exposure (PDE) limits have not been established. As a result of this, these elements have not been included in this manuscript. Regarding the most toxic elements, the Q3D(R1) guideline also reports the PDE limits by oral, parenteral, and inhalation administration routes [30]. PDE is the maximum acceptable intake of the elemental impurity per day. Although this guideline is not specific for cosmetics, the fact that it deals with elemental impurities of drugs (which are intended to reach the bloodstream) makes it useful to also ensure the safety of cosmetics.

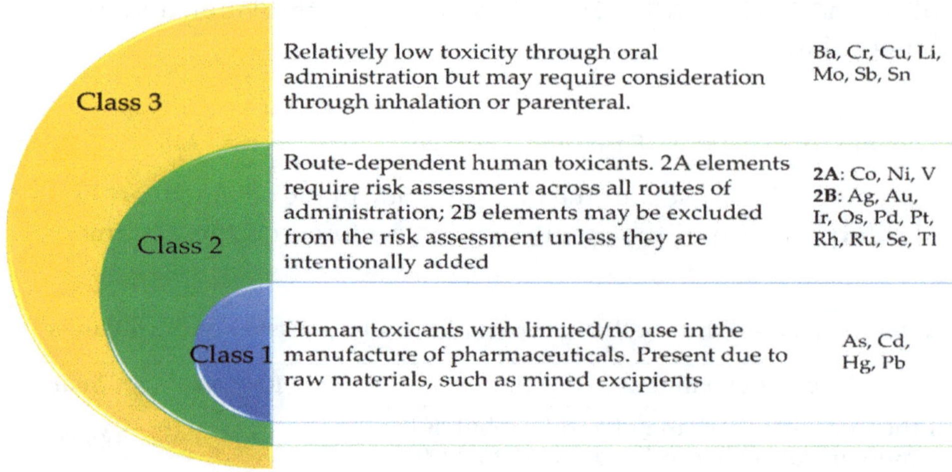

Figure 2. Element classification of the ICH Q3D(R1) guideline. Based on ICH Q3D(R1) [30].

Finally, the European Regulation EC 1223/2009, from all the documents and guidelines included in this study, is the most restricting one in terms of impurities present in cosmetics [3]. Only those elements considered safe and innocuous for the human being are allowed in cosmetics, while the rest of them are banned without any limit or maximum dose established. Furthermore, according to article 17 of this regulation, "the presence of traces of banned substances will only be allowed if they are technically inevitable and do not impair the safety of the cosmetic product". In this regard, in vitro studies such as Franz cells could help to discern and discuss this point since they allow the study of the mobility of the elements present in the ingredients.

Dose of Nanoclay/Natural Spring Water Hydrogels

The toxicity of elemental impurities obviously depends on the administration route of the dosage form. Nanoclay hydrogels prepared in this study are intended to be topically applied over either the healthy or wounded skin of patients subjected to balneotherapy treatments. In thermal stations, natural or artificial clay-based/spring water formulations could be applied in different forms. The most common one includes the administration of semisolid systems at 45–50 °C on restricted body regions (mainly isolated joints) with 210 cm of thickness or in the form of total/partial baths. Most of these treatments usually last for 15 to 30 min [40–42]. The density of the hydrogels was obtained by the Minimum Square Method applied to experimental volume, and mass hydrogels measurements (R^2 were >0.998 in both cases): ϱALIPS9 = 1.0606 g/mL; ϱALIG30 = 1.0992 g/mL. These data would be used to calculate safe doses of hydrogels in order to not exceed the PDE limits defined in the Guideline for Elemental Impurities [30] for each element. Moreover, despite the bioavailability of topically administered dosage forms hardly reaching 100%, in the discussion, we will systematically consider the maximum potential bioavailability in order to guarantee safe doses.

3. Results

3.1. Elemental Composition of Pristine Ingredients

The elemental composition of PS9, G30 nanoclays, and natural spring water (ALI) is summarized in Table 2. Below, the results will be discussed from the most innocuous to the most dangerous elements, as well as by the amount in which they were detected.

Regarding PS9 and G30, Ba, Cr, and Li (Class 3) and V (class 2A), were detected in remarkable amounts. The presence of Zr and Nd was also reported. Except for Li, the amount of the aforementioned elements was higher in G30 than in PS9, thus highlighting the presence of more impurities in G30. This statement is in agreement with the solid-state characterization of G30 made by García-Villén et al. [32]. The presence of hazardous elements such as Pb, As, and Cd in fibrous clay minerals have been reported as a common feature of natural deposits, though the present values are minimal with respect to previously reported levels [43].

Table 2. Elemental composition of pristine ingredients (PS9 and G30 nanoclays and ALI spring water) determined by ICP-MS. The elements are classified depending on regulations [3,30]. "ND" stands for "Not detected".

Element	PS9 (ppm)	G30 (ppm)	ALI (ppb)	Comments
Ba	56.2	144.8	18.8	Class 3 in Q3D(R1) [30]; Not listed as element in EC 1223/2009 [3]
Cr	14.0	391.8	4.3	Class 3 in Q3D(R1) [30]; Not allowed in EC 1223/2009 [3]
Cu	8.1	11.3	2.5	Class 3 in Q3D(R1) [30]; Allowed in EC 1223/2009 [3]
Li	149.0	30.4	244.2	Class 3 in Q3D(R1) [30]; Not listed in EC 1223/2009 [3]
Mo	0.2	0.2	3.8	
Sb	0.3	2.1	0.1	Class 3 in Q3D(R1) [30]; Not allowed in EC 1223/2009 [3]
Sn	10.8	3.3	ND	Class 3 in Q3D(R1) [30]; Not listed in EC 1223/2009 [3]
Ag	0.04	0.2	0.1	Class 2B in Q3D(R1) [30]; Allowed in EC 1223/2009 [3]
Au	ND	ND	ND	
Ir	0.2	0.9	ND	Class 2B in Q3D(R1) [30]; Not listed in EC 1223/2009 [3]
Se	0.9	1.5	2.3	Class 2B in Q3D(R1) [30]; Not allowed in EC 1223/2009 [3]
Tl	0.2	0.1	0.1	
Co	2.3	7.4	0.4	Class 2A in Q3D(R1) [30]; Not listed in EC 1223/2009 [3]
Ni	3.7	50.7	9.4	Class 2A in Q3D(R1) [30]; Not allowed in EC 1223/2009 [3]
V	24.9	249.1	ND	Class 2A in Q3D(R1) [30]; Not listed in EC 1223/2009 [3]
As	2.0	1.3	0.2	Class 1 in Q3D(R1) [30]; Not allowed in EC 1223/2009 [3]
Cd	0.02	1.5	ND	
Hg	ND	ND	ND	
Pb	3.2	4.1	ND	
P	0.3	8.5	0.1	Not allowed in EC 1223/2009 [3]
Be	1.8	3.6	0.01	
Zr	21.5	50.3	0.2	
Te	ND	ND	ND	
Nd	8.0	30.2	ND	
Ta	0.9	0.7	0.005	

With respect to the ALI spring water, the main hazardous impurities detected were Li and Ba, followed by Cr (class 3 elements in all cases). Therefore, the major elements detected (Table 2) belong to class 3 or class 2A [30], which indicates that they are elements whose presence in the raw materials should be borne in mind, though with relatively low toxicity. Additionally, the presence of Cr, Zr, and Nd is not allowed in cosmetics, according to the EC 1223/2009 [3]. From class 2B, only the presence of Se and Tl is banned in cosmetics, though the three of them were detected as traces (Table 2). Ni, which belongs to class 2A and its not allowed in cosmetics, was detected in significant amounts in G30, unlike PS9 and ALI.

Class 1 element group is formed by hazardous elements As, Cd, Hg, nd Pb (Figure 1), all of them prohibited according to EC 1223/2009 [3,30]. As, Cd, and Pb were similar to the ones reported for natural products used in cosmetics [8]. Unlike class 1 and EC 1223/2009, the NNHPD [39] specifies the acceptable limits for heavy metals in topical products (Figure 1), including Sb (class 3). All the aforementioned elements were below the limits established by the NNHPD.

The rest of the elements (from P onwards, Table 2) are not classified in Q3D(R1), thus not belonging to any specific group previously mentioned. Among them, Zr highlights due to the high amount present both in PS9 and G30 in comparison with the rest of the non-allowed elements.

3.2. *In Vitro Release of Hazardous Elements from Hydrogels*

The results obtained after the Franz cell studies regarding the release of the elements from nanoclay hydrogels at 48 h and after one month are summarized in Table 3.

Table 3. Mobility of hazardous elements after Franz diffusion cell tests. The concentrations are expressed in μg/100 g of hydrogel. Elements have been placed in the same order as in Table 2. Mean values ± s.e. ($n = 6$). "ND" stands for "not detected".

Elements	ALIPS9		ALIG30	
	48h	1 Month	48h	1 Month
Ba	5.6 ± 1.55	1.8 ± 0.934	8.3 ± 0.944	1.2 ± 0.360
Cr	ND		ND	
Cu	10.8 ± 3.293	3.6 ± 2.17	20.6 ± 3.725	0.91 ± 0.608
Li	20.5 ± 3.293	17.7 ± 3.214	4.3 ± 0.362	1.7 ± 0.379
Mo	0.7 ± 0.095	0.61 ± 0.125	1.8 ± 0.0572	0.21 ± 0.123
Sb	ND		ND	
Sn	28.7 ± 8.232	10.4 ± 2.138	50.4 ± 4.866	6.5 ± 1.945
Ag, Au, Ir, Se, Tl	ND		ND	
Co	0.26 ± 0.206	0.6 ± 0.093	1.1 ± 0.660	0.58 ± 0.237
Ni	ND		ND	
V	1.7 ± 0.310	1.8 ± 0.492	5.9 ± 0.306	7.5 ± 0.315
As	0.1 ± 0.010	0.4 ± 0.039	0.08 ± 0.050	0.1 ± 0.063
Cd	ND	ND	0.1 ± 0.064	0.2 ± 0.0087
Hg, Pb P, Be, Zr, Te, Nd, Ta	ND		ND	

Ba release was very variable between ALIPS9 and ALIG30, though the higher values detected in ALIG30 could be ascribed to higher Ba presence in the pristine material G30 in comparison with PS9 (Table 2). Cu mobility, which was higher in ALIG30 due to a higher amount in G30, significantly decreased after one month for both ALIG30 and ALIPS9.

The Li release was higher in ALIPS9 due to the higher Li levels in PS9 and maintained constant with time (no significant differences between 48h and 1 month). On the other hand, ALIG30 hydrogels showed a reduction in Li release as time passed. The highest Mo was found in ALIG30—48 h and significantly decreased after one month. On the other hand, ALIPS9 demonstrated a constant release of Mo through time. Sn, V, and Cd released from both hydrogels came from clay minerals since none of these elements were detected in ALI (Table 2). The V release increased with time, while Sn showed the opposite trend.

Heavy metals Hg, Pb, and Sb, though present in the pristine materials, were not released. Other not-allowed elements, such as Cr, Se, Tl, Ni, P, Be, Zr, Te, Nd, and Ta were neither release elements, which means that they do not pose any problem in terms of safety. On the other hand, Cd and As were slightly released, with higher results in the case of ALIG30 hydrogels. The absence of Cd in ALIPS9 is due to the extremely low amounts detected in PS9 and its absence in ALI. On the contrary, G30 possessed a higher amount of Cd (Table 2), which explains the release results (Table 3). In conclusion, Cd and As are the most crucial elements determining the safety of the hydrogels. It is worth mentioning that with respect to the As and Cd amounts and release, ALIPS9 hydrogel is considered the safest formulation.

4. Discussion

4.1. In Vitro Release of Elements: Safety Concerns and Doses

The toxicity of elemental impurities obviously depends on the administration route of the dosage form. The studied hydrogels are topically administered, and the bioavailability of a certain element hardly reached 100%. Tateo et al. [9], in previous studies regarding elemental percutaneous mobility, stated that the major part of the elements could cross the skin. Nonetheless, they reported that "none of these elements reaches concentrations so high as to represent hazardous conditions". In the discussion, we systematically will consider a theoretical 100% bioavailability in order to guarantee safe doses in any case.

According to the results, the maximum amount of Ba released came from ALIG30, 48 h, and it counted for 8.3 μg/100 g of hydrogel. The oral PDE of barium was established as 730 μg/day [30]. If we consider the maximum mobility and a 100% bioavailability of Ba through the skin, the administration of ALIG30 and ALIPS9 hydrogels would be considered safe if doses are less than 8.79 kg hydrogel/day (Table 4). In view of the high amounts of hydrogels needed to pose a risk regarding Ba, it is possible to state that both ALIPS9 and ALIG30 are safe with respect to this element.

Table 4. Theoretical safe doses of ALIPS9 and ALIG30 hydrogels based on elements with defined parenteral Permitted Daily Exposure (PDE) levels. Calculations have been made by using the higher mobility value reported by Franz cells (either ALIPS9 or ALIG30). Additionally, safety doses are calculated assuming a theoretical dermal bioavailability of 100%.

Element	PDE_{parent} Limits [29]	Maximum Release Detected	Hydrogel Safe Dose/Day
Ba	730 µg/day	8.3 µg/100 g (ALIPS9–1 month)	≤8.79 kg
Cu	340 µg/day	20.6 µg/100 g (ALIG30–48 h)	≤1.65 kg
Li	280 µg/day	20.5 µg/100 g (ALIPS9–48 h)	≤1.37 kg
Mo	1700 µg/day	1.8 µg/100 g (ALIG30–48 h)	≤94.4 kg
Sn	640 µg/day	50.4 µg/100 g (ALIG30–48 h)	≤1.27 kg
Co	5 µg/day	1.1 µg/100 g (ALIG30–48 h)	≤454 g
V	12 µg/day	7.5 µg/100 g (ALIG30–1 month)	≤160 g
As	15 µg/day	0.4 µg/100 g (ALIPS9–1 month)	≤3.75 kg
Cd	1.7 µg/day	0.2 µg/100 g (ALIG30–1 month)	≤850 g

Among the possible adverse effects associated with Cu, allergic dermatitis is the most commonly experienced [44]. Safe amounts of hydrogels regarding Cu release (Table 3) have been calculated according to parenteral PDE (Table 4). In view of the results, hydrogels aged for one month could be considered safe in terms of allergenic copper effects, since its mobility practically disappears. Moreover, ALIPS9 would be more advisable than ALIG30; the amount of Cu being lower in the former one. The amount of Cu released from extemporaneous formulated hydrogels could limit their use in general baths, as the calculated safe dose (Table 4) should be lesser than two kilograms of hydrogel.

Li is of relatively low toxicity by the oral route. Is a common metal present in animal tissues and is used in certain kinds of treatments, such as bipolar disorder or depression, among others. Recently, Yuan et al. [45] prepared a sponge scaffold with LiCl and evaluated wound healing activity in vitro. The presence of Li reduced inflammation and improved angiogenesis, re-epithelialization, and expression of β-catenin. Seborrheic dermatitis is another skin disorder that has been addressed by Li as an active lithium gluconate/succinate, with successful results [46–49]. The main problem of Li is the narrow therapeutic margin it possesses [50,51]. Parenteral Li PDE was established to be 280 µg/day [30]. Considering that all the released Li would be able to reach the bloodstream once the hydrogel is applied, the administration of ≤ 1.37 kg hydrogel/day would guarantee safe doses of Li (below the parenteral PDE, Table 4).

Mo could be considered as an essential element since its deficiencies have been related to night-blindness, nausea, disorientation, coma, tachycardia, tachypnea, and other biochemical abnormalities [30]. Nonetheless, excessive accumulation of Mo could also produce toxicity, so its limits need to be controlled. In particular, Mo could be accumulated in the skin, bound to dermal collagen. The amount of Mo released from ALIPS9 was constant with time, while it significantly reduced after one month in ALIG30 (Table 3). Parenteral PDE levels of Mo are 1700 µg/day. Considering the highest released amount of Mo (ALIG30—48 h), and supposing 100% of bioavailability, 94 kg/day of hydrogels would be necessary to reach PDE limits (Table 4). In view of these calculations, it is possible to guarantee that ALIPS9 and ALIG30 are safe with respect to Mo levels.

Tin is an element widely used nowadays [52]. The PDE limits of Sn have been established since it has been reported to increase in vitro oxidative stress or DNA breakage [53]. In view of tin's released amounts in ALIPS9 and ALIG30, its toxicity and PDE limits should be borne in mind. In particular, this element showed lower release from both hydrogels after one month of preparation. The inhalation and oral consumption of Sn are the main routes for Sn intoxication [54–56], thus meaning that the topical application of these hydrogels would be a safe administration route. In fact, in vitro cytotoxicity studies of these hydrogels were not shown to hinder normal dermal human fibroblast growth nor cell motility during in vitro wound healing [57].

Ni has been widely detected in cosmetic products, together with Co and Cr, among others [8,58]. The attention paid to Ni, Co, and Cr is based mainly on skin conditions, such as contact allergic dermatitis, itching, and edema, among others [59–64]. What is more, these elements can be solubilized by sweat during prolonged contact [60,65]. Pristine materials possessed higher amounts of Ni than Co. Nonetheless, no Ni and Cr mobility was detected in Franz cell tests, thus reducing the risk of contact skin alterations produced by ALIPS9 and ALIG30 hydrogels. The Co mobility in ALIPS9 increased with time, while in ALIG30, it maintained constant (Table 3). The application of young hydrogels (ALIPS9) would entail the lowest risk of skin allergies related to cobalt. Co is an integral component of vitamin B_{12}, which means that it is essential for the human body. It is estimated that the average person receives about 11 μg Co/day with normal diet, and the parenteral PDE is established to be 5 μg/day [3]. Additionally, it has been demonstrated that Co is able to pass the skin [65,66], though its percutaneous absorption was found to be very low (0.0123 $\mu g \cdot cm^{-2} \cdot h^{-1}$). Time of hydrogels application in thermal stations takes at about 20–30 min, which is not enough time for all the mobile Co (Table 3) to cross the human skin, thus making the "hydrogel safe dose/day" (calculated assuming a 100% of bioavailability, Table 4) to be remarkably higher in real conditions.

V is a ubiquitous element in the human body, though no essential role has been found yet for this element. Although systemic toxicity of V has already been accepted, its deficiency has also proved to be problematic since it is associated to thyroid, glucose, and lipid metabolism malfunctions. It also participates in the regulation of several genes and has been demonstrated to influence cancer development, including skin cancers such as malignant melanoma [67,68]. V was a mobile element in both hydrogels prepared. No V was detected in the ALI, Franz cells results ascribable to pristine clay minerals composition (Table 2). In ALIG30, the mobility of V was higher due to the higher amount of this element in G30 in comparison with ALIPS9 (Table 3). Although antiproliferative properties of V ions have been found [68], neither ALIPS9 nor ALIG30 hydrogels impaired normal human fibroblasts in vitro proliferation, according to previous studies [57].

As is a forbidden element in cosmetics [3]. Arsenic mobility is reported to be very low in both hydrogels. It maintains constant through time in ALIG30, while it increases in ALIPS9 after one month. This element is very ubiquitous in the environment, so it is expected to be present in natural ingredients such as clay minerals. This element is classified in the category 1A in view of its carcinogenicity, as reported in the European Regulation EC 1272/2008 [69]. For greater clarity, substances belonging to the 1A category are known to have carcinogenic potential to humans. It possesses a pronounced affinity for skin and keratinizing structures, although it does not act as a sensitizer due to poor skin penetrating ability. According to article 1 of the EC 1223/2009, "prohibited substances should be acceptable at trace levels only if they are technologically inevitable with correct manufacturing processes and provided that the product is safe". Assuming 100% bioavailability and using parenteral PDE levels, the maximum dose of hydrogels that could be used without exceeding these levels is 3.75 $kg \cdot day^{-1}$ (Table 4) [30]. Moreover, the maximum mobility of As is far less than the maximum permissible concentration of inorganic As in drinking water (10 μg/L [70,71] vs. 4.24 μg/L in ALIPS9 one month).

Cd is another element whose presence in cosmetics is forbidden. Cd did not show mobility from ALIPS9. Higher amounts of Cd in G30 justified the higher mobility of this element in ALIG30. The low release of Cd from fibrous clay minerals is in agreement with previous studies, which reported irreversible interaction between Cd and the solid phase, thus hindering the mobility of this element [72]. Regarding toxicity, Cd is classified in the category 2 (suspected human carcinogen). It can accumulate in the skin, having deleterious effects on this organ, as recently demonstrated by an in vivo study [73]. Nonetheless, the in vitro percutaneous bioavailability of cadmium chloride salt tested through human skin was determined to be among 0.07% (from water) and 0.01% (from soil) [74].

Other heavy metals such as Pb and Sb, though present in the pristine materials (Table 2), were not mobile (Table 3). Hg and Au were not detected in the pristine materials, and their absence after Franz cell diffusion guaranteed the absence of contamination during preparation, conservation, packaging, and manipulation of the hydrogels (art. 17 of the EC 1223/2009 [3]). Additionally, the cytotoxicity of these hydrogels has been previously tested in vitro [57], obtaining very positive results, which supports the hypothesis of product safety.

4.2. Mobility of Hazardous Elements

The presence in a product of an elemental impurity will have safety concerns only once released, with different mechanisms underlying the release of each particular element, mainly depending on its position in the structure of the hydrogel components. Nevertheless, it is possible to calculate a parameter of general comparative interest; mobility of the elements from the dosage form. The mobility of an element could be calculated as the ratio between the element content/element released.

In view of the previously shown results, the mobility of hazardous elements from ALIPS9 and ALIG30 hydrogels was minimal in the major part of the cases (Figure 3). These results could be explained by the high adsorption capacity of palygorskite and sepiolite clay minerals, their low cation exchange capacity, and the gel network of hydrogels. The mobility of tracers has been explained due to the formation of inner-sphere complexes with clay and other associated mineral surfaces [75–77]. It also seems clear that different ionic equilibriums are established through time in both hydrogels (Figure 4). For instance, Co, Ba, and Sn reduce their mobility while As and Cd increase it, thus demonstrating that elements established different equilibriums within the hydrogel.

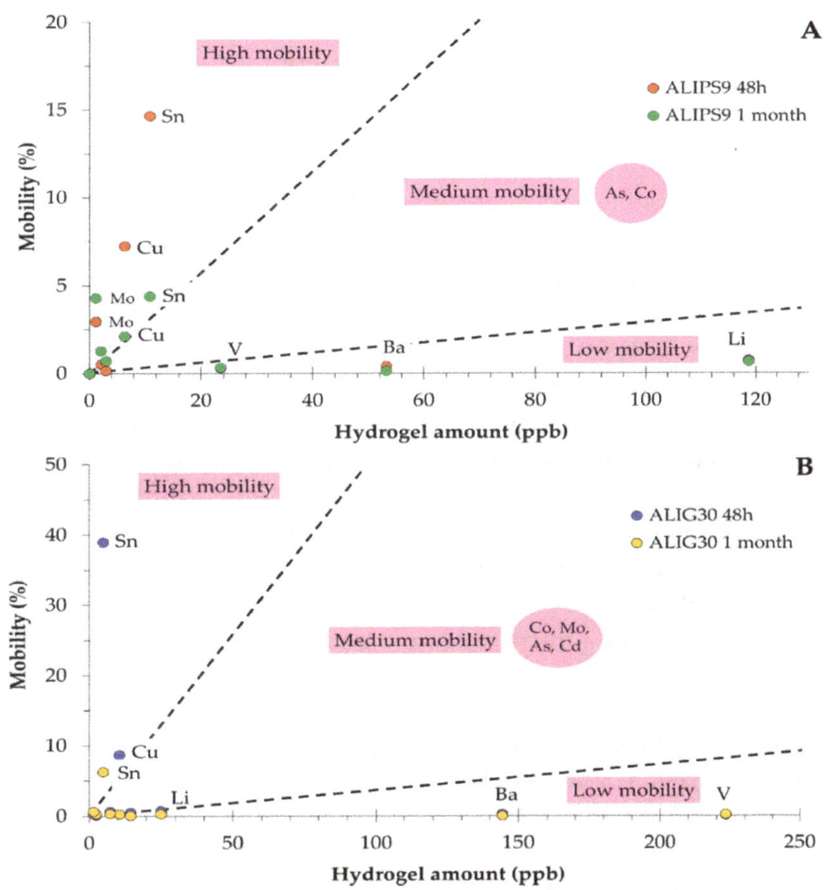

Figure 3. Element mobility (%) versus the total amount of element in ALIPS9 (**A**) and ALIG30 (**B**). Only mobile elements are shown.

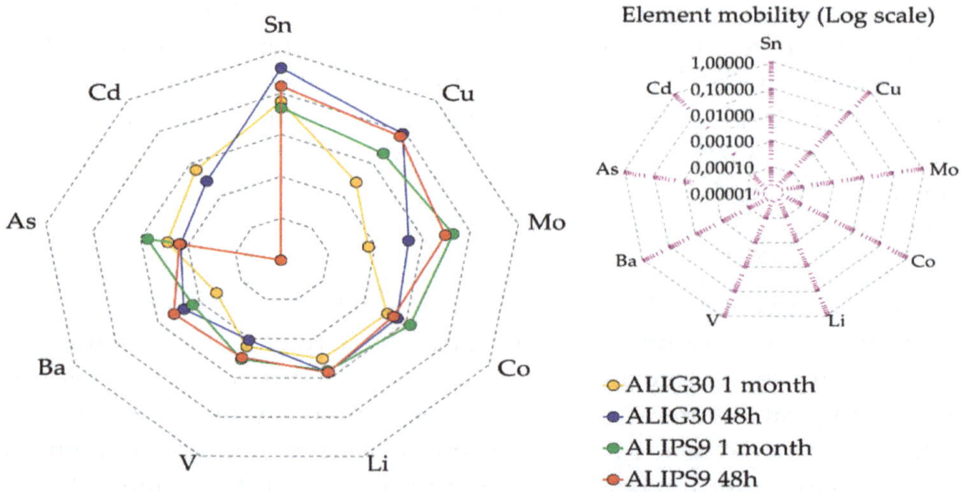

Figure 4. Spider diagram of element mobility. Only mobile elements are shown. The logarithmic scale was used, though not included in the spider diagram for simplicity and clarity.

Sn showed to be the most mobile element, followed by Cu (Figure 3). Sn was not detected in ALI, which indicates that the release of this element came from PS9 and G30. On the other hand, Cu was detected in the three ingredients. In ALIPS9, the third element with significant mobility was Mo (Figure 3A). Molybdenum was also detected as an element with remarkable mobility in ALIPS9, while the mobility in ALIG30 was significantly smaller. The differences in Mo amounts released (Table 3) could be ascribed to the differential solid-liquid equilibrium established within both hydrogels since both PS9 and G30 presented the same amount of this element (Table 2). The reduction of Mo mobility in ALIG30 indicates that the G30 clay mineral has a better ability to retain the Mo in ALI.

Li, Ba, V, and Cd were the elements with the smaller mobility. V was not detected in ALI, which means that the released amount was due to the clay minerals. V and Li did not participate in the solid-liquid equilibrium established between solid and liquid phases since their mobility was constant with time. Although Ba was an element with minimal mobility, it reduced with time in both hydrogels. The fact that G30 showed higher Ba amount than PS9 together with the fact that Ba mobility in this hydrogel was smaller than in ALIPS9 indicates that it is a structural element of G30. Moreover, the similar release of Ba from ALIPS9 and ALIG30 means that, probably, the major part of the Ba released came from ALI instead of PS9 and G30.

Cd and As were slightly mobile, with higher results in the case of ALIG30 hydrogels. The absence of Cd mobility in ALIPS9 was due to the extremely low amounts detected in PS9 and its absence in ALI. On the contrary, G30 possessed higher amounts of Cd (Table 2), which explains the mobility results (Table 3). Cd and As were the most crucial elements determining the safety of the hydrogels. It is worth to mention that, with respect to the As and Cd amounts and mobility, ALIPS9 hydrogels could be considered the safest formulation.

The mobility of Sn, Cu, Mo, and Ba from hydrogels reduced as time passed. The mobility reduction could be explained by the irreversible adsorption of the elements by PS9 and G30. In fact, fibrous clay minerals have been proposed as environmental remediation ingredients and wastewater treatments aiming to eliminate heavy metals with promising results [78–81].

The spider diagram (Figure 4) clearly shows that, as a general trend, palygorskite hydrogels reduced the mobility of hazardous elements with time (with a reduction in area), whereas this was not obvious for sepiolite hydrogels.

Finally, previous studies on elemental mobility from clay minerals, spring waters, and thermal muds have reported that the amount of released elements highly depends on their concentration in spring water, the release of elements from the solid phase being negligible [9]. Nonetheless, in view of the results of the present study suggest that solid-phase composition did play a crucial role. This discordance could be due to the high structuration of the present hydrogels.

At this point of the study, and looking at the safe dose calculations (Table 4), the way to guarantee the absence of any intoxication risk would be to apply the hydrogels locally (over restricted areas of the skin, wounds, joints, etc. That is, hydrogel bath treatment should be avoided if potentially toxic doses of the elemental impurities want to be minimized. Nonetheless, bioavailability and percutaneous permeation studies would be highly useful and valuable to establish safe usage guidelines for these formulations.

5. Conclusions

Elemental impurities in medicinal products have to be controlled within safety limits with different guidelines and normatives being useful from a pharmaceutical quality perspective. The essential role of clay minerals in drug products and cosmetics is widely known. Nanoclay/natural spring water hydrogels have been prepared by mixing a sepiolite and a palygorskite with local spring water (Alicún de las Torres, Granada, Spain). Clay hydrogels are traditionally used in balneotherapy or as natural cosmetics (masks, shampoos, etc.). Since these formulations are intended to establish an intimate contact with the skin (either healthy, sensitive, or damaged skin) their composition is of high importance in terms of safety. In this study, special attention has been paid to the presence of heavy metals and other hazardous elements. As expected, pristine materials possessed a wide variety of hazardous elements such as Cd, Pb, or P, among others. Since these elements are specifically forbidden in cosmetics according to the European Regulation (EC 1223/2009), pristine materials do not accomplish cosmetic regulations on their own. Nonetheless, the presence of certain substances in a cosmetic does not imply that they are able to be absorbed or enter in contact with the skin. In order to discern the potential bioavailability of these elements, their mobility was evaluated by using Franz cells in vitro tests. Among all the specifically forbidden elements in cosmetics, only As and Cd were detected as mobile, though in very low amounts. Their mobility was so low that, taking into account the corresponding PDE for the parenteral route and assuming 100% of bioavailability through the skin, the calculated safe doses were approximately 1 kg of hydrogel per day. In conclusion, the present study demonstrates that the composition and nature of the solid phases of the hydrogel determine the mobility of the elements. Legally speaking, the mobility of As and Cd could hinder the authorization of ALIPS9 and ALIG30 hydrogels as cosmetic products. Nonetheless, there is no sufficient evidence to confirm that the presence of these elements is detrimental to their safety and, though further studies are still necessary, ALIPS9 and ALIG30 hydrogels could be used in practice. Finally, it is worth to mention that, despite that ALIG30 showed higher ability to reduce the elements mobility, the ALIPS9 hydrogel would be easier to authorize as a medicine or cosmetic, since the mobility of As and Cd in this hydrogel was minimum or absent. Future perspectives of this particular study include the assessment of the percutaneous mobility of the elements (bioavailability) both in vitro and in vivo. These kinds of studies would help to better define the best techniques to apply fibrous clay-based hydrogels to maximize benefits by minimizing the risks.

Author Contributions: Data curation, F.G.-V.; Funding acquisition, P.C. and C.V.; Investigation, F.G.-V.; Methodology, R.S.-E.; Supervision, C.V.; Writing–original draft, F.G.-V.; Writing–review & editing, R.S.-E., A.B.-S., L.P. and C.V. All authors have read and agreed to the published version of the manuscript.

Acknowledgments: This project was supported by the Spanish research group CTS-946. Technical support was provided by the CIC (Centro de Instrumentación Científica, University of Granada) and the IACT (Instituto Andaluz de Ciencias de la Tierra, CSIS-UGR). Special thanks to TOLSA group (Madrid), who kindly gifted clay minerals samples, and Alicún de las Torres thermal station, who provided spring water samples for the study.

References

1. Government of Canada Guidance on Heavy Metal Impurities in Cosmetics—Canada. Available online: https://www.canada.ca/en/health-canada/services/consumer-product-safety/reports-publications/industry-professionals/guidance-heavy-metal-impurities-cosmetics.html#a32 (accessed on 3 May 2018).
2. FDA Prohibited and Restricted Ingredients in Cosmetics. Available online: https://www.fda.gov/cosmetics/cosmetics-laws-regulations/prohibited-restricted-ingredients-cosmetics (accessed on 12 December 2019).
3. EU. *Regulation (EC) No 1223/2009 on Cosmetic Products*; European Union: Brussels, Belgium, 2009; pp. 1–151.
4. EU. *Manual of the Working Group on Cosmetic Products (Sub-Group on Borderline Products) on the Scope of Application of the Cosmetics Regulation (EC) No 1223/2009 (Art. 2(1)(A))*; European Union: Brussels, Belgium, 2017; pp. 1–33.
5. *Annual Growth of the Global Cosmetics Market from 2004 to 2018*; L'Oréal: Clichy/Paris, France, 2019; Available online: https://www.statista.com/statistics/297070/growth-rate-of-the-global-cosmetics-market/ (accessed on 1 July 2020).
6. Directive 2003/15/EC of the European Parliament and of the Council Amending Council Directive 76/768/EEC on the Approximation of the Laws of the Member States Relating to Cosmetic Products 2003, 26–35. Available online: https://eur-lex.europa.eu/LexUriServ/LexUriServ.do?uri=OJ:L:2003:066:0026:0035:EN:PDF (accessed on 22 November 2019).
7. *United States Code—Federal Food, Drug, and Cosmetic Act*; Office of the Law Revision Counsel: Washington, DC, USA, 2006. Available online: https://uscode.house.gov/browse/prelim@title21/chapter9/subchapter2&edition=prelim (accessed on 1 July 2020).
8. Borowska, S.; Brzóska, M.M. Metals in cosmetics: Implications for human health. *J. Appl. Toxicol.* **2015**, *35*, 551–572. [CrossRef] [PubMed]
9. Tateo, F.; Ravaglioli, A.; Andreoli, C.; Bonina, F.; Coiro, V.; Degetto, S.; Giaretta, A.; Menconi Orsini, A.; Puglia, C.; Summa, V. The in-vitro percutaneous migration of chemical elements from a thermal mud for healing use. *Appl. Clay Sci.* **2009**, *44*, 83–94. [CrossRef]
10. Hostynek, J.J. Factors determining percutaneous metal absorption. *Food Chem. Toxicol.* **2003**, *41*, 327–345. [CrossRef]
11. Sánchez-Espejo, R.; Aguzzi, C.; Salcedo, I.; Cerezo, P.; Viseras, C. Clays in complementary and alternative medicine. *Mater. Technol.* **2014**, *29*, B78–B81. [CrossRef]
12. Natural Health Products Ingredients Database. Available online: http://webprod.hc-sc.gc.ca/nhpid-bdipsn/search-rechercheReq.do (accessed on 18 December 2019).
13. López-Galindo, A.; Viseras, C. Pharmaceutical and Cosmetic Application of Clays. In *Clay Surfaces: Fundamentals and Applications*; Wypyc, F., Satyanarayana, K.G., Eds.; Elsevier Ltd.: Berlin, Germany, 2004; pp. 267–289. Available online: https://www.sciencedirect.com/science/article/pii/B978044453607500013X (accessed on 1 July 2020).
14. Viseras, C.; López-Galindo, A. Pharmaceutical applications of some spanish clays (sepiolite, palygorskite, bentonite): Some preformulation studies. *Appl. Clay Sci.* **1999**, *14*, 69–82. [CrossRef]
15. Viseras, C.; Lopez-Galindo, A.; Yebra, A. Characteristics of pharmaceutical grade phyllosilicate compacts. *Pharm Dev. Technol.* **2000**, *5*, 53–58. [CrossRef]
16. López-Galindo, A.; Viseras, C.; Aguzzi, C.; Cerezo, P. Pharmaceutical and cosmetic uses of fibrous clays. In *Developments in Clay Science*; Galán, E., Singer, A., Eds.; Elsevier Ltd.: Berlin, Germany, 2011; Volume 3, pp. 299–324, ISBN 9780444536075.
17. López-Galindo, A.; Viseras, C.; Cerezo, P. Compositional, technical and safety specifications of clays to be used as pharmaceutical and cosmetic products. *Appl. Clay Sci.* **2007**, *36*, 51–63. [CrossRef]
18. Potpara, Z.; Duborija-Kovacevic, N. Effects of the peloid cream from the Montenegrin Adriatic coast on skin humidity, transepidermal water loss and erythema index, examined with skin bioengeneering in vivo methods. *Farmacia* **2012**, *60*, 524–534.
19. Centini, M.; Tredici, M.R.; Biondi, N.; Buonocore, A.; Maffei Facino, R.; Anselmi, C. Thermal mud maturation: Organic matter and biological activity. *Int. J. Cosmet. Sci.* **2015**, *37*, 339–347. [CrossRef]
20. Khiari, I.; Sánchez-Espejo, R.; García-Villén, F.; Cerezo, P.; Aguzzi, C.; López-Galindo, A.; Jamoussi, F.; Viseras, C. Rheology and cation release of tunisian medina mud-packs intended for topical applications. *Appl. Clay Sci.* **2019**, *171*, 110–117. [CrossRef]

21. Elkayam, O.; Ophir, J.; Brener, S.; Paran, D.; Wigler, I.; Efron, D.; Even-Paz, Z.; Politi, Y.; Yaron, M. Immediate and delayed effects of treatment at the Dead Sea in patients with psoriatic arthritis. *Rheumatol. Int.* **2000**, *19*, 77–82. [CrossRef] [PubMed]
22. Delfino, M.; Russo, N.; Migliaccio, G.; Carraturo, N. Experimental study on efficacy of thermal muds of Ischia Island combined with balneotherapy in the treatment of psoriasis vulgaris with plaques. *Clin. Ter.* **2003**, *154*, 167–171. [PubMed]
23. Cozzi, F.; Raffeiner, B.; Beltrame, V.; Ciprian, L.; Coran, A.; Botsios, C.; Perissinotto, E.; Grisan, E.; Ramonda, R.; Oliviero, F.; et al. Effects of mud-bath therapy in psoriatic arthritis patients treated with TNF inhibitors. Clinical evaluation and assessment of synovial inflammation by contrast-enhanced ultrasound (CEUS). *Jt. Bone Spine* **2015**, *82*, 104–108. [CrossRef] [PubMed]
24. Riyaz, N.; Arakkal, F. Spa therapy in dermatology. *Indian J. Dermatol. Venereol. Leprol.* **2011**, *77*, 128. [CrossRef]
25. Harari, M. Beauty is not only skin deep: The Dead Sea features and cosmetics. *Anales de Hidrología Médica* **2012**, *5*, 75–88.
26. Williams, L.B.; Haydel, S.E.; Giese, R.F., Jr.; Eberl, D.D. Chemical and mineralogical characteristics of french green clays used for healing. *Clays Clay Miner.* **2008**, *56*, 437–452. [CrossRef]
27. Comacchi, C.; Hercogova, J. A single mud treatment induces normalization of stratum corneum hydration, transepidermal water loss, skin surface pH and sebum content in patients with seborrhoeic dermatitis. *J. Eur. Acad. Dermatol. Venereol.* **2004**, *18*, 372–374. [CrossRef]
28. Argenziano, G.; Delfino, M.; Russo, N. Mud and baththerapy in the acne cure. *Clin. Ter.* **2004**, *155*, 125.
29. Masiero, S.; Maccarone, M.C.; Magro, G. Balneotherapy and human immune function in the era of COVID-19. *Int. J. Biometeorol.* **2020**, *1*, 1–2. [CrossRef]
30. *Guideline for Elemental Impurities Q3D(R1)*; European Medicines Agency: Amsterdam, The Netherlands, 2019.
31. Bocca, B.; Pino, A.; Alimonti, A.; Forte, G. Toxic metals contained in cosmetics: A status report. *Regul. Toxicol. Pharmacol.* **2014**, *68*, 447–467. [CrossRef]
32. García-Villén, F.; Sánchez-Espejo, R.; López-Galindo, A.; Cerezo, P.; Viseras, C. Design and characterization of spring water hydrogels with natural inorganic excipients. *Appl. Clay Sci.* **2020**, *197*, 105772. [CrossRef]
33. *United States Pharmacopeia and National Formulary, 2019*; United States Pharmacopeial Convention: Rockville, MD, USA, 2016.
34. Ph. Eur. 9th. Magnesium trisilicate monograph. In *European Pharmacopoeia*; Council of Europe: Strasbourg, France, 2018.
35. Ph. Eur. 9th. Magnesium Aluminium silicate monograph. In *European Pharmacopoeia*; Council of Europe: Strasbourg, France, 2018.
36. Diputación Provincial de Granada; Instituto Tecnológico Geominero de España Atlas Hidrogeológico de la Provincia de Granada. Available online: http://aguas.igme.es/igme/publica/libro75/lib_75.htm (accessed on 10 September 2018).
37. Maraver Eyzaguirre, F.; Armijo de Castro, F. *Vademécum II de Aguas Mineromedicinales Españolas*; Maraver Eyzaguirre, F., Armijo Castro, F., Eds.; Editorial Complutense: Madrid, Spain, 2010; ISBN 9788474919981.
38. The European Cosmetic and Perfumeryn Association. *Guidelines for Percutaneous Absorption/Penetration*; COLIPA: Brussels, Belgium, 1997; pp. 1–36.
39. *Quality of Natural Health Products Guide*; Natural and Non-Prescription Health Products Directorate: Ottawa, ON, Canada, 2015.
40. Sánchez-Espejo, R.M. *Suspensions of Special Clays in Mineromedicinal Waters to Be Used in Therapeutics*; Andalusian Institute of Earth Science and University of Granada: Granada, Spain, 2014.
41. Meijide Faílde, R.; Mourelle Mosqueira, L.; Vela Anero, Á.; Muíños López, E.; Fernández Burguera, E.; Gómez Pérez, C.P. Aplicación a pacientes: Peloterapia en patologías dermatológicas. In *Peloterapia: Aplicaciones Médicas y Cosméticas de Fangos Termales*; Fundación BILBILIS para la Investigación e Innovación en Hidrología Médica y Balneaoterapia: Madrid, Spain, 2013; pp. 169–183.
42. Gomes, C.; Silva, J.; Gomes, J. Natural peloids versus designed and engineered peloids. *Bol. Soc. Española Hidrol. Medica* **2015**, *30*, 15–36. [CrossRef]
43. Post, J.L.; Crawford, S. Varied forms of palygorskite and sepiolite from different geologic systems. *Appl. Clay Sci.* **2007**, *36*, 232–244. [CrossRef]

44. Ababneh, F.A.; Abu-Sbeih, K.A.; Al-Momani, I.F. Evaluation of allergenic metals and other trace elements in personal care products. *Jordan J. Chem.* **2013**, *8*, 179–190. [CrossRef]
45. Yuan, J.; Hou, Q.; Chen, D.; Zhong, L.; Dai, X.; Zhu, Z.; Li, M.; Fu, X. Chitosan/LiCl composite scaffolds promote skin regeneration in full-thickness loss. *Sci. China Life Sci.* **2019**, *28*, 1–11. [CrossRef] [PubMed]
46. Leeming, J.P. Use of topical lithium succinate in the treatment of seborrhoeic dermatitis. *Dermatology* **1993**, *187*, 149. [CrossRef]
47. Dreno, B.; Moyse, D. Lithium gluconate in the treatment of seborrhoeic dermatitis: A multicenter, randomised, double-blind study versus placebo. *Eur. J. Dermatol.* **2002**, *12*, 549–552.
48. Dreno, B.; Chosidow, O.; Revuz, J.; Moyse, D. Lithium gluconate 8% vs. ketoconazole 2% in the treatment of seborrhoeic dermatitis: A multicentre, randomized study. *Br. J. Dermatol.* **2003**, *148*, 1230–1236. [CrossRef]
49. Gupta, A.K.; Versteeg, S.G. Topical treatment of facial seborrheic dermatitis: A systematic review. *Am. J. Clin. Dermatol.* **2017**, *18*, 193–213. [CrossRef]
50. McKnight, R.; Adida, M.; Budge, K.; Stockton, S.; Goodwin, G.; Gedded, J. Lithium toxicity profile: A systematic review and meta-analysis. *Lancet* **2012**, *379*, 721–728. [CrossRef]
51. Grandjean, E.; Aubry, J. Lithium: Updated human knowledge using an evidence-based approach. Part II: Clinical pharmacology and therapeutic monitoring. *CNS Drugs* **2009**, *23*, 331–349. [CrossRef] [PubMed]
52. Granjeiro, J.M.; Cruz, R.; Leite, P.E.; Gemini-Piperni, S.; Boldrini, L.C.; Ribeiro, A.R. Health and environment perspective of tin nanocompounds: A safety approach. In *Tin Oxide Materials. Synthesis, Properties, and Applications*; Ornaghi-Orlandi, M., Ed.; Elsevier: Berlin, Germany, 2020; pp. 133–162.
53. Bai, D.; Li, Q.; Xiong, Y.; Zhao, J.; Bai, L.; Shen, P.; Yuan, L. Editor's highlight: Effects of intraperitoneal injection of SnS2 flowers on mouse testicle. *Toxicol. Sci.* **2018**, *161*, 388–400. [CrossRef] [PubMed]
54. Tabei, Y.; Sonoda, A.; Nakajima, Y.; Biju, V.; Makita, Y.; Yoshida, Y.; Horie, M. In vitro evaluation of the cellular effect of indium tin oxide nanoparticles using the human lung adenocarcinoma A549 cells. *Metallomics* **2015**, *7*, 816–827. [CrossRef] [PubMed]
55. Roopan, S.M.; Kumar, S.H.S.; Madhumitha, G.; Suthindhiran, K. Biogenic-production of SnO2 nanoparticles and its cytotoxic effect against hepatocellular carcinoma cell line (HepG2). *Appl. Biochem. Biotechnol.* **2014**, *175*, 1567–1575. [CrossRef]
56. Boogaard, P.J.; Boisset, M.; Blunden, S.; Davies, S.; Ong, T.J.; Taverne, J.P. Comparative assessment of gastrointestinal irritant potency in man of tin (II) chloride and tin migrated from packaging. *Food Chem. Toxicol.* **2003**, *41*, 1663–1670. [CrossRef]
57. García-Villén, F.; Faccendini, A.; Miele, D.; Ruggeri, M.; Sánchez-Espejo, R.; Borrego-Sánchez, A.; Cerezo, P.; Rossi, S.; Viseras, C.; Sandri, G. Wound healing activity of nanoclay/spring water hydrogels. *Pharmaceutics* **2020**, *12*, 467. [CrossRef]
58. Hepp, N.M.; Mindak, W.R.; Gasper, J.W.; Thompson, C.B.; Barrows, J.N. Survey of cosmetics for arsenic, cadmium, chromium, cobalt, lead, mercury, and nickel content. *J. Cosmet. Sci.* **2014**, *65*, 125–145.
59. Zulaikha, S.; Syed Ismail, S.N.; Praveena, S.M. Hazardous ingredients in cosmetics and personal care products and health concern: A review. *Public Health Res.* **2015**, *5*, 7–15.
60. Schaumlöffel, D. Nickel species: Analysis and toxic effects. *J. Trace Elem. Med. Biol.* **2012**, *26*, 1–6. [CrossRef]
61. Román-Razo, E.A.; O'Farrill, P.M.; Cambray, C.; Herrera, A.; Mendoza-Revilla, D.A.; Aguirre, D. Allergic contact dermatitis to cobalt and nickel in a metal industry worker. Case report and literature review. *Rev. Alerg. Mex.* **2019**, *66*, 371–374.
62. Chou, T.C.; Wang, P.C.; De Wu, J.; Sheu, S.C. Chromium-induced skin damage among Taiwanese cement workers. *Toxicol. Ind. Health* **2016**, *32*, 1745–1751. [CrossRef] [PubMed]
63. Pathania, Y.S.; Budania, A. Chrome Ulcers: An occupational hazard. *J. Eur. Acad. Dermatol. Venereol.* **2019**, *34*, e180–e182. [CrossRef] [PubMed]
64. Al Hossain, M.M.A.; Yajima, I.; Tazaki, A.; Xu, H.; Saheduzzaman, M.; Ohgami, N.; Ahsan, N.; Akhand, A.A.; Kato, M. Chromium-mediated hyperpigmentation of skin in male tannery workers in Bangladesh. *Chemosphere* **2019**, *229*, 611–617. [CrossRef] [PubMed]
65. Larese Filon, F.; Maina, G.; Adami, G.; Venier, M.; Coceani, N.; Bussani, R.; Massiccio, M.; Barbieri, P.; Spinelli, P. In vitro percutaneous absorption of cobalt. *Int. Arch. Occup. Environ. Health* **2004**, *77*, 85–89. [CrossRef] [PubMed]
66. Filon, F.L.; D'Agostin, F.; Crosera, M.; Adami, G.; Bovenzi, M.; Maina, G. In vitro absorption of metal powders through intact and damaged human skin. *Toxicol. In Vitro* **2009**, *23*, 574–579. [CrossRef] [PubMed]

67. Mukherjee, B.; Patra, B.; Mahapatra, S.; Banerjee, P.; Tiwari, A.; Chatterjee, M. Vanadium—An element of atypical biological significance. *Toxicol. Lett.* **2004**, *150*, 135–143. [CrossRef]
68. Pisano, M.; Arru, C.; Serra, M.; Galleri, G.; Sanna, D.; Garribba, E.; Palmieri, G.; Rozzo, C. Antiproliferative activity of vanadium compounds: Effects on the major malignant melanoma molecular pathways. *Metallomics* **2019**, *11*, 1687–1699. [CrossRef]
69. EU. *Regulation (EC) No 1272/2008 on Classification, Labelling and Packaging of Substances and Mixtures, Amending and Repealing Directives 67/548/EEC and 1999/45/EC, and Amending Regulation (EC) No 1907/2006*; Official Journal of the European Union, 2008; pp. 1–1355. Available online: https://osha.europa.eu/es/legislation/directives/regulation-ec-no-1272-2008-classification-labelling-and-packaging-of-substances-and-mixtures (accessed on 10 August 2020).
70. US Environmental Protection Agency. Technical Fact Sheet: Final Rule for Arsenic in Drinking Water; Office of Water; United States. 2001. Available online: https://nepis.epa.gov/Exe/ZyNET.exe/20001XXE.TXT?ZyActionD=ZyDocument&Client=EPA&Index=2000+Thru+2005&Docs=&Query=&Time=&EndTime=&SearchMethod=1&TocRestrict=n&Toc=&TocEntry=&QField=&QFieldYear=&QFieldMonth=&QFieldDay=&IntQFieldOp=0&ExtQFieldOp=0&XmlQuery=&File=D%3A%5Czyfiles%5CIndex%20Data%5C00thru05%5CTxt%5C00000001%5C20001XXE.txt&User=ANONYMOUS&Password=anonymous&SortMethod=h%7C-&MaximumDocuments=1&FuzzyDegree=0&ImageQuality=r75g8/r75g8/x150y150g16/i425&Display=hpfr&DefSeekPage=x&SearchBack=ZyActionL&Back=ZyActionS&BackDesc=Results%20page&MaximumPages=1&ZyEntry=1&SeekPage=x&ZyPURL (accessed on 10 August 2020).
71. WHO. *Guidelines for Drinking-Water Quality*, 4th ed.; World Health Organization: Geneva, Switzerland, 2017; ISBN 978-92-4-154995-0.
72. Shirvani, M.; Kalbasi, M.; Shariatmadari, H.; Nourbakhsh, F.; Najafi, B. Sorption-desorption of cadmium in aqueous palygorskite, sepiolite, and calcite suspensions: Isotherm hysteresis. *Chemosphere* **2006**, *65*, 2178–2184. [CrossRef]
73. Tucovic, D.; Popov Aleksandrov, A.; Mirkov, I.; Ninkov, M.; Kulas, J.; Zolotarevski, L.; Vukojevic, V.; Mutic, J.; Tatalovic, N.; Kataranovski, M. Oral cadmium exposure affects skin immune reactivity in rats. *Ecotoxicol. Environ. Saf.* **2018**, *164*, 12–20. [CrossRef]
74. Wester, R.C.; Maibach, H.I.; Sedik, L.; Melendres, J.; DiZio, S.; Wade, M. In vitro percutaneous absorption of cadmium from water and soil into human skin. *Fundam. Appl. Toxicol.* **1992**, *19*, 1–5. [CrossRef]
75. Bradbury, M.H.; Baeyens, B.; Geckeis, H.; Rabung, T. Sorption of Eu(III)/Cm(III) on Ca-montmorillonite and Na-illite. Part 2: Surface complexation modelling. *Geochim. Cosmochim. Acta* **2005**, *69*, 5403–5412. [CrossRef]
76. Elzinga, E.J.; Rouff, A.A.; Reeder, R.J. The long-term fate of Cu^{2+}, Zn^{2+}, and Pb^{2+} adsorption complexes at the calcite surface: An X-ray absorption spectroscopy study. *Geochim. Cosmochim. Acta* **2006**, *70*, 2715–2725. [CrossRef]
77. Altmann, S.; Tournassat, C.; Goutelard, F.; Parneix, J.C.; Gimmi, T.; Maes, N. Diffusion-driven transport in clayrock formations. *Appl. Geochemistry* **2012**, *27*, 463–478. [CrossRef]
78. Guo, N.; Wang, J.S.; Li, J.; Teng, Y.G.; Zhai, Y.Z. Dynamic adsorption of Cd^{2+} onto acid-modified attapulgite from aqueous solution. *Clays Clay Miner.* **2014**, *62*, 415–424. [CrossRef]
79. Cheng, Q.; Ye, R. A Kind of Hydrogel Expanded Material for Handling Heavy Metal Containing Sewage and Preparation Method Thereof. 2015. Available online: https://patents.google.com/patent/CN105542095B/en (accessed on 1 July 2020).
80. Zhang, J.; Jin, Y.; Wang, A. Rapid removal of Pb(II) from aqueous solution by chitosan-*g*-poly(acrylic acid)/attapulgite/sodium humate composite hydrogels. *Environ. Technol.* **2011**, *32*, 523–531. [CrossRef] [PubMed]
81. Wang, X.; Wang, A. Removal of Cd(II) from aqueous solution by a composite hydrogel based on attapulgite. *Environ. Technol.* **2010**, *31*, 745–753. [CrossRef]

2

Halloysite- and Montmorillonite-Loaded Scaffolds as Enhancers of Chronic Wound Healing

Giuseppina Sandri [1,*], Angela Faccendini [1], Marysol Longo [1,2], Marco Ruggeri [1], Silvia Rossi [1], Maria Cristina Bonferoni [1], Dalila Miele [1], Adriele Prina-Mello [2], Carola Aguzzi [3], Cesar Viseras [3] and Franca Ferrari [1]

1 Department of Drug Sciences, University of Pavia, Viale Taramelli 12, 27100 Pavia, Italy; angela.faccendini@gmail.com (A.F.); marysol.longo01@universitadipavia.it (M.L.); marco.ruggeri02@universitadipavia.it (M.R.); silvia.rossi@unipv.it (S.R.); cbonferoni@unipv.it (M.C.B.); dalila.miele@gmail.com (D.M.); franca.ferrari@unipv.it (F.F.)

2 Trinity Translational Medicine Institute, Trinity College Dublin, Dublin 8, Dublin, Ireland; prinamea@tcd.ie

3 Department of Pharmacy and Pharmaceutical Technology, Faculty of Pharmacy, University of Granada, Campus of Cartuja s/n, 18071 Granada, Spain; carola@ugr.es (C.A.); cviseras@ugr.es (C.V.)

* Correspondence: giuseppina.sandri@unipv.it

Abstract: The increase in life expectancy and the increasing prevalence of diabetic disease and venous insufficiency lead to the increase of chronic wounds. The prevalence of ulcers ranges from 1% in the adult population to 3–5% in the over 65 years population, with 3–5.5% of the total healthcare expenditure, as recently estimated. The aim of this work was the design and the development of electrospun scaffolds, entirely based on biopolymers, loaded with montmorillonite (MMT) or halloysite (HNT) and intended for skin reparation and regeneration, as a 3D substrate mimicking the dermal ECM. The scaffolds were manufactured by means of electrospinning and were characterized for their chemico-physical and preclinical properties. The scaffolds proved to possess the capability to enhance fibroblast cells attachment and proliferation with negligible proinflammatory activity. The capability to facilitate the cell adhesion is probably due to their unique 3D structure which are assisting cell homing and would facilitate wound healing in vivo.

Keywords: electrospinning; chitosan; chondroitin sulfate; scaffolds; montmorillonite; halloysite; fibroblasts proliferation; immune response

---

1. Introduction

The skin is the largest organ of the body and plays a pivotal role in maintaining physiological homeostasis against fluid imbalance, thermal dysregulation, and infections. It is formed by the epidermis, consisting of keratinocytes, and by the dermis, mainly based on the extracellular matrix (ECM) (collagen, elastin, glycosaminoglycans) and sparse fibroblasts. Damage or loss of integrity of the skin caused by a wound, may impair skin functions, exposing the body to potentially challenging situations. Wound healing is a complex event based on overlapping but well-orchestrated cellular and molecular processes to repair damaged tissue and restore skin function. Healing is divided in different phases (hemostasis, inflammatory, proliferative, and remodeling) and is accomplished by ECM molecules, soluble mediators, as cytokines and growth factors, various resident cells, and infiltrating leucocytes [1].

Acute wounds are mainly traumatic or surgical and generally heal within few weeks without any significant interventions, whereas in chronic wounds, the healing process remains frozen in the inflammatory state. These, commonly defined as wounds that fail to proceed through an orderly and timely process to restore skin anatomical and functional integrity. These include venous leg ulcers, arterial ulcers, diabetic ulcers, and pressure ulcers, such as bed sores. The increase in life expectancy and the increasing prevalence of diabetic disease and venous insufficiency lead to an increase in chronic wounds. Although assessing the prevalence of chronic wounds is problematic because of the disparities in study design and their evaluation, they have become a major challenge to healthcare systems worldwide. It is estimated that the prevalence of ulcers ranges from 1% in the adult population to 3–5% in the over 65 years population; whereas globally it accounts for the 3–5.5% of the total healthcare expenditure as recently estimated [2,3].

Recently, clay minerals have been proposed in the biomedical field in tissue engineering as enhancers of cell attachment, proliferation and differentiation [4,5], and also as antimicrobials [6]. In particular, montmorillonite (MMT, M_x (Al_2-yMg_y) Si_4O_{10} $(OH)_2$ nH_2O) and halloysite (HNT, Al_2O_3 $2SiO_2$ $2H_2O$) have been recently described as biocompatible and as proliferation enhancers [7]. Both MMT and HNT are phyllosilicates, having a planar and rolled structure, respectively. Nanocomposites, based on these biomaterials, have been developed to tune cell adhesion and their biocompatibility [8–11]. The cell interaction with clays remain unclear and not fully understood, and only a few recent studies have attempted to shed light on this interaction [7,12].

However, there are many evidences in literature related to the combination of nanostructured materials with nanoscale fabrication processes, to achieve high levels of morphological control, surface and mechanical properties [13–15]. In light of these, layered silicates are characterized by a high aspect ratio with the ability to confer high strength to 3D structures. Moreover, unlike most inorganic fillers, layered silicates are hydrophilic, and capable to interact with the polymer matrix, by changing surface tension, conductivity, and shear viscosity. Thus, the combination of clay minerals and nanofibrous scaffolds should lead to 3D architectures which facilitate cell homing, but also enhance the cell attachment and proliferation thanks to the enhancing properties provided by biopolymers. In particular, chitosan and chondroitin sulfate are polysaccharides capable to aid cell proliferation, and moreover, the latter is also providing protection against growth factor degradation by electrostatic interaction [16]. Having previously assessed the scaffold composition in the basic biopolymers [16]; these made of pullulan, chitosan, and chondroitin sulfate; the manufacturing processing was then addressed by means of electrospinning in a one-pot process to obtain a nanofibrous scaffold which proved to enhance the mechanical properties of the scaffold.

Given the advances achieved on these materials and their manufacturing processes, the aim of this work was the design, development and characterization of electrospun 3D scaffolds, entirely based on biopolymers, loaded with MMT or HNT, as a dermal substitute for skin reparation and regeneration tested in a preclinical model, leading to tissue reparation towards a complete skin restore.

2. Materials and Methods

2.1. Materials

The following polysaccharides were used: chitosan (CH) (β-(1-4)-linked D-glucosamine and N-acetyl-D-glucosamine) low MW 251 kDa, deacetylation degree 98%, (ChitoClear, Iceland); chondroitin sodium sulfate (CS) (β-1,4-linked D-glucuronic acid and β-1,3-linked N-acetyl galactosamine) bovine 100 EP, low MW 14 kDa, and a mixture of chondroitin A (chondroitin 4 sulfate) and chondroitin C (chondroitin 6 sulfate) (Bioiberica, Italy); pullulan (P) (based on maltotriose repeating units, linear α 1–4 and α 1–6 glucan, produced by *Aureobasidium pullulans*) low MW ~200–300 kDa (food grade, Hayashibara, Giusto Faravelli, Italy). Citric Acid (CA) (monohydrated citric acid, EP grade, Carlo Erba, I) was used as the crosslinking agent. Pharmaceutical grade clay minerals were considered: montmorillonite (MMT) (particle size: 1352 nm (±17); polydispersity index: 0.696 (±0.184)) (Veegum® HS, Vanderbilt, Nashville, TN, USA) or halloysite (particle size: 563 nm (±70); polydispersity index: 0.647 (±0.077); internal diameter = 28 ± 5.1 nm and external diameter = 70 ± 8.3 nm) (Halloysite Nanotubes—HTNs) (Sigma-Aldrich, St. Louis, MO, USA).

2.2. Methods

2.2.1. Preparation of Polymeric Blends

P and CS were solubilized in water while the CH solution was prepared in 90% v/v acetic acid and CA was added. A polymeric blend was prepared by mixing P and CS with a CH solution at a 1:1 weight ratio. The preparation schematic is reported in Figure 1.

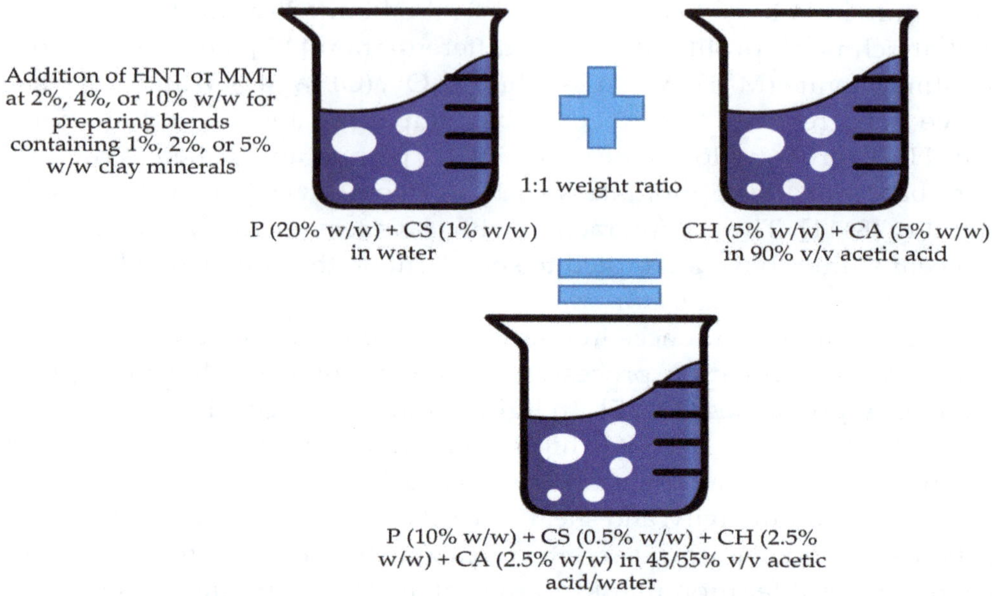

Figure 1. Schematic of the blend preparation.

The hybrid blends were then prepared by the addition of MMT or HNT to the polymeric blend, prepared as previously described [16]. For this purpose, clay minerals were grounded in a mortar and sieved with a 75 µm sieve. Either MMT or HNT were added to the P and CS blend at different concentrations. All the blends prepared had the same composition in polysaccharides while they were based on different concentrations of clay minerals. The composition of all the systems prepared is reported in Table 1.

Table 1. Composition (% w/w) of the polymeric blends.

% w/w	MMT	HNT	P	CH	CA	CS	H_2O/CH_3COOH
Blank	-	-					
MMT1	1	-					
MMT2	2	-					
MMT5	5	-	10	2.5	2.5	0.5	55/45
HNT1	-	1					
HNT2	-	2					
HNT5	-	5					

2.2.2. Characterization of Polymeric Blends

The surface tension of the blends was measured at T = 30 °C with a tensiometer (DY-300, Kyowa, Japan) (measurement range 0–300 mN/m) equipped with a platinum plate of 2.5 cm × 1 cm.

The electrical conductivity was determined by a conductometer (FiveGoTM-Mettler Toledo, Italy) equipped with the LE703-IP67 sensor.

The penetrometry was measured using the Texture Analyzer TA-XT plus (ENCO, Italy), equipped with an A/TG measuring system and a 5 kg load cell. The analysis was performed employing a Perspex 20 mm cylinder probe (P/20P; Batch N° 11434). The measuring probe was lowered at a 0.50 mm/s speed up to a 3 mm penetration distance. The penetration force was recorded as a function of probe displacement.

2.2.3. Preparation of Electrospun Scaffolds

Scaffolds were obtained using an electrospinning apparatus (STKIT-40, Linari Engineering, Italy), equipped with a high-voltage power supply (40 kV), a volumetric pump (Razel R99-E), a 10 mL syringe, and a conductive static collector, covered by aluminum foil. The following parameters were used: ΔV (voltage) = 22 kV, collector spinneret distance = 24 cm, polymeric solution flow = 0.4 mL/h, spinning time = 1.30 h, temperature = 30 °C, relative humidity = 30%; and needle dimensions: 0.5 × 20 mm for MMT and 0.4 × 20 mm for HNT. The obtained scaffolds were then crosslinked by heating at 150 °C for 1 h, to prevent their solubilization in aqueous media and to allow cell homing. The heating process is also reported as able to dry sterilize the products [17].

2.2.4. Scaffold Characterizations

Chemico-Physical Characterization

Scaffold morphology was assessed by means of SEM (Tescan, Mira3XMU, CISRIC, University of Pavia) after graphite sputtering. The scaffolds were analyzed before and after the crosslinking procedure and after 6 days of hydration in distilled water. Nanofiber diameters and pores sizes were measured by image analysis software (DiameterJ plugin, Image J, NIH).

X-ray powder diffraction (XRPD) analysis was carried out using a diffractometer (X-Pert Pro model, Malven Panalytical, Italy) equipped with a solid-state detector (X-Celerator) and a spinning sample holder. The diffractogram patterns were recorded using random oriented mounts with CuKα radiation, operating at 45 kV and 40 mA, in the range 4–60° 2θ. The diffraction data were analyzed using the XPOWDER® software (www.xpowder.com).

Fourier-transform infrared spectroscopy (FT-IR) spectra were recorded using spectrophotometer (JASCO 6200) with a Ge ATR. All samples were analyzed from 400 to 4000 cm^{-1} with a resolution of 0.25 cm^{-1} and the results were processed with Spectra Manager v2 software.

Thermogravimetric analysis (TGA) (TGA-50H, Shimadzu, Kyoto, Japan) was performed using a vertical oven and a precision of 0.001 mg. Approximately 40 mg of each sample were placed in aluminum pans. The experiments were performed at the 30–950 °C range and using a 10 °C/min heating rate. Additionally, differential scanning calorimetry (DSC) analyses were performed (Mettler Toledo, Columbus, OH, USA) using aluminum crucibles, a 30–400 °C temperature range, at a heating rate of 10 °C/min. All the analyses were performed in atmospheric air.

High-resolution Transmission Electron Microscopy (TEM) was performed by means of an analytical electron microscope (AEM) (Titan G2 60–300, FEI Company, Thermo Fisher Scientific, Waltham, MA, USA) with a SUPER-X silicon-drift windowless energy dispersive X-ray spectroscopy detector. X-ray chemical element maps were also collected. The samples were directly deposited onto copper grids (300 mesh coated by formvar/carbon film, Agar Scientific, Italy).

Mechanical Properties

Mechanical properties of nanofibrous scaffolds were measured using a TA-XT plus Texture Analyzer (Stable Microsystems, ENCO, Italy) equipped with a 5.0 kg load cell. Before testing, nanofibrous scaffolds were cut 30 × 10 mm and the strips (thickness ranging from 150 to 200 μm, thickness gauge apparatus, Mitutoyo) were clamped between two tensile grips (A/TG probe) setting an initial distance between the grips of 10.0 mm. Mechanical properties were evaluated in the dry and hydrated state. The hydration was performed by dipping the scaffolds in water up to complete hydration (1 h). Then, the upper grip was moved forward at a constant speed of 5.0 mm/s up to break. The force at break was recorded (force at break) (TS, N/mm^2) and the elongation (%) was calculated as follows:

$$E\% = 100 \times (L_{break} - L_0)/L_{break} \tag{1}$$

where L_{break} is the distance of the two grips at scaffold breaking and L_0 is the initial distance of the two grips.

Moreover, Young's Modulus (mN/cm^2) was calculated as the slope of the initial linear portion of force vs. grip displacement [10,18,19].

Fibroblasts Biocompatibility and Adhesion

NHDFs (normal human dermal fibroblasts from juvenile foreskin, Promocell WVR, Italy) were grown with Dulbecco's Modified Eagle Medium (Sigma, I) supplemented with 10% fetal bovine serum (FBS, Sigma, Italy) and with 200 IU/mL penicillin/0.2 mg/mL streptomycin (Sigma-Aldrich, Italy), kept at 37 °C in a 5% CO_2 atmosphere with 95% relative humidity (RH).

Preliminarily, the cytocompatibility and proliferation in the presence of pure components were assessed. Fibroblasts were seeded with a seeding density of 25×10^3 cells/well in 96-well plates. After 24 h of growth (at sub-confluence), the following samples (in growth medium, GM) were considered: CS (0.08 mg/mL), P (1.5 mg/mL), CA (0.4 mg/mL), CH (0.4 mg/mL), MMT (MMT1: 0.2 mg/mL; MMT2: 0.8 mg/mL; MMT5: 1.2 mg/mL), and HNT (HNT1: 0.2 mg/mL; HNT 2: 0.8 mg/mL; HNT5: 1.2 mg/mL). Valinomycin (Val, Fisher Scientific, Ireland) (final concentration 120 μM) was used as the cytotoxic control and GM (growth medium) as the biocompatible control.

After 24 or 72 h of contact, the MTT test was performed. Briefly, the MTT test evaluates the activity of mitochondrial dehydrogenase of vital cells that convert MTT into formazan salts. The MTT was solubilized in PBS at a concentration of 5 mg/mL per well. A total of 50 μL of the MTT solution and 100 μL of the DMEM (DMEM w/o phenol red, Sigma, Italy) were dispensed into each well and subsequently the plates were placed in an incubator at 37 °C for 3 h. The reagent was then removed from each well and the cells were washed with 150 μL of PBS to remove the samples and the un-reacted MTT solution. After PBS removal, 100 μL of DMSO were added to each well and the absorbance was detected with an ELISA plate reader (ELISA plate reader, Biorad, Italy; Epoch, Microplate Spectrophotometer, BioTek, Ireland) at a wavelength of 570 nm with a wavelength of reference of 690 nm.

Subsequently the scaffold cytocompatibility was assessed. For this purpose, scaffolds were cut to have an area of 0.36 cm^2 to cover the bottom of a well in a 96 well-plate and fibroblasts were seeded onto each scaffold with 35×10^3 cells/well and grown for 3, 6, and 10 days. An MTT assay was performed, as previously described. In addition, SEM and CLSM analysis were performed to visualize the fibroblasts adhered and proliferated to each scaffold.

Fibroblasts grown onto the scaffolds were fixed with a 3% glutaraldehyde solution for 1 h at 4 °C (glutaraldehyde 50%—Sigma Aldrich, Italy), and washed twice with PBS. As for SEM, scaffolds were dehydrated in increasing concentrations of ethanol, placed onto stub and sputtered with graphite. The images were acquired at a high voltage of 8 kV, in high vacuum, at room temperature and different magnifications (5.00 kX; 10.00 kX; 20.00 kX) (SEM: Tescan, Mira3XMU, CISRIC, University of Pavia).

As for CLSM the fixed scaffolds were stained by dipping the scaffolds in contact with 50 μL of phalloidin Atto 488 (50 μg/mL in PBS) (Sigma Aldrich, Italy) for 40 min. Cell nuclei were subsequently stained by dipping the scaffolds in 100 μL of Hoechst 33258 solution (0.5 μg/mL in PBS) (Sigma Aldrich, Italy) for 10 min. Subsequently, the samples were washed twice for 10 min with PBS and placed on microscope slide and analyzed by using a CLSM (Leica TCS SP2, Leica Microsystems, Italy) using $\lambda ex = 346$ nm and $\lambda em = 460$ nm for Hoechst 33342 (Sigma, Italy) and $\lambda ex = 501$ nm and $\lambda em = 523$ nm for phalloidin Atto 488 (Sigma, Italy).

Cytocompatibility of Macrophages and Pro-Inflammatory Immune Response

Human monocytic cell line THP-1 (American Type Culture Collection, Manassas, VA, USA) was cultured in RPMI-1640 medium (Gibco, Thermo Fisher, Ireland) supplemented with 10% fetal bovine serum (FBS, Sigma, Ireland), and with 200 IU/mL penicillin/0.2 mg/mL streptomycin kept at 37 °C in a 5% CO_2 atmosphere with 95% relative humidity (RH). A total of 1×10^5 cells/mL were treated with

100 nM phorbol-12-myristate-13-acetate (PMA, Sigma Aldrich, Germany) for 48 h. After 48 h the cells were differentiated into macrophages and let to rest for 24 h before being treated.

Preliminarily, the cytocompatibility of the pure components was assessed considering sample concentrations as previously described in Section "Fibroblasts Biocompatibility and Adhesion" paragraph. Valinomycin (Val, Fisher Scientific, Ireland) or cysplatinum (Cys, Sigma Aldrich, Ireland) (final concentration 120 μM) was used as the cytotoxic control and GM (growth medium) as the biocompatible control.

THP-1 was differentiated using PMA and 20×10^3 cells were seeded in each well of the 96-well plates. After 24 h rest, the components were added to each well and the biocompatibility was assessed after 24 or 72 h of contact time, using MTT test, as previously described.

Subsequently, the scaffold cytocompatibility was assessed. Scaffolds were cut to have an area of 7.65 cm^2 (diameters of 1.5 cm) and placed on a cell crown (Sigma, Italy). THP-1 cells were differentiated by seeding 200×10^3 cells on the bottom of each well of the 24-well plates. After 24 h rest, the scaffold placed on the cell crown was inserted in the well. The cytocompatibility was assessed using an MTT assay (Sigma Aldrich, Ireland) after 24 or 72 h of contact time, as previously described.

TNF-α, pro-inflammatory cytokine, was assayed to evaluate the pro-inflammatory immune response using the commercially available ELISA kit (BioLegend, Medical Supply Co. Ltd., Ireland). Supernatants were collected from the cultures at 24 or 72 h after the treatment with the components or the scaffolds.

The cytokine secretion by macrophages was assayed at 450 nm with 570 nm as the reference wavelength (Epoch microplate reader, Biotek, Mason Technologies, Ireland). The method was linear in the concentration range from 7.8 to 500 pg/mL with the R^2 always higher than 0.995. Lipopolysaccharide (LPS, 100 ng/mL for 24 h) was used as the positive control.

2.2.5. Statistical Analysis

Statistical differences were evaluated using a non-parametric test: the Mann–Whitney (Wilcoxon) W test, (Statgraphics Centurion XV, Statistical Graphics Corporation, MD, USA). Differences were considered significant at $p < 0.05$.

3. Results and Discussion

3.1. Polymeric Blend Characterization

The characterization of the polymers in terms of conductivity (μS/cm), surface tension (N/m), and consistency (mN × mm) of all the polymeric blends is reported in Table 2.

The increase in clay mineral concentration caused an increase in conductivity, surface tension, and consistency. In particular, MMT at concentrations higher than 1% increased conductivity, surface tension, and consistency to values greater than those of the blank (blend without MMT). This behavior was less evident when HNT was blended with the polymeric mixture, probably due to the diff particle sizes of the two clays. It is conceivable that the addition of HNT or MMT to the polymer blend caused a partial immobilization of the polymer chains due to charge–charge or hydrophobic interaction. In case of a lower amount of clay minerals added (1%), this determined a decrease in consistency and conductivity, while higher amounts (2% or 5%) had the opposite behavior probably due to an excess of charges from MMT or HNT not counterbalanced from the polymers in the solution [14].

Table 2. Conductivity, surface tension, and consistency of the polymer blends (blank) and polymer blends containing MMT or HNT at 1%, 2%, or 5% w/w (mean values ± SD; n = 3).

Sample	Conductivity (μS/cm)	Surface Tension (N/m)	Consistency (mN × mm)
Blank	1363 ± 11	36.6 ± 0.2	188 ± 2
HNT1s	1271 ± 3	37.7 ± 0.2	155 ± 3
HNT2s	1303 ± 4	38.1 ± 0.1	175 ± 2
HNT5s	1352 ± 9	38.6 ± 0.2	203 ± 5
MMT1s	1255 ± 23	38.7 ± 0.4	171 ± 2
MMT2s	1527 ± 17	40.8 ± 0.2	308 ± 8
MMT5s	1663 ± 9	41.3 ± 0.1	338 ± 4

3.2. Scaffold Characterizations

3.2.1. Chemico-Physical Characterization

Advanced images such as SEM microphotographs of MMT- or HNT-based scaffolds and a blank scaffold in the dry or hydrated state are presented in Figure 2. The pore size evaluated for each scaffold is reported in an inset. Furthermore, in each image, the fiber diameter is reported.

In the dry state, the blank scaffold was characterized by fibers with a smooth surface, and fiber diameters with a coarse distribution around 1500 nm. HNT scaffolds were therefore characterized by the nanofibers' regular structure and smooth surface, where the addition of the clay minerals in the scaffolds provided a significant decrease in the fiber dimensions. The scaffolds containing 2% and 5% HNT had halved the diameter size compared to the blank scaffolds. Moreover, HNT determined a much more regular structure compared to the blank scaffolds. This was probably due to the unique structure of HNT, which are nanotubes with a high aspect ratio of 10 [9,20], thus capable of aligning along the fiber length and providing increasing surface tension. This allowed to obtain a more regular polymer solution jet during the electrospinning process. MMT scaffolds were characterized by nanofiber portions with a regular, smooth surface spaced out in a broaden interwoven, resembling knots, and with a wider structure organisation. These conceivably could be related to montmorillonite [9,21]. The increase of MMT concentration, especially in the 5% MMT scaffold, caused an increase in the surface roughness of the fibers, while the fiber diameters were significantly lower than those of the blank scaffold, although this was not influenced from the clay concentration. It is reported that clay minerals could act as a compatibilizer and this could positively affect the electrospinning of a polymer blend, containing positively and negatively charged polymers, as chitosan and chondroitin sulfate. Therefore, MMT or HNT could conceivably reduce the interfacial tension in the polymer blend, thus facilitating electrospinning, to obtain finer and more homogeneous nanofibers with respect to the blank [22]. Moreover, it is reported that the conductivity of the solution, influenced by the clay content, could increase the charge on the surface of the droplet to form a Taylor cone, and consequently could cause the decrease in the fiber diameter [23].

The presence of HNT or MMT in the scaffolds increased the systems porosity, and although there were not significant differences, the increase of clay mineral concentration increased the pore dimensions: this seems inversely related to the decrease of fiber dimensions. Porosity and fiber dimensions seem to have a crucial role for facilitating cell adhesion in the scaffold: The porosity could convert the scaffold from a surface to a fiber network, which could act as a sieve to the home cells.

The hydration significantly increased the fiber dimension, however no solubilization of the scaffold occurred thanks to the cross-linking by heating: The structural analysis (FTIR and SAXS) and the water holding capacity suggested that no new chemical bond was formed upon heating treatment while a polymer chain felting occurred when water was released due to thermal treatment, resulting in local physical multi-entanglement between the fibers, which could not be released by simple hydration. When HNT or MMT were at lower concentrations, up to 2%, the hydration did not alter the fibrous structure of the scaffolds, while when HNT or MMT were at a 5% concentration, the fibers were fused although the morphology was preserved. The higher content of hydrophilic clay minerals could weaken the overall scaffold structure, since the polymer chains in the matrix loosened their tightness causing a higher fiber swelling.

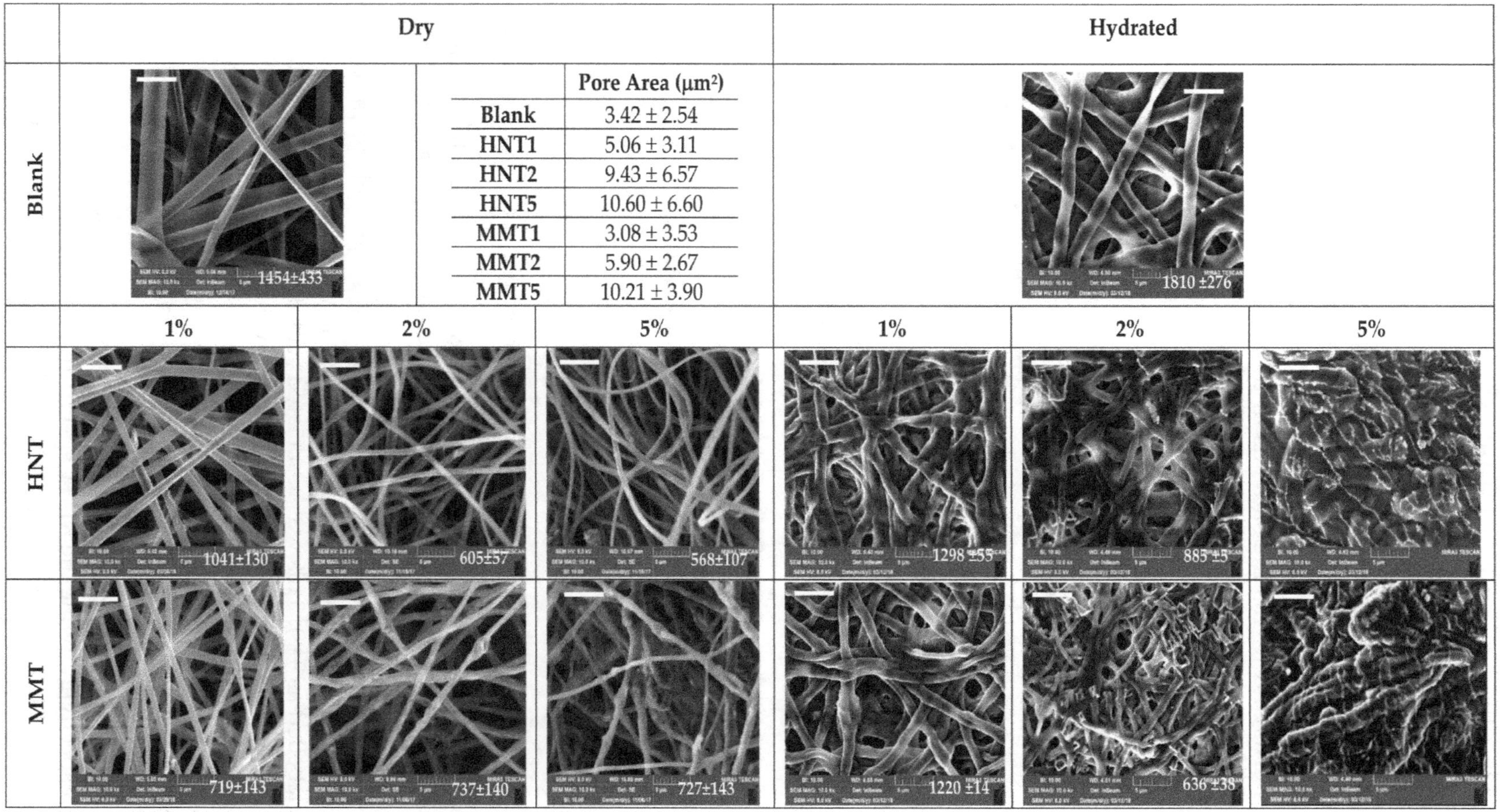

	Pore Area (μm²)
Blank	3.42 ± 2.54
HNT1	5.06 ± 3.11
HNT2	9.43 ± 6.57
HNT5	10.60 ± 6.60
MMT1	3.08 ± 3.53
MMT2	5.90 ± 2.67
MMT5	10.21 ± 3.90

Figure 2. SEM images of the scaffolds: blank (scaffold without clay) and montmorillonite (MMT) or halloysite (HNT) scaffolds containing 1%, 2%, or 5% of the clay mineral in the dry and hydrated state (the bar in each image is 5 μm). In the inset the fiber diameters (nm) are reported (mean values ± SD; n = 100).

XRPD of all the scaffolds developed is presented as comparison to the pristine HNT and MMT, in Figure 3. A blank scaffold was characterized by an amorphous pattern and no crystalline or paracrystalline behavior could be detected. Pristine HNT was characterized by a peak at 12.25° 2θ corresponding to 7.24 Å, a typical height of the dehydrated HNT interlaminar spaces (Figure 3, peak labelled as #). The peaks at 20.14° 2θ and at 25.03° 2θ confirmed the HNT tubular structure and its phyllosilicate nature (Figure 3, peak labelled as ##) [24]. HNT-loaded scaffolds were characterized by patterns more similar to that of the blank scaffold rather than those of pristine HNT: In these patterns, only the peaks attributable to the phyllosilicate nature of HNT (peaks at 25.03° 2θ) were present and there was a signal increase directly related to HNT concentration. Since the diffraction angle remained constant in all the patterns and it was the same as in the pristine HNT, it could be argued that no enlargement of the interlaminar space of the rolled structure occurred.

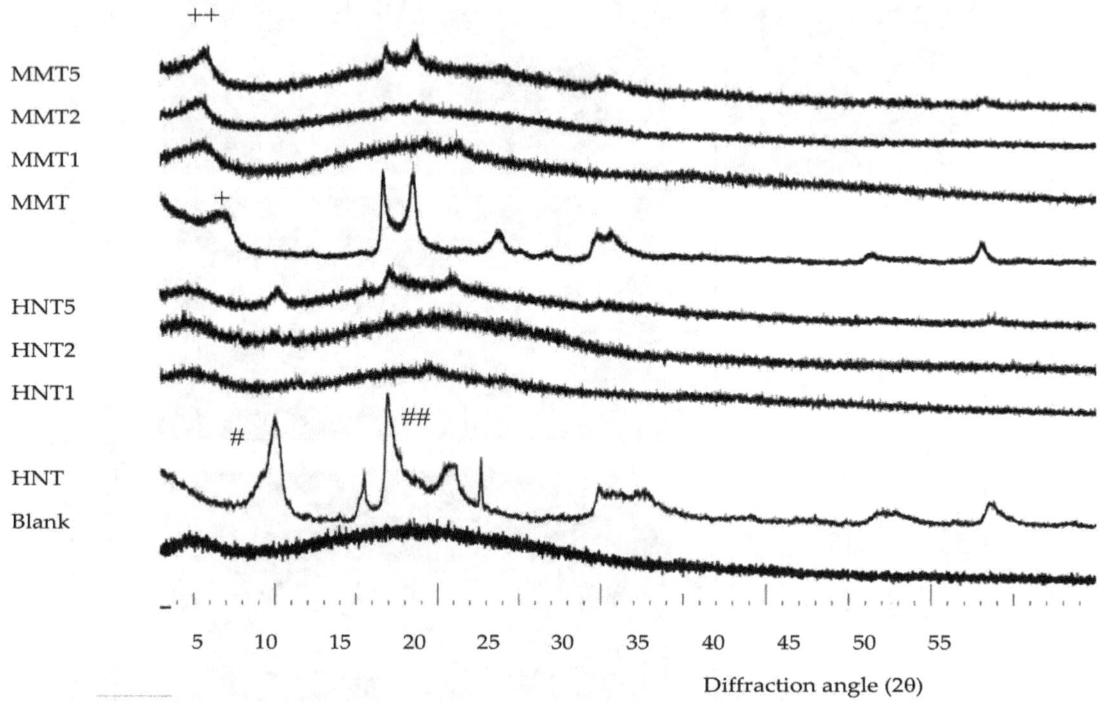

Figure 3. Comparison of XRPD patterns of all the scaffolds developed against pristine HNT and MMT.

The pattern of pristine MMT was characterized by a peak at 7° 2θ due to the distance of the d001 basal reflection, corresponding to 12.2 Å, characteristic of predominantly Na+ smectites (Figure 3 peak labelled as +).

In the MMT scaffolds, the d001 basal reflection was shifted to approximately 6° 2θ. This corresponded to a distance of 14.0 Å, suggesting that there was an enlargement of the interlayer space (Figure 3, peak labelled as ++). This was associated with the intercalation of the biopolymer into MMT layers, probably as monolayer between the silicate layers [10,25].

FTIR spectra of all the scaffolds developed is presented as comparison to the pristine HNT and MMT in Figure 4. In the spectrum of the blank scaffold, the signals related to pullulan (P) and citric acid (CA) are marked. These characteristic signals were present also in all the scaffolds containing either MMT or HNT.

HNT spectrum was characterized by two signals at 3696 cm^{-1} and 3622 cm^{-1}, due to OH inner and outer stretching, respectively, while the MMT spectrum was characterized by a signal at 3624 cm^{-1} caused by the Al–OH stretching. The characteristic peaks of both the clay minerals were hidden by a broad band due to a typical polysaccharide signal (hydrogen bonds of –OH and –NH_2 groups). (pullulan: 3331 cm^{-1} and chitosan: 3355 cm^{-1}). Moreover, the vibrational band of NH_3^+ groups of chitosan could be identified at 1550 cm^{-1}, as a shoulder [26,27].

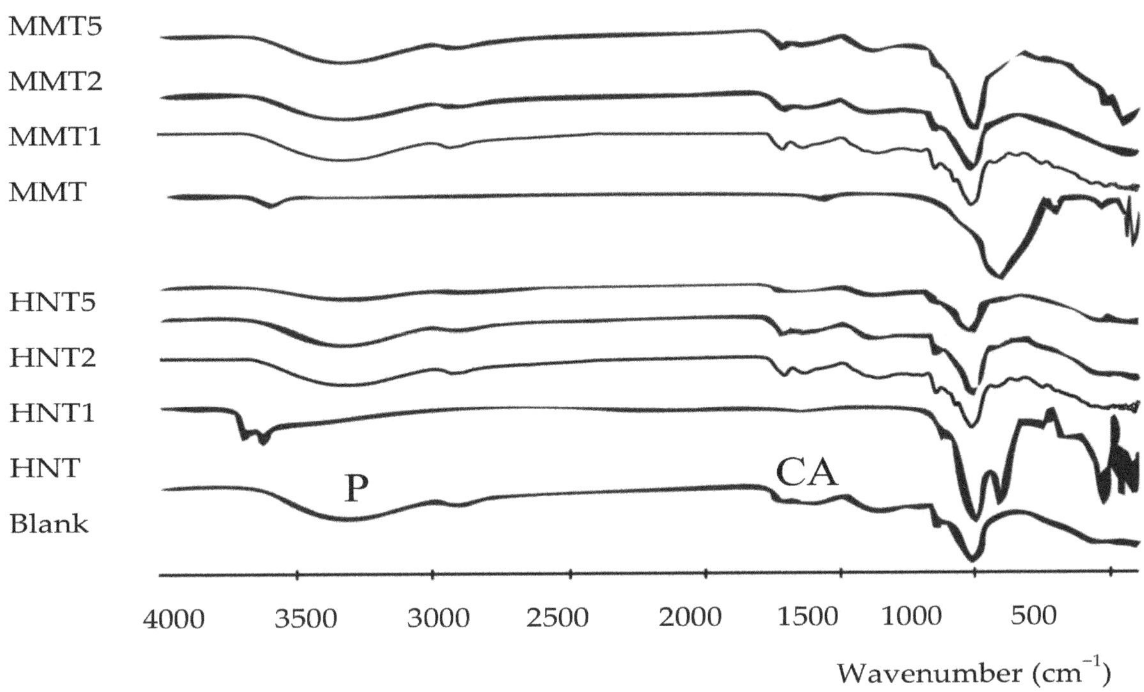

Figure 4. Comparison of the FTIR spectra of all the scaffolds developed against to the pristine HNT and MMT. In the blank spectrum the signals related to P (pullulan) and CA (citric acid) are marked.

TGA (a,b) and DSC (c) profiles of all the scaffolds, compared to pristine HNT and MMT is reported in Figure 5. Thermal analysis was performed to characterize the role of the clay minerals in the scaffold structure. TGA and DCS profiles suggested than both HNT and MMT had high thermal stability.

TGA analysis suggested that all the scaffolds, independently of the clay mineral loaded and its concentration, were subjected to a slight weight loss corresponding to the evaporation of hydration water. This accounted for about 7% of the scaffolds weight (30–101 °C) (Figure 5a). DSC analysis (Figure 5b,c) showed a slight endothermic event between 30 and 110 °C, confirming the TGA results.

Additionally, characterization showed that all the scaffolds reported a more prominent weight loss (onset: about 230 °C; offset: about 400 °C) with greater mass loss to reach 26%, 12%, and 7% of residual weight for the MMT 5, MMT2, and MMT1, respectively. These coincided with two endothermic events in the DSC thermograms and these could be conceivably caused by the decomposition [28,29].

The clay minerals loaded into the scaffolds, independently from the types and concentrations used, maintained their thermal stability and were able to slightly stabilize the scaffolds towards thermal degradation, increasing the onset temperatures of each thermal event; this is particularly evident in the TGA profiles (Figure 5a,b).

The residual mass was related to the clay mineral concentration in each scaffold: HNT: 5.56% for 1% loading; 11.40% for 2%, and 21.02% for 5%; MMT: 5.46% for 1% loading; 11.02% for 2%, and 22.36% for 5%.

HRTEM microphotographs of the broadened parts of the fibers is presented in Figure 6, and Figure 7 reports their EDX spectra.

The HRTEM and EDX analysis evidenced that the broadened parts were based on clay mineral particles: The tubular structure of HNT and laminar one of MMT could be identified. Moreover, the elemental analysis showed the presence of Al and Si typical in the case of HNT and the presence of Al, Si, and Mg in the case of MMT, but also of S and C, to indicate that the inorganic material was embedded into the organic component.

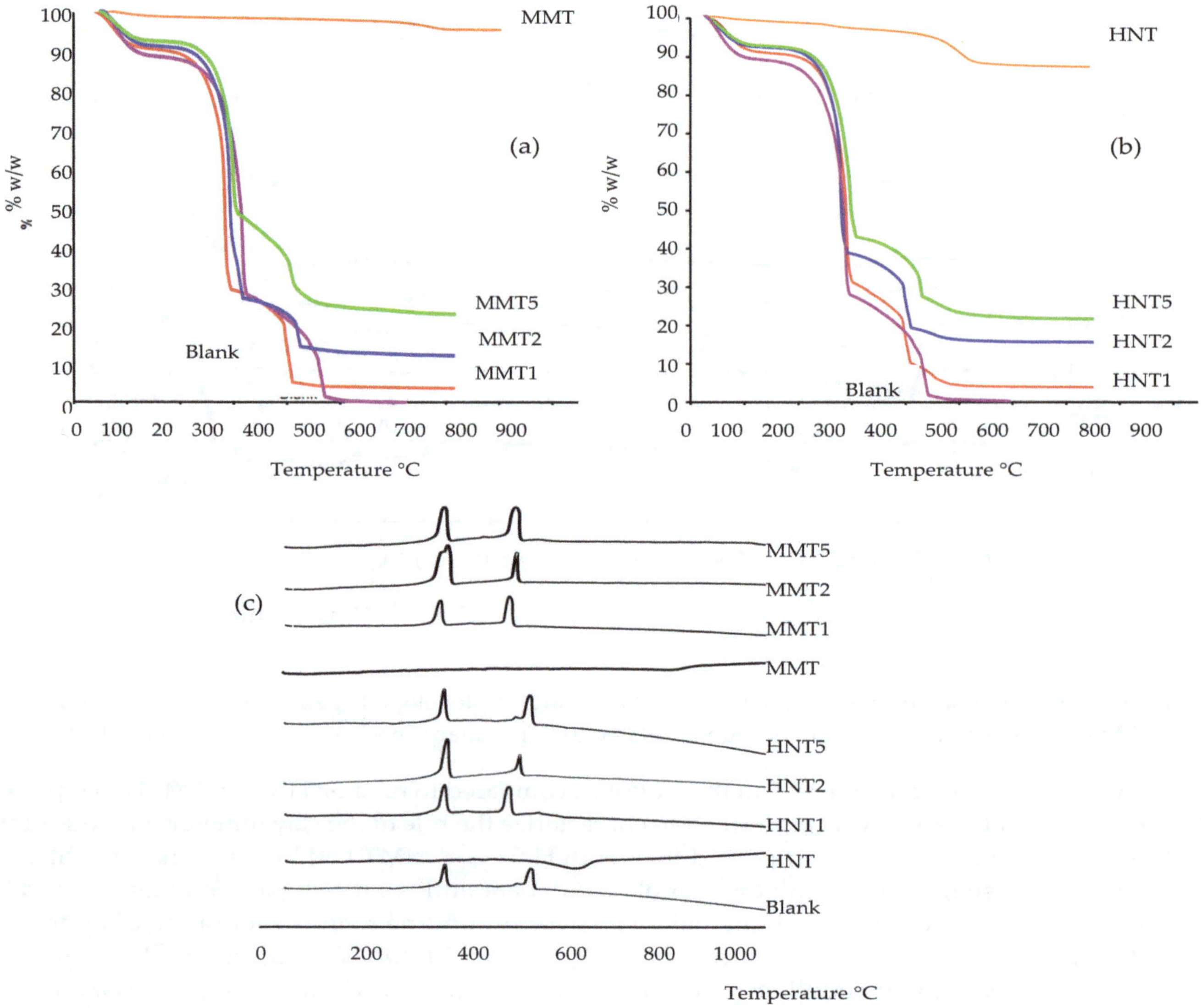

Figure 5. Comparison of TGA (**a**,**b**) and DSC (**c**) profiles of all the scaffolds against pristine HNT and MMT.

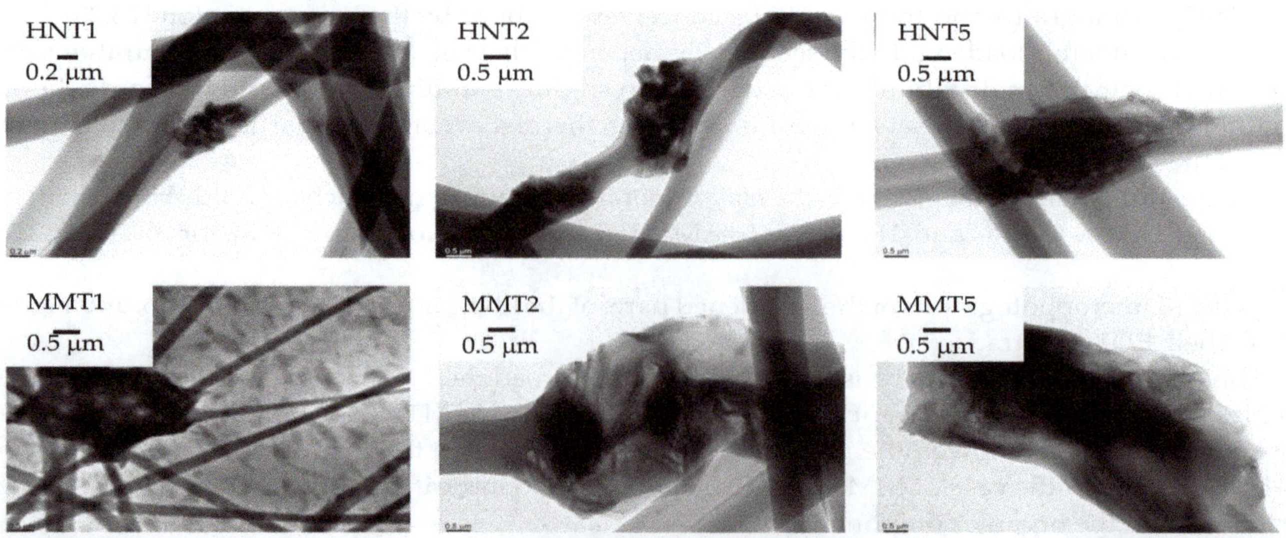

Figure 6. HRTEM microphotographs of the broadened parts of the fibers.

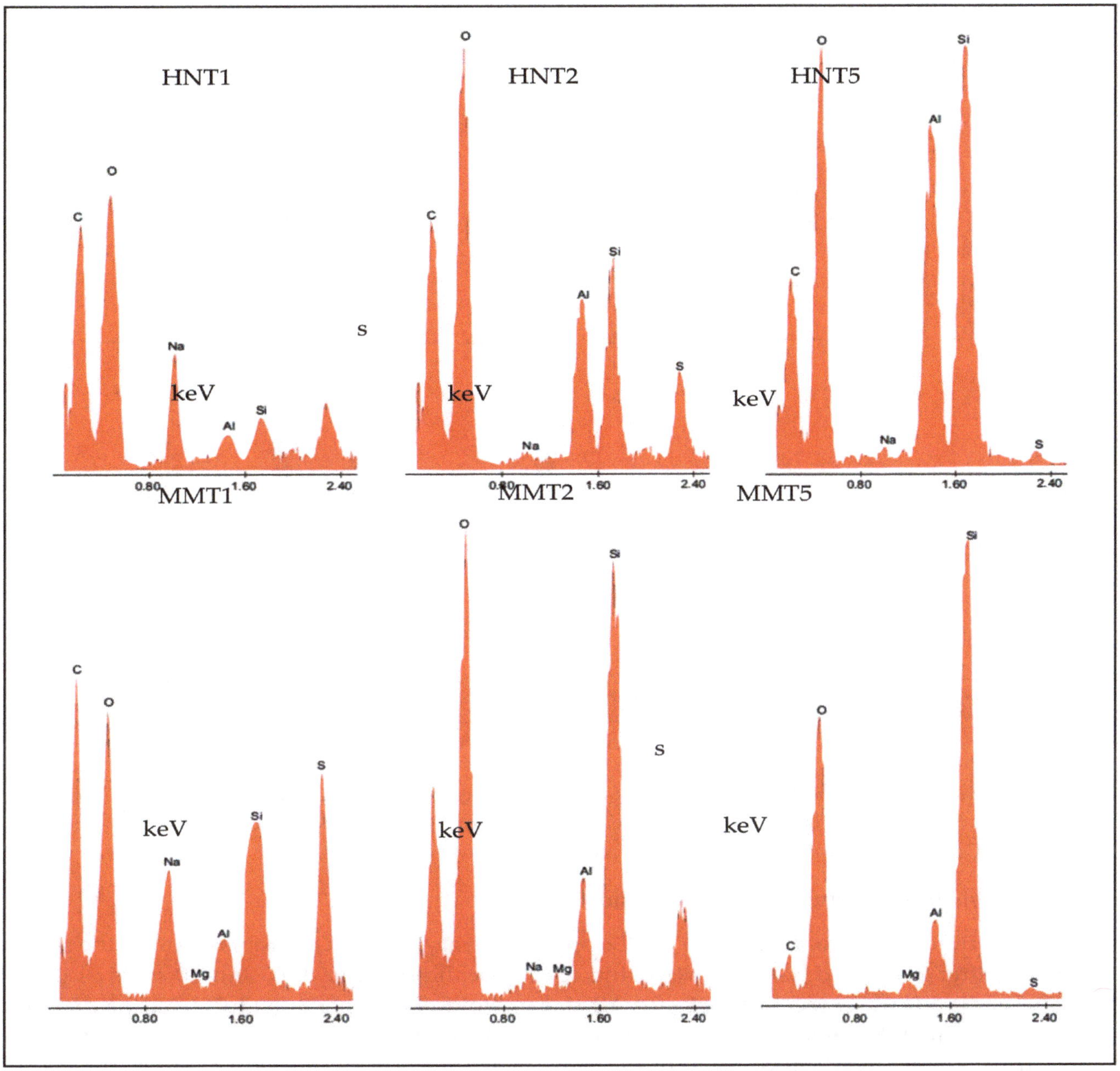

Figure 7. EDX spectra of the broadened parts of the fibers.

3.2.2. Mechanical Properties

The mechanical properties (force at break mN, a,b; elongation %, c,d; Young's Modulus mN cm^2, e,f) of scaffolds loaded with HNT or MMT, in dry (a,c,e) or wet (b,d,f) conditions are presented in Figure 8.

In the dry state, the increase of HNT caused a decrease of force at break (Figure 8a) and of system elasticity (Figure 8c), while MMT reinforced the scaffold structure increasing the resistance to break (Figure 8a) and the system elasticity (Figure 8c) up to the 2% concentration; a further increase weakened the scaffold. The scaffolds were characterized by moderate deformability higher than that of the blank scaffolds (Figure 8b). The hydration caused a remarkable decrease in resistance to break, an increase of deformability, and a loss of elasticity (Figure 8d–f). Clay minerals seem to reinforce the scaffold structure; however, if their concentration exceeded a certain threshold, the presence of particles embedded into the polymeric matrix could disrupt the polymer chain entanglements, weakening the scaffolds.

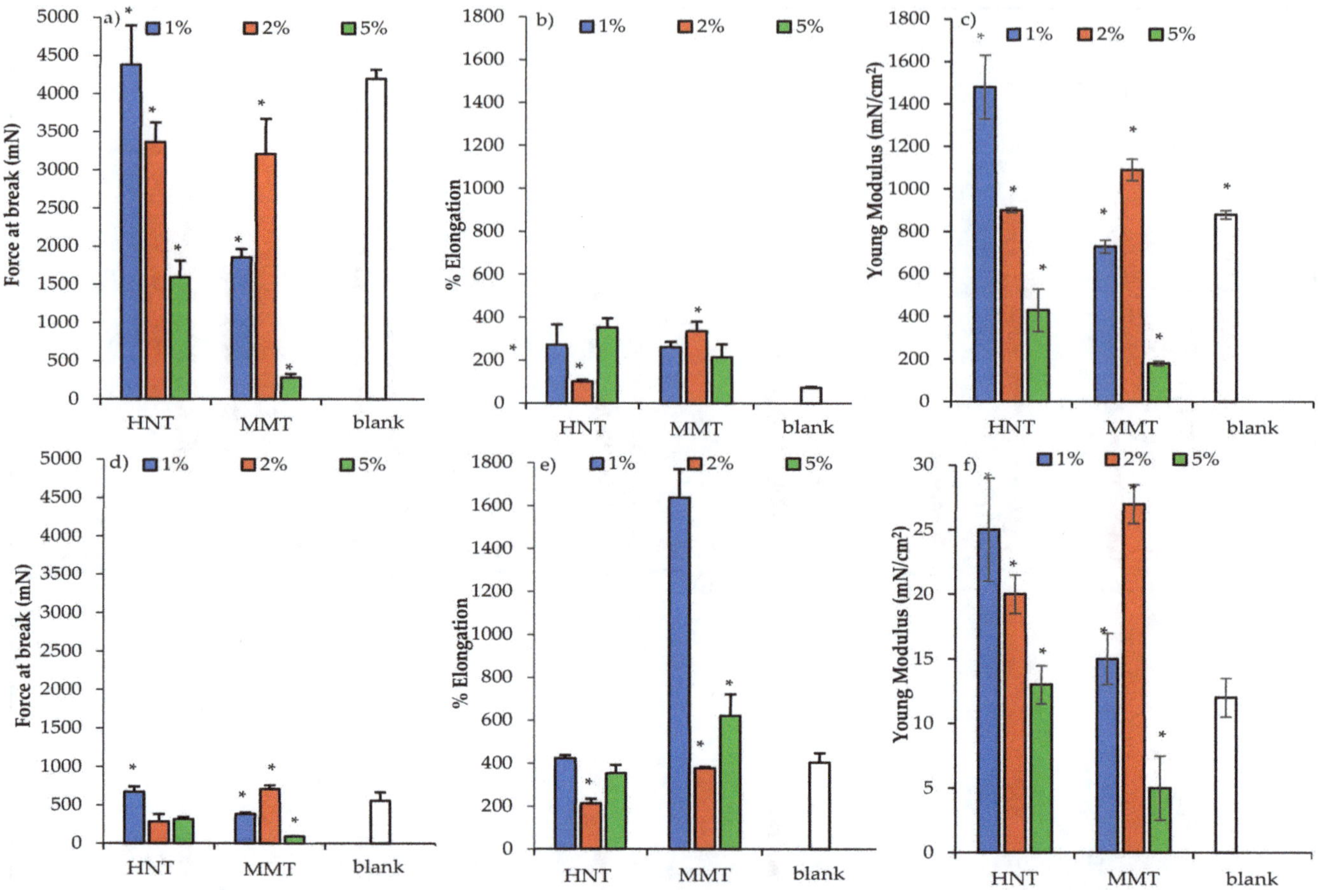

Figure 8. Mechanical properties (force at break mN, **a–c**; elongation %, **b–e**; Young's Modulus mN/cm^2, **c–f**) for dry (**a–c**) and wet (**d–f**) scaffolds loaded with HNT or MMT at different concentrations (mean values ± SD; n = 3). Statistics: * = Mann–Whitney (Wilcoxon) W test $p < 0.05$.

3.2.3. Fibroblasts Biocompatibility and Adhesion

Assessment for the cytocompatibility (OD, optical density) towards fibroblasts of (a) the scaffold components after 3 and 6 days of growth, and (b) the scaffolds after 3, 6, and 10 days of growth is summarized and presented in Figure 9. All the scaffold components (solubilized or dispersed in growth medium, GM) were characterized by similar biocompatibility considering 3 or 6 days of interaction, attachment and exposure with the fibroblasts (Figure 9a). Both HNT and MMT showed good biocompatibility. Of note, the fibroblast cytocompatibility decreased with their concentrations: in these conditions, clay minerals as powders (not soluble in GM) could negatively influence cell viability due to their sedimentation.

Fibroblast cells showed to grow onto the scaffolds, and these were compared to those of the control (GM, cell growth in standard conditions) (Figure 9b). After 3 days of cell growth onto the scaffolds loaded with either 2% HNT or 2% MMT, these were able to proliferate similarly to that seen when in simple substrate exposed to growth medium (as reference control). Conversely, all the other compositions caused a significant decrease in cell viability, as shown in Figure 9a,b. After 6 days, the blank scaffold and the scaffolds loaded with MMT (at all the concentrations) and HNT (at 2% and 5%) enhanced cell proliferation similarly to control samples, and only the scaffolds loaded with HNT at 1% was not able to show any proliferation as the control. After 10 days, the GM was unable to progress into further cell growth due to the extensive cytotoxicity issues. Nonetheless, the scaffolds loaded with both the clay minerals at 2% and 5% showed increased cell proliferation, and HNT and MMT at 2% showed the best proliferative responses. A possible explanation could be due to the specific properties of halloysite and montmorillonite which showed the enhancing fibroblast proliferation [9,10].

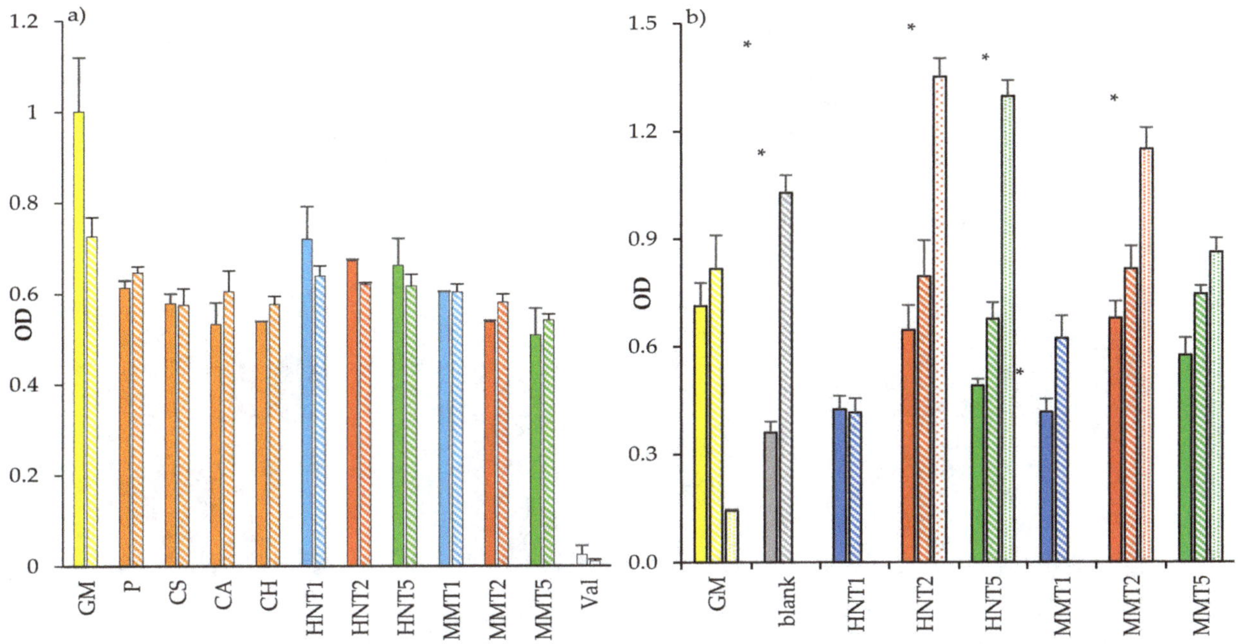

Figure 9. Cytocompatibility (OD, optical density) towards fibroblasts of (**a**) the scaffold components (GM: growth medium; P: pullulan; CS: chondroitin sulfate; CA: citric acid; CH: chitosan; Val: valinomycin) after 3 days (plain color) and 6 days (oblique line) of growth, and (**b**) of the scaffolds loaded with HNT or MMT after 3 days (plain colors), 6 days (oblique lines), and 10 days (spotted) of growth (**b**) (mean values ± SD; n = 8). Statistics: * = Mann–Whitney (Wilcoxon) W test $p < 0.05$.

These results are in agreement with the analysis carried out on the observed CLSM and the SEM images (Figure 10). In particular, from the SEM and CLSM analysis it could be suggested that the loading of clay minerals in the scaffolds allowed homogeneous fibroblast attachment, spreading and growth all over the scaffolds. Interestingly, only the scaffold containing MMT at 5% caused cell growth in clusters and this could be associated with the irregular surface and morphology of the scaffold fibers, which prevented cell attachment and surface adhesion. However, the scaffolds loaded with HNT or MMT at 2% allowed the fibroblasts to maintain their fusiform structure and aligned and elongated the cytoskeleton filaments, enhancing cell confluency.

In a previous work [16], a blank scaffold was characterized for surface zeta potential by means of the measurements of a streaming current and streaming potential. Such a scaffold possessed 2.9 isoelectric point with a zeta potential plateau above pH 5, at about −13.8 mV, and this was related to the strong interaction between CS and the amino groups of CH. Moreover, the structural features at the mesoscale were characterized by means of SAXS analysis [16]. These evidenced that nanofibers in the scaffold were characterized by tubular structures and that the hydration caused polymer chains protruding and stretching out from the fibers surface. The scaffold swelling was due to the dilatation of the scaffold mesh rather than single fiber swelling [16]. In addition, the blank scaffold possessed a certain degree of antibacterial activity against *Staphylococcus aureus*, and this was attributable to chitosan that retained its antimicrobial properties although entangled in the scaffold structure. Furthermore, the blank scaffold demonstrated to be resorbed in vivo in a preclinical (burn excisional murine) model after the lesion healing [16]: the evaluation of the degradation pathway evidenced that lysozyme, continuously secreted by white cells (macrophages and neutrophils) during the inflammatory phase of wound healing, played a crucial role in scaffold degradation [30].

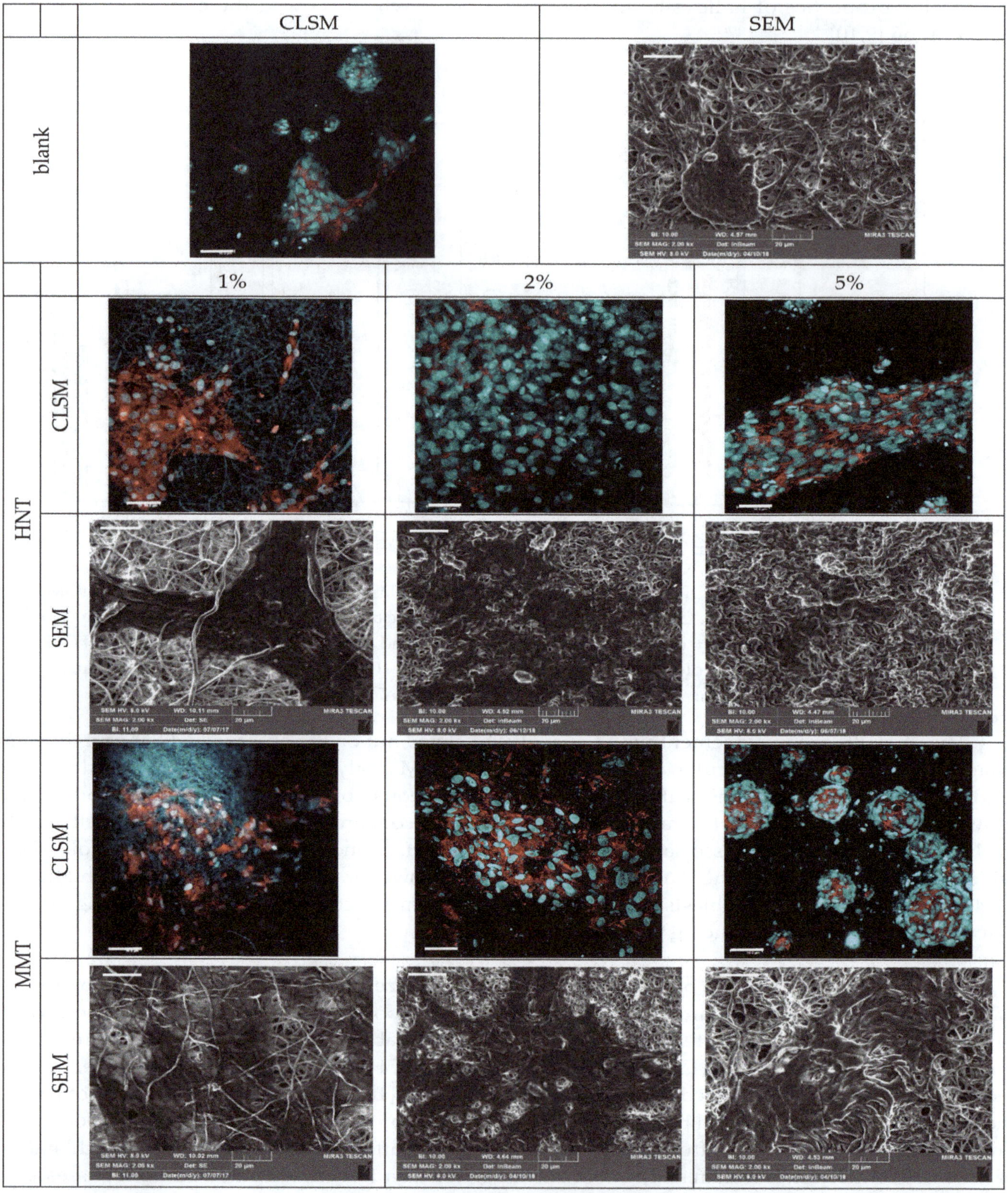

Figure 10. CLSM (scale bar: 50 μm) and SEM (scale bar: 20 μm) representative images of fibroblasts grown for 6 days onto the scaffolds loaded with HNT or MMT at 1%, 2%, and 5% (CLSM: in blue: nuclei; in red: cytoskeleton). Cell proliferation pattern showed by the nuclear staining increased frequencies in the HNT and MMT.

3.2.4. Cytocompatibility of Macrophages and Pro-Inflammatory Immune Response

Cytocompatibility was carried out by means of MTT assessment, recorded as intensity profile, analysed and presented on the macrophages in response to the scaffold components (a), the exposure and interaction with scaffolds after 24 and 72 h time points (b), as shown in Figure 11a,b. Moreover, TNFα concentrations (pg/mL), secreted by the macrophages after the contact with the components or the scaffolds are reported, in parallel to the MTT intensity readouts, in response to the components (Figure 11c); and the scaffolds (Figure 11d). From the collective results, it emerges that for all the cell substrates exposed to the components of the scaffold prepared in solution and for the LPS, at higher concentration (used as proinflammatory control) presented a full biocompatibility range when considering the two time points 24 or 72 h of contact with the macrophages (Figure 11a). Both HNT and MMT showed comparable biocompatibility although the macrophages' cytocompatibility decreased with MMT concentrations probably due to their different degradation profile up to 72 h.

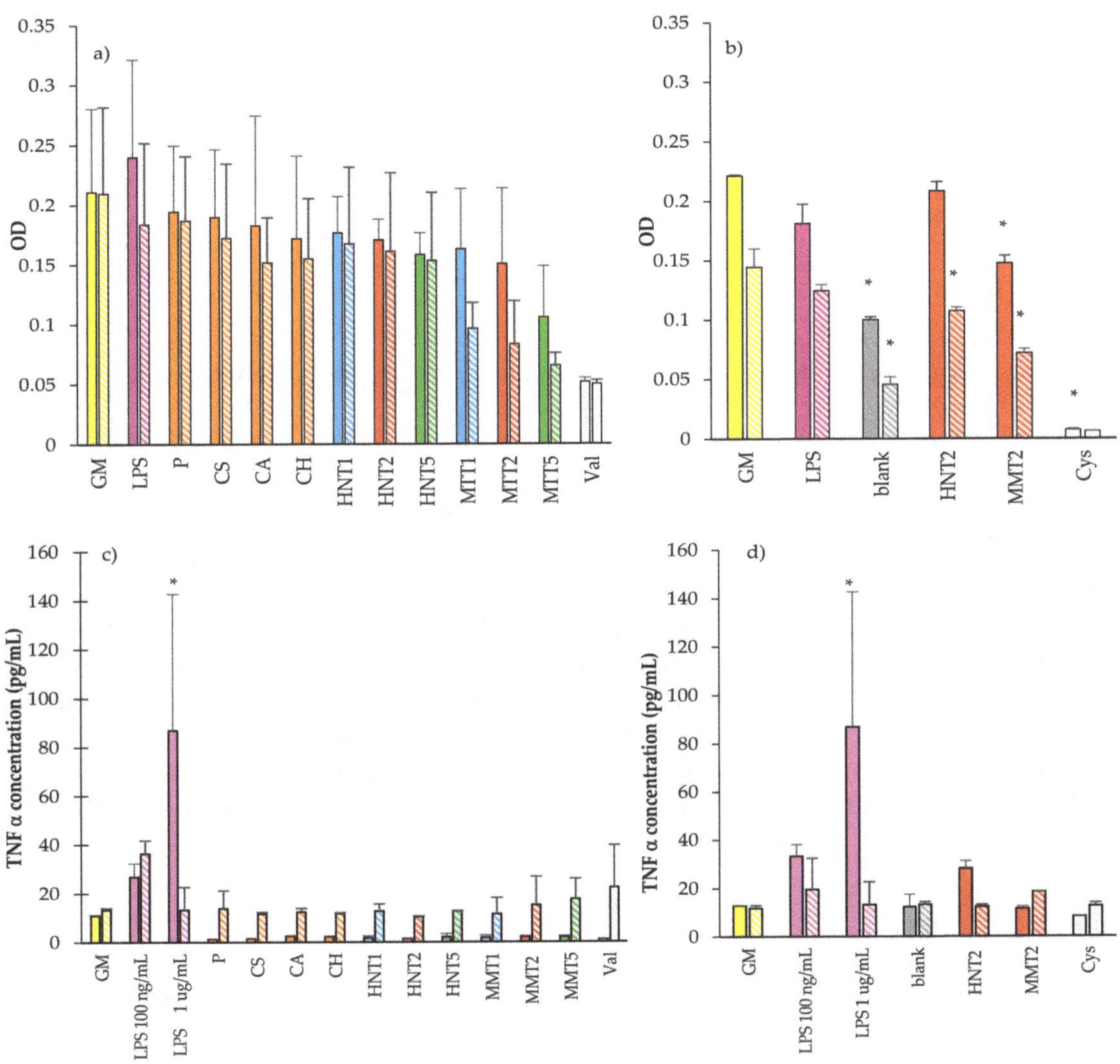

Figure 11. Cytocompatibility of THP-1 macrophages of the scaffold components (**a**), and the scaffolds after 24 (plain color) and 72 h (oblique lines) of exposure and contact (**b**). TNFα cytokine expression and concentrations (pg/mL) for THP-1 cells exposed to components (**c**); and (**d**) scaffolds (mean values ± SD; n = 8) (GM: growth medium; LPS: lipopolysaccharide; P = pullulan; CS: chondroitin sulfate; CA: citric acid; CH: chitosan; HNT1: 1% w/w halloysite; HNT2: 2% w/w halloysite; HNT5: 5% w/w halloysite; MMT1: 1% w/w montmorillonite; MMT2: 2% w/w montmorillonite; MMT: 5% w/w montmorillonite; blank: unloaded scaffold; Val: valinomycin; Cys: cysplatinum) Statistics: * = Mann–Whitney (Wilcoxon) W test $p < 0.05$.

The scaffold cytocompatibility towards fibroblasts and their proinflammatory response were evaluated only in the case of 2% clay mineral loading. In fact, the results obtained from mechanical properties and cell adhesion and proliferation capacity suggest that 2% clay mineral conferred to the scaffolds suitable stiffness/elasticity combined with the capability to support cell homing. After 24 and 72 h of growth, the scaffolds loaded with either HNT or MMT at 2% allowed macrophage viability similarly to that of their negative controls (GM, cell growth in standard conditions) (close to 75% of viability) (Figure 11b). However, the blank scaffold showed 50% cell viability with respect to the GM. The increase in the exposure time at 72 h also shows a decreased viability of the macrophages, when compared to their negative controls (GM).

Interestingly when looking at cytokine secretion, TNFα was secreted in significantly lower amounts from the cells in exposed and in contact with scaffold components for 24 h, while after 72 h of contact, the TNFα secretions were similar to the negative control, GM. The LPS positive controls provided the evidence that the cells were responsive to stimuli (proinflammatory agent) (Figure 11c). Considering 24 h exposure, the scaffolds caused a TNFα secretion similar to that of the GM. The scaffold loaded with HNT induced the TNFα secretion similar to those obtained when LPS was at a lower concentration but significantly lower than those observed for LPS at a higher concentration (Figure 11d). After 72 h of exposure time, all the scaffolds were assessed in their TNFα secretions that were not significantly different to the GM. This could be possibly also linked to the decrease in macrophage viability after 72 h in standard growth conditions. These results showed that HNT and MMT scaffolds did not show any significant proinflammatory activity compared to controls.

4. Conclusions

Halloysite or montmorillonite were loaded in an electrospun polysaccharidic scaffold in a one-pot process. Halloysite scaffolds were characterized by a fiber regular structure and smooth surface, and did not show any structural alterations when embedded in the polymeric matrix, probably due to the nanotubular structure of this clay mineral. MMT scaffolds were characterized by nanofiber portions with a regular, smooth surface, spaced out in broadened parts as knots with a scattered structure, possibly due to its structure. Moreover, MMT inclusion in the polymeric matrix of the scaffold caused interlayer space enlargement, causing the biopolymer intercalation into the MMT galleries, resulting in a deep interaction between the scaffold matrix and clay mineral. HNT or MMT (2% concentration) in the scaffolds were able to sustain homogeneous fibroblast spreading all over the scaffolds and their growth up to confluency, maintaining a cell fusiform structure and aligned and elongated cytoskeleton filaments. HNT and MMT (2% concentration) scaffolds. Due to their capability to support and enhance fibroblasts proliferation with negligible proinflammatory activity, these scaffolds are promising for applications in wound healing: Their capability to enable cell attachmnent and adhesion is probably due to their morphological 3D structure-assisted cell homing, and this could facilitate wound healing in vivo.

5. Patents

Sandri: G.: Bonferoni, M.C.; Rossi, S.; Ferrari, F. Electrospun nanofibers and membranes, PCT/IT2017/000160, 2017.

Author Contributions: Conceptualization, G.S., A.P.-M. (Cytocompatibility of Macrophages and Pro-inflammatory Immune Response); methodology, G.S.; A.P.-M. (Cytocompatibility of Macrophages and Pro-inflammatory Immune Response); software, F.F. and M.C.B.; validation, C.V.; investigation, M.L., A.F., D.M., M.R.; data curation, G.S., C.A. A.P.-M. (Cytocompatibility of Macrophages and Pro-inflammatory Immune Response); writing—original draft preparation, G.S., M.R., A.F.; writing—review and editing, G.S., A.P.-M. (Cytocompatibility of Macrophages and Pro-inflammatory Immune Response); supervision, G.S., A.P.-M. (Cytocompatibility of Macrophages and Pro-inflammatory Immune Response); project administration, G.S.; funding acquisition, G.S., S.R., F.F., M.C.B., A.P.-M. (Cytocompatibility of Macrophages and Pro-inflammatory Immune Response). All authors have read and agreed to the published version of the manuscript.

Acknowledgments: The authors wish to thank Giusto Faravelli SpA for supplying the polymers.

References

1. Sorg, H.; Tilkorn, D.J.; Hager, S.; Hauser, J.; Mirastschijski, U. Skin Wound Healing: An Update on the Current Knowledge and Concepts. *Eur. Surg. Res.* **2017**, *58*, 81–94. [CrossRef]
2. Järbrink, K.; Ni, G.; Sönnergren, H.; Schmidtchen, A.; Pang, C.; Bajpai, R.; Car, J. The humanistic and economic burden of chronic wounds: A protocol for a systematic review. *Syst. Rev.* **2017**, *6*, 15. [CrossRef]
3. Sen, C.K. Human Wounds and Its Burden: An Updated Compendium of Estimates. *Adv. Wound Care* **2019**, *8*, 39–48. [CrossRef]
4. Naumenko, E.A.; Guryanov, I.D.; Yendluri, R.; Lvov, Y.M.; Fakhrullin, R.F. Clay nanotube–biopolymer composite scaffolds for tissue engineering. *Nanoscale* **2016**, *8*, 7257–7271. [CrossRef]
5. Dawson, J.I.; Oreffo, R.O.C. Clay: New Opportunities for Tissue Regeneration and Biomaterial Design. *Adv. Mater.* **2013**, *25*, 4069–4086. [CrossRef] [PubMed]
6. Williams, L.B.; Metge, D.W.; Eberl, D.D.; Harvey, R.W.; Turner, A.G.; Prapaipong, P.; Poret-Peterson, A.T. What Makes a Natural Clay Antibacterial? *Environ. Sci. Technol.* **2011**, *45*, 3768–3773. [CrossRef]
7. Sandri, G.; Bonferoni, M.C.; Rossi, S.; Ferrari, F.; Aguzzi, C.; Viseras, C.; Caramella, C. *Clay Minerals for Tissue Regeneration, Repair, and Engineering*; Ågren, M.S., Ed.; Elsevier: Amsterdam, The Netherlands, 2016; pp. 385–402.
8. Garcia-Villen, F.; Faccendini, A.; Aguzzi, C.; Cerezo, P.; Bonferoni, M.C.; Rossi, S.; Grisoli, P.; Ruggeri, M.; Ferrari, F.; Sandri, G.; et al. Montmorillonite-norfloxacin nanocomposite intended for healing of infected wounds. *Int. J. Nanomed.* **2019**, *14*, 5051–5060. [CrossRef]
9. Sandri, G.; Aguzzi, C.; Rossi, S.; Bonferoni, M.C.; Bruni, G.; Boselli, C.; Cornaglia, A.I.; Riva, F.; Viseras, C.; Caramella, C.; et al. Halloysite and chitosan oligosaccharide nanocomposite for wound healing. *Acta Biomater.* **2017**, *57*, 216–224. [CrossRef] [PubMed]
10. Aguzzi, C.; Sandri, G.; Viseras, C.; Bonferoni, M.C.; Cerezo, P.; Rossi, S.; Ferrari, F.; Caramella, C. Solid state characterization of silver sulfadiazine loaded on montmorillonite/chitosan nanocomposite for wound healing. *Colloid Surf. B* **2014**, *113*, 152–157. [CrossRef] [PubMed]
11. Sandri, G.; Bonferoni, M.C.; Ferrari, F.; Rossi, S.; Aguzzi, C.; Mori, M.; Grisoli, P.; Cerezo, P.; Tenci, M.; Viseras, C.; et al. Montmorillonite-chitosan-silver sulfadiazine nanocomposites for topical treatment of chronic skin lesions: In vitro biocompatibility, antibacterial efficacy and gap closure cell motility properties. *Carbohyd. Polym.* **2014**, *102*, 970–977. [CrossRef]
12. Gaharwar, A.K.; Cross, L.M.; Peak, C.W.; Gold, K.; Carrow, J.K.; Brokesh, A.; Singh, K.A. 2D Nanoclay for Biomedical Applications: Regenerative Medicine, Therapeutic Delivery, and Additive Manufacturing. *Adv. Mater.* **2019**, *31*, 1900332. [CrossRef] [PubMed]
13. Mousa, M.; Evans, N.D.; Oreffo, R.O.C.; Dawson, J.I. Clay nanoparticles for regenerative medicine and biomaterial design: A review of clay bioactivity. *Biomaterials* **2018**, *159*, 204–214. [CrossRef] [PubMed]
14. Vivekanandhan, S.; Schreiber, M.; Mohanty, A.K.; Misra, M. *Advanced Electrospun Nanofibers of Layered Silicate Nanocomposites: A Review of Processing, Properties, and Applications*; Pandey, J., Reddy, K., Mohanty, A., Misra, M., Eds.; Springer: Berlin/Heidelberg, Germany, 2014; pp. 361–388.
15. Lvov, Y.; Abdullayev, E. Functional polymer–clay nanotube composites with sustained release of chemical agents. *Prog. Polym. Sci.* **2013**, *38*, 1690–1719. [CrossRef]
16. Sandri, G.; Rossi, S.; Bonferoni, M.C.; Miele, D.; Faccendini, A.; Del Favero, E.; Di Cola, E.; Icaro Cornaglia, A.; Boselli, C.; Luxbacher, T.; et al. Chitosan/glycosaminoglycan scaffolds for skin reparation. *Carbohydr. Polym.* **2019**, *220*, 219–227. [CrossRef] [PubMed]
17. Kupiec, T.C.; Matthews, P.; Ahmad, R. Dry-heat sterilization of parenteral oil vehicles. *Int. J. Pharm. Compd.* **2000**, *4*, 223–224. [PubMed]
18. Malgarim Cordenonsi, L.; Faccendini, A.; Rossi, S.; Bonferoni, M.C.; Malavasi, L.; Raffin, R.; Scherman Schapoval, E.E.; Del Fante, C.; Vigani, B.; Miele, D.; et al. Platelet lysate loaded electrospun scaffolds: Effect of nanofiber types on wound healing. *Eur. J. Pharm. Biopharm.* **2019**, *142*, 247–257. [CrossRef]
19. Saporito, F.; Sandri, G.; Bonferoni, M.C.; Rossi, S.; Malavasi, L.; Del Fante, C.; Vigani, B.; Black, L.; Ferrari, F. Electrospun gelatin-chondroitin sulfate scaffolds loaded with platelet lysate promote immature cardiomyocyte proliferation. *Polymers* **2018**, *10*, 208. [CrossRef]

20. Cravero, F.; Churchman, G.J. The origin of spheroidal halloysites: A review of the literature. *Clay Miner.* **2016**, *51*, 417–427. [CrossRef]
21. Faccendini, A.; Ruggeri, M.; Rossi, S.; Bonferoni, M.C.; Aguzzi, C.; Grisoli, P.; Viseras, C.; Sandri, G.; Ferrari, F. Norfloxacin loaded electrospun scaffolds: Montmorillonite nanocomposite vs. free drug. *Pharmaceutics* **2020**, in press.
22. Habibi, S.; Saket, M.; Nazockdast, H.; Hajinasrollah, K. Fabrication and characterization of exfoliated chitosan–gelatin–montmorillonite nanocomposite nanofibers. *J. Text. I* **2019**, *110*, 1672–1677. [CrossRef]
23. Sandri, G.; Rossi, S.; Bonferoni, M.C.; Caramella, C.; Ferrari, F. Electrospinning Technologies in Wound Dressing Applications. *Ther. Dress. Wound Health Appl.* **2020**, *14*, 315–366.
24. Falcón, J.M.; Sawczen, T.; Aoki, I.V. Dodecylamine-Loaded Halloysite Nanocontainers for Active Anticorrosion Coatings. *Front. Mater.* **2015**, *2*, 69. [CrossRef]
25. Darder, M.; Colilla, M.; Ruiz-Hitzky, E. Biopolymer–clay nanocomposites based on chitosan intercalated in montmorillonite. *Chem. Mater.* **2003**, *15*, 3774–3780. [CrossRef]
26. Deb Nath, S.; Abueva, C.; Kim, B.; Taek Lee, B. Chitosan–hyaluronic acid polyelectrolyte complex scaffold crosslinked with genipin for immobilization and controlled release of BMP-2. *Carbohydr. Polym.* **2015**, *115*, 160–169. [CrossRef] [PubMed]
27. Sedghi, R.; Sayyari, N.; Shaabani, A.; Niknejad, H.; Tahereh, T. Novel biocompatible zinc-curcumin loaded coaxial nanofibers for bone tissue engineering application. *Polymers* **2018**, *142*, 244–255. [CrossRef]
28. Drosou, C.; Krokida, M.; Biliaderis, C.G. Composite pullulan-whey protein nanofibers made by electrospinning: Impact of process parameters on fiber morphology and physical properties. *Food Hydrocoll.* **2017**, *17*, 726–735. [CrossRef]
29. Islam, S.; Rahaman, S.; Yeum, J.H. Electrospun novel super-absorbent based on polysaccharide–polyvinyl alcohol–montmorillonite clay nanocomposites. *Carbohydr. Polym.* **2015**, *115*, 69–77. [CrossRef]
30. Sandri, G.; Miele, D.; Faccendini, A.; Bonferoni, M.C.; Rossi, S.; Grisoli, P.; Taglietti, A.; Ruggeri, M.; Bruni, G.; Vigani, B.; et al. Chitosan/Glycosaminoglycan Scaffolds: The Role of Silver Nanoparticles to Control Microbial Infections in Wound Healing. *Polymers* **2019**, *11*, 1207. [CrossRef]

3

Polymeric Bioadhesive Patch Based on Ketoprofen-Hydrotalcite Hybrid for Local Treatments

Cinzia Pagano [1], Loredana Latterini [2], Alessandro Di Michele [3], Francesca Luzi [4], Debora Puglia [4], Maurizio Ricci [1], César Antonio Viseras Iborra [5] and Luana Perioli [1,*]

1 Department of Pharmaceutical Sciences, University of Perugia, 06123 Perugia Italy; cinzia.pagano@unipg.it (C.P.); maurizio.ricci@unipg.it (M.R.)
2 Department of Chemistry, Biology and Biotechnology, University of Perugia, 06123 Perugia, Italy; loredana.latterini@unipg.it
3 Department of Physics and Geology, University of Perugia, 06123 Perugia, Italy; alessandro.dimichele@collaboratori.unipg.it
4 Civil and Environmental Engineering Department, University of Perugia, UdR INSTM, 05100 Terni, Italy; francesca.luzi@unipg.it (F.L.); debora.puglia@unipg.it (D.P.)
5 Department of Pharmacy and Pharmaceutical Technology, Faculty of Pharmacy, University of Granada, Campus of Cartuja, 18071 Granada, Spain; cviseras@ugr.es
* Correspondence: luana.perioli@unipg.it

Abstract: Ketoprofen (KET) represents one of the most common drugs used in the topical treatment of pain and inflammations. However, its potential is rather limited due to the very low solubility and photochemical instability. The local administration of KET by conventional products, such as gels, emulgels, creams, and foams, does not guarantee an efficacious and safe treatment because of its low absorption (due to low solubility) and its sensitivity to UV rays. The photodegradation of KET makes many photoproducts responsible for different adverse effects. In the present work, KET was intercalated into the lamellar anionic clay ZnAl-hydrotalcite (ZnAl-HTlc), obtaining the hybrid ZnAl-KET with improved stability to UV rays and water solubility in comparison to the crystalline form (not intercalated KET). The hybrid was then formulated in autoadhesive patches for local pain treatment. The patches were prepared by casting method starting from a hydrogel based on the biocompatible and bioadhesive polymer NaCMC (Sodium carboxymethycellulose) and glycerol as a plasticizing agent. The introduction of ZnAl-KET in the patch composition demonstrated the improvement in the mechanical properties of the formulation. Moreover, a sustained and complete KET release was obtained within 8 h. This allowed reducing the frequency of anti-inflammatory administration, compared to the conventional formulations.

Keywords: hydrotalcite; ketoprofen; hybrid; photostability; hydrogel film; bioadhesion

1. Introduction

Ketoprofen (KET) is one of the most common NSAIDs (Nonsteroidal anti-inflammatory drugs) used for relieving pain in many acute and chronic conditions as musculoskeletal, tendinitis, strain, sprain, trauma, and arthritis [1,2]. However, its efficacy, especially in topical therapies, is impaired due to both the very poor water solubility (KET is labeled in class II of the biopharmaceutics classification system, BCS) and photochemical instability [3,4].

KET exposition to UV radiations, especially UVA, is responsible for phototoxic and photoallergic reactions [5,6]. These reactions are due to radical intermediates generated by KET-UV rays interactions responsible for DNA damage, mitochondria depolarization, and lysosomes destabilization [6–8]. Thus, KET topical administration by conventional formulations, such as gels, emulgels, creams, sprays, and foams, does not guarantee protection from UV radiation, exposing the patient to serious health problems [9]. Moreover, conventional formulations are responsible for a limited residence time of the drug in the application site.

Thus, in order to exploit the benefits of KET and to overcome these problems, it is necessary to find a suitable formulation able to protect it from sunlight and to improve the residence time.

With this aim, many approaches have been purposed mainly based on KET entrapment in supramolecular structures as cyclodextrins, liposomes, niosomes, microparticles [10–12]. A further interesting approach is represented by the realization of host-guest complexes using an inorganic matrix as the anionic clay hydrotalcite (HTlc) [13]. This material shows the typical lamellar structure able to store anionic molecules (guest) in the nanosized interlamellar space (host) [14].

The general formula of synthetic HTlc is $[M(II)_{1-x}M(III)_x(OH)_2]^{x+}(A^{n-}{}_{x/n})^{x-}$ mS, where M(II) is a divalent metal cation (usually Mg, Zn); M(III) is a trivalent metal cation (usually Al, Fe); generally, the x value, M(III)/M(II) + M(III), ranges between 0.25 and 0.33; A^{n-} is an exchangeable inorganic or organic anion, which compensates the positive charge of the layer; m is the mol of solvent S, usually water, co-intercalated per mole of compound [13]. The intercalation of an organic molecule (drug) into HTlc lamellae allows obtaining a new inorganic-organic hybrid product with enhanced properties in terms of solubility [15,16], photoprotection [17–19], and physical and chemical stability [20]. These lamellar materials represent a valuable strategy in developing formulations with prolonged efficacy, thanks to the double control of the release and protection of the guest.

The aim of this work was to purpose a new formulation in which KET is stabilized from UV light, able to be applied on skin without adhesives, and to stay there for a prolonged time. Therefore, the photoprotective effect of the lamellar clay ZnAl-HTlc towards KET, once intercalated into the lamellae (ZnAl-KET), was investigated. Moreover, the performances of a self-adhesive/biocompatible patch loaded with the intercalation product ZnAl-KET were evaluated in terms of mechanical properties, bioadhesion, and drug release capability.

2. Materials and Methods

2.1. Materials

Ketoprofen acid form (KETH) and sodium salt (KET-Na) were purchased from Sigma-Aldrich (Milano, Italy). Glycerol and urea were purchased from Acef S.p.A. (Fiorenzuola D'Arda, Piacenza, Italy). Aluminum chloride esahydrate, calcium chloride, potassium dihydrogen phosphate, sodium hydrogen phosphate, polyvinilpyrrolidone, potassium carbonate (Carlo Erba, Cornaredo, Milano, Italy) were supplied by DueM (Perugia, Italy). Zinc oxide was supplied by Caelo (Hilden, North-Rhine Westphalia, Germany). Sodium carboxymethycellulose (NaCMC) was supplied by Hercules Inc.—Aqualon division (Wilmington, DE, USA).

Ultrapure water was obtained by reverse osmosis process in a MilliQ system Millipore (Roma, Italy). Other reagents and solvents were of analytical grade and used without further purification.

2.2. Hydrotalcite Synthesis

ZnAl-HTlc in carbonate form was obtained by coprecipitation of Zn(II)-Al(III), accomplished by the hydrolysis of urea. The nitrate form ZnAl-HTlc-NO_3 (ZnAl-NO_3) was obtained, treating the solid with a diluted solution of the corresponding mineral acid [21].

2.3. Hybrid Preparation

The hybrid ZnAl-KET was prepared by ion-exchange mechanism according to previous work [15]. A carbon dioxide-free NaOH water solution 0.1 M was added to a suspension of KET (0.1 M). Then, ZnAl-NO_3 was added to the obtained salt solution (molar ratio HTlc/KET 1:2). The suspension was kept under magnetic stirring (600 rpm) for 24 h at room temperature. The solid (ZnAl-KET) was recovered by centrifugation (A.L.C. centrifuge. mod. 4236A. Milano, Italy), washed with carbonate free water, and dried at room temperature under P_2O_5.

2.4. Hybrid Characterization

2.4.1. X-ray Analysis

Powder X-ray diffraction patterns (XRPD) of powders were registered with a Philips X'Pert PRO MPD diffractometer (Malvern Panalytical, Royston, United Kingdom) operating at 40 kV and 40 mA, with a step size 0.03° 2theta and step scan 40 s, using Cu Kα radiation and an X'Celerator detector (Malvern Panalytical, Royston, United Kingdom).

2.4.2. Metal Composition

Metal analyses were performed by Varian 700-ES series Inductively-Coupled Plasma-Optical Emission Spectrometers (ICP-OES, Varian Inc., Santa Clara, CA, USA) using solutions prepared by dissolving the samples in some drops of concentrated HNO_3 solution and properly diluted.

2.4.3. Thermogravimetric Analysis (TGA)

Thermogravimetric analysis (TGA) was performed by a Netzsch STA 449C apparatus (NETZSCH-Gerätebau GmbH, Selb, Germany) in air flow and heating rate of 10 °C/min to determine the weight loss (water and drug) as a function of increasing temperature.

2.4.4. Differential Scanning Calorimetry (DSC) Analysis

DSC analyses were performed using an automatic thermal analyzer Mettler Toledo DSC821e (Mettler-Toledo S.p.A., Milano, Italy) and an indium standard for temperature calibrations. Holed aluminum pans were employed in the experiments for all samples, and an empty pan, prepared in the same way, was used as a reference. Samples of 3–6 mg were weighted directly into the aluminum pans, and the thermal analyses of samples were conducted, at a heating rate of 5 °C/min, from 25 to 200 °C.

2.4.5. Scanning Electron Microscopy Analysis (SEM)

SEM micrographs were acquired by FE-SEM LEO 1525 ZEISS (Carl Zeiss Microscopy, Jena, Germany). The samples were prepared by deposition of the sample on conductive carbon adhesive tape and then metalized with chromium (8 nm) by sputtering. Elemental mapping was determined by energy dispersive X-ray analysis (EDX, Bruker Quantax, Billerica, MA, USA).

2.4.6. Solubility Studies

The solubility of KET from the crystalline acid form (KETH) and ZnAl-KET was measured in water, and the samples were prepared as follows: an excess of the sample (10 mg KETH and 24.10 mg of ZnAl-KET corresponding to 10 mg of KETH) was dispersed in 10 mL of ultrapure water under magnetic stirring (600 rpm) at 25 °C until equilibrium was achieved (48 h). The samples were filtered through a 0.45 μm nylon filter, suitably diluted, and analyzed by UV-VIS spectrophotometry.

2.4.7. Photochemical Analysis

The photostability of the samples was spectrophotometrically investigated. Absorption spectra of the powder samples were recorded by a Varian Cary 4000 spectrophotometer (Varian, East Lyme, CT, USA), equipped with a 150-mm integration sphere, and a barium sulfate tablet was used as a reference. The recorded spectra were analyzed by the Kubelka-Munk equation.

Steady-state irradiation experiments were performed using a Xenon lamp 150 W(Agilent, Santa Clara, CA, USA) as light source, the irradiation wavelength was selected by a monochromator, and a band-pass slit of 35 nm was used. The spectra analysis was carried out at different irradiation times.

2.5. Patches Preparation

The hybrid ZnAl-KET was formulated in patches by casting method [22] starting from the hydrogel composition optimized in previous work [23]:

ZnAl-KET: 1% *wt./wt.*
NaCMC: 2% *wt./wt.*
Glycerol: 10% *wt./wt.*
Water (CO_2 free): 87% *wt./wt.*

The hybrid was mixed with NaCMC powder by mortar and pestle and then wetted with glycerol. The water, free from CO_2 in order to avoid KET deintercalation, was added slowly until complete hydrogel formation. In order to remove the air incorporated during the mixing, the hydrogel was degassed in a conditioning planetary mixer (Thinky mixer ARE-250, Intertronics, Kidlington, England) at 2000 rpm for 10 min. The patches were prepared by casting 3.5 g of the hydrogel in circular silicon molds (diameter 3 cm) and then placed in a ventilated oven at 37 °C for 24 h.

2.6. Patches Characterization

2.6.1. Weight and Thickness Measurement

Patches (circles, area: 7.065 cm^2) were weighted by a Mettler-Toledo weighing balance, model XS205 (Milano, Italy). The thickness was measured in three different points of the patch by an electronic micrometer (QuantuMike IP 65 Coolant Proof, Mitutoyo, Takatsu-ku, Japan).

2.6.2. Mechanical Characterization

The tensile tests were performed by using a digital microprocessor instrument Llyod LR30K (Lloyd instruments, Bognor Regis, UK). The patches were cut in portions 100 × 10 mm (UNI ISO 527) to have a useful length of 50 mm. The experiment was performed at 5 mm/min, cell load 50 N. The two ends of the patch were fixed with clamps to the dynamometer. The sample was subjected to tensile stress until deformation and break. Maximum stress (σ_{max}), deformation at the break for maximum stress ($\varepsilon_{\ at\ \sigma max}$), and elastic modulus ($E_{Young}$) values were calculated from the stress-strain curves. Before the test, the patches were equilibrated for 1 week under silica gel (relative humidity, RH 30%). The results were an average of five measurements (n = 5).

2.6.3. Ex Vivo Adhesion Studies

Patch adhesion force was assessed using pig skin samples (from shoulder region), obtained from large white pigs weighing ~165–175 kg, furnished by Veterinary Service of ASL N.1 Città di Castello (Perugia, Italy), and used within 12 h from pig death [22]. The ex vivo adhesion force was measured by a dynamometer (Didatronic, Treni, Italy). The patch (2 × 2 cm) was attached to support, connected to the dynamometer, using cyanoacrylate glue. A piece of porcine skin tissue (4 × 4 cm) was fixed with cyanoacrylate glue on the surface of glass support placed in a thermostatic bath at 32 °C ± 0.5. The free side of the patch was wetted with 100 µL of phosphate buffer pH 5.50 and put in contact with the skin sample by applying a light force for 20 s. The force necessary for patch detachment to skin was measured and expressed as the average of three measurements (n = 3).

2.6.4. In Vitro Release

In vitro KET release, from ZnAl-KET and ZnAl-KET dispersed in the patch, was evaluated by dissolution testing for transdermal patches according to the European Pharmacopoeia (Ph. Eur. 10th

Ed.). Precisely, the apparatus II of the dissolution test was used, positioning an extraction cell (Ph. Eur. 10th Ed.) at the bottom of the vessel.

The central part of the cell formed a cavity (depth of 2.6 mm, diameter 27.0 mm) to hold the patch. On the top of the cell was positioned a cover with a central opening of 20.0 mm obtaining a release surface of 3.14 cm^2. The cell was positioned at the bottom of the vessel with the cover facing upwards and at a distance of 25.0 ± 2.0 mm from the paddle blade. The test was carried out for 24 h by working at 40 rpm at 32.0 ± 0.5 °C in sink conditions and using phosphate buffer pH 5.50 (Ph. Eur. 10th Ed.) as a dissolution medium (400 mL). At predetermined intervals, 2 mL of sample was withdrawn from the vessel and replaced by the same amount of fresh dissolution medium.

2.6.5. Quantitative Analysis

KET quantification was performed using a UV-VIS spectrophotometer (8453 Agilent, Santa Clara, CA, USA). The quantification was made using a calibration curve in phosphate buffer pH 5.50 previously prepared (λ_{max} = 261 nm, r = 0.99), using phosphate buffer pH 5.50 as blank. Experiments were performed in triplicate, and the error expressed as standard deviation (±SD).

2.6.6. Statistical Analysis

Results were reported as mean ± standard deviation (mean ± SD). A one-way ANOVA test was used for statistical analysis. Differences were considered statistically significant for $p < 0.05$.

3. Results

3.1. Hybrid Preparation and Characterization

The hybrid ZnAl-KET was obtained by ion exchange mechanism (Scheme 1) using ZnAl-NO_3, having the following formula obtained by ICP-OES analysis: $[Zn_{0.70}\ Al_{0.30}\ (OH)_2](NO_3)_{0.30}\cdot 0.4\ H_2O$.

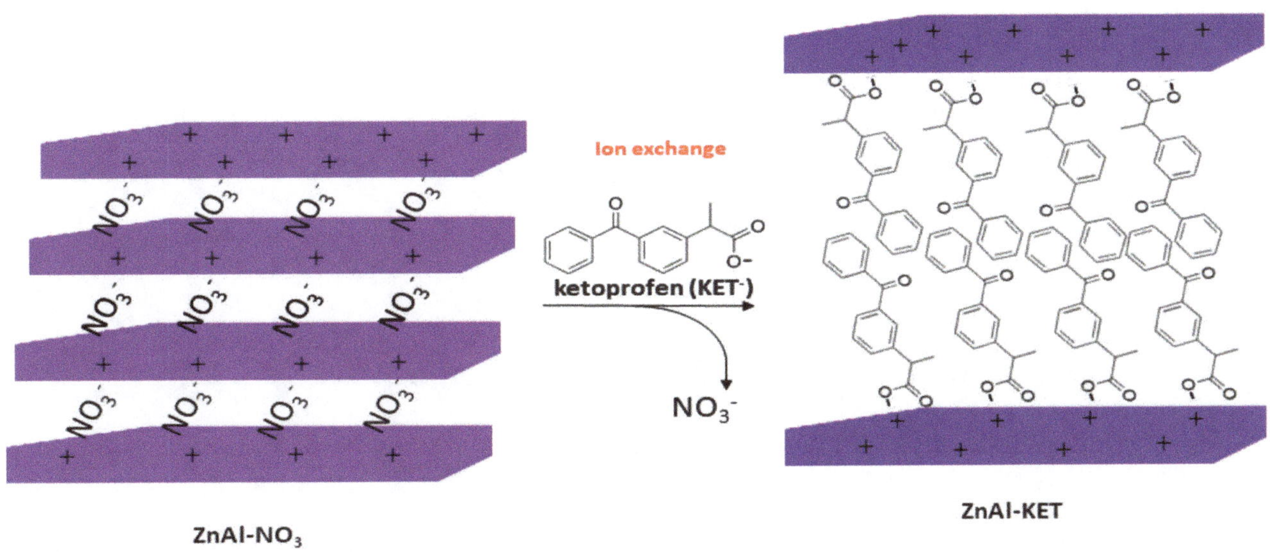

Scheme 1. Schematic representation of the ion exchange between NO_3^- ions in the pristine ZnAl-HTlc (ZnAl-hydrotalcite) and KET^- (ketoprofen).

The XRPD analysis confirmed KET^- intercalation into HTlc lamellae. In fact, the hybrid pattern showed a reflection at 2.19 nm, which was increased in comparison to pristine ZnAl-NO_3 that shows a reflection at 0.89 nm, typical of nitrate anion (Figure 1A). Combining the results coming from ICP-OES and TGA analyses, the final formula was calculated as $[Zn_{0.70}\ Al_{0.30}\ (OH)_2]\ (KET)_{0.30}\cdot 0.98\ H_2O$ (ZnAl-KET); drug loading was 41.89% *wt./wt*.

KET intercalated into HTlc in the anionic form (KET^-) showed a different solid-state compared to the pristine crystalline form. In fact, the reflection of the crystalline form disappeared in the intercalation product XRPD spectrum, testifying the lack of the crystalline form (Figure 1A). This was confirmed also by the thermal profile obtained by differential scanning calorimetry analysis. In fact, while crystalline KETH (alone) showed a sharp endothermic peak at 94 °C, corresponding to the melting point, this was not detectable in the ZnAl-KET profile, meaning that the crystallinity form was not present in this product (Figure 1B).

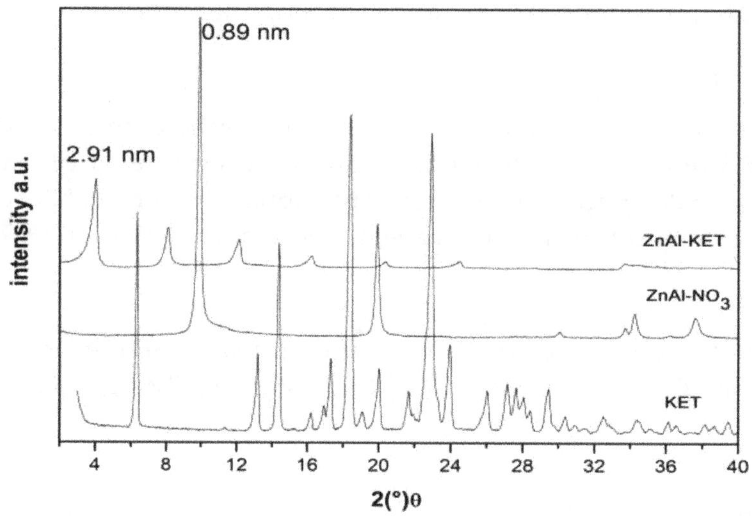

(A)

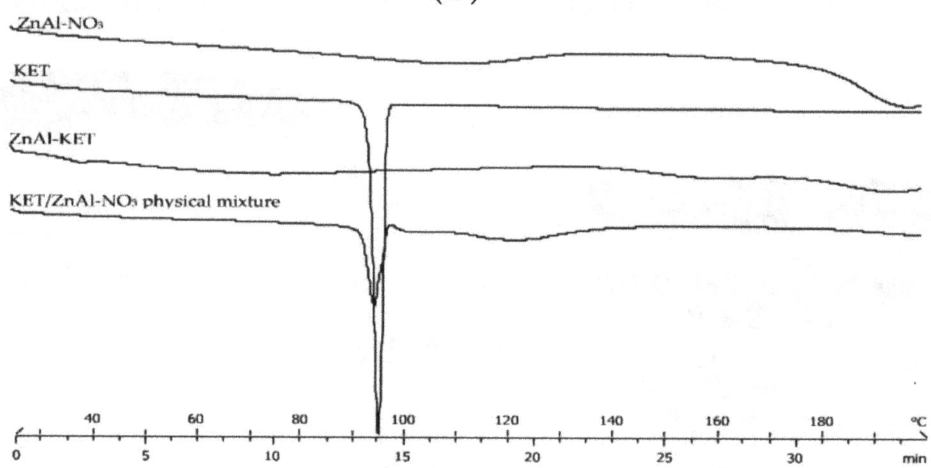

(B)

Figure 1. (**A**) XRPD pattern (X-ray diffraction patterns) of crystalline ketoprofen (KET) (acid form), pristine ZnAl-NO_3, and the hybrid ZnAl-KET. (**B**) Thermal profiles measured by differential scanning calorimetry of ZnAl-NO_3, crystalline KET, ZnAl-KET, and KET/ZnAl-NO_3 physical mixture.

The morphological analysis carried out by scanning electron microscopy (SEM) showed the typical desert-like rose structure of pristine ZnAl-NO_3 crystals (Figure 2A,B) [24] having dimensions in the range of 1–10 μm. The intercalation procedure induced the modification of this morphology, as can be observed from the micrographs reported in Figure 2C,D appearing fragmented with rounded edges, while the dimensions were maintained in the same range of the raw ZnAl-NO_3.

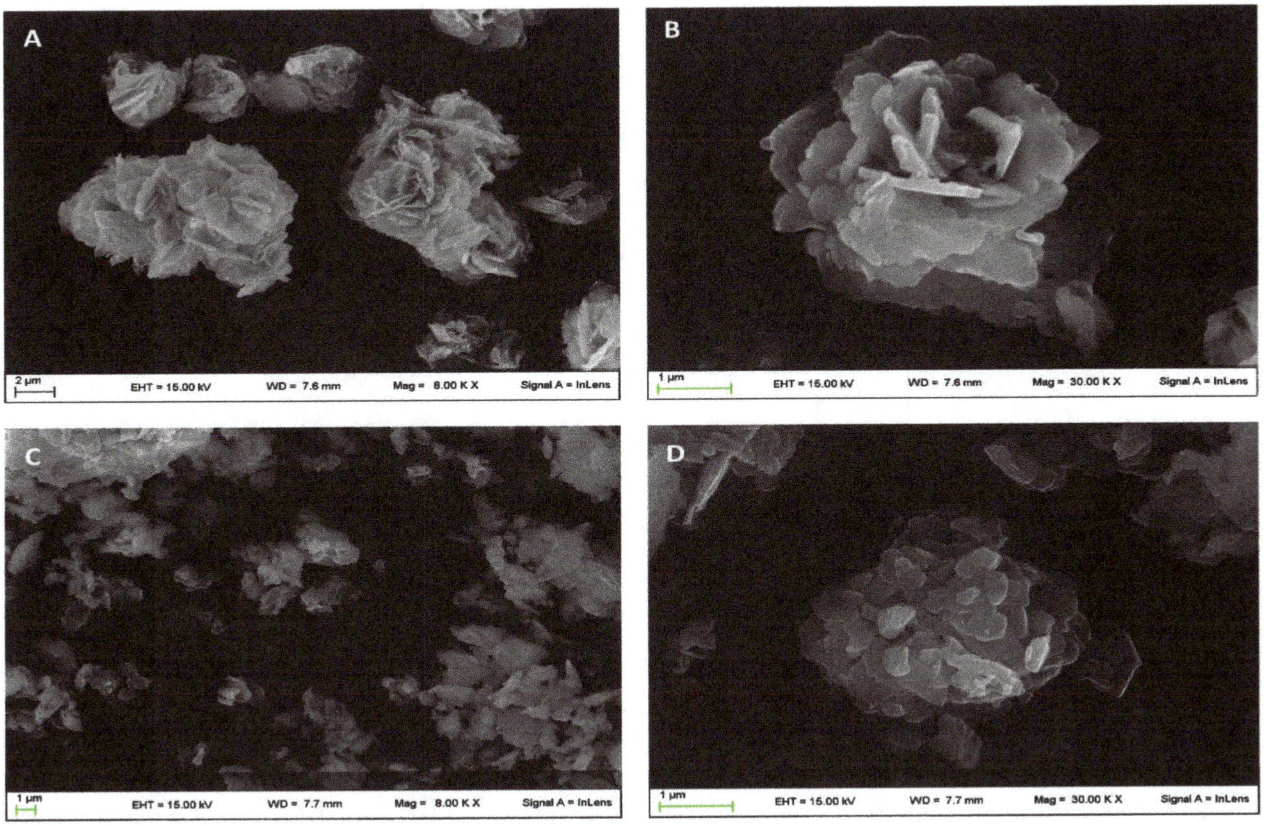

Figure 2. Micrographs obtained by scanning electron microscopy of pristine ZnAl-NO_3 (**A**,**B**) and ZnAl-KET (**C**,**D**).

3.2. Apparent Solubility Studies

The solubilization rate of KET from the crystalline form (acid form) from the hybrid (ZnAl-KET) was evaluated in vitro method in order to evaluate if the intercalation procedure allows enhancing this property. The obtained results showed that crystalline KET (acid form) had a limited solubilization rate, as testified by the concentration value measured (12 ± 0.15 µg/mL). This result was in accordance with the literature data [25]. On the other hand, the results obtained from ZnAl-KET were very different; in fact, a concentration of 106.00 ± 0.20 µg/mL was measured. This result can be explained by taking into account that KET is intercalated into HTlc lamellae as an anion in the molecular form. Thus, when ZnAl-KET makes contact with the water, KET^- anions are exchanged and replaced by OH^- (deriving from water molecules dissociation) in the interlayer space. Once in the medium, KET^- anions are protonated obtaining a free dissolved molecules.

3.3. Photochemical Characterization

Spectrophotometric measurements gave insight into the radiation frequencies absorbed by the drug and its intercalated compound and could be used to achieve information on the photostability of the materials. The absorption spectrum of crystalline KET in acid form (KETH) presented a maximum at 280 nm and a broad and structured band in the 320–390 nm (Figure 3). Deprotonation of the drug did not change its absorption spectrum; in fact, the KET-Na (Figure 3) showed a spectrum very similar to that obtained for KETH, probably because the acid functionality is not conjugated with the chromophoric moiety. On the other hand, the spectrum of the intercalated sample ZnAl-KET showed the main band centered at 280 nm and a shoulder without any structures at about 330 nm (Figure 3). The different spectra recorded for KET-Na and ZnAl-KET indicated that the interactions with the inorganic matrices and/or the interactions between chromophores modified the electronic distribution in the drug.

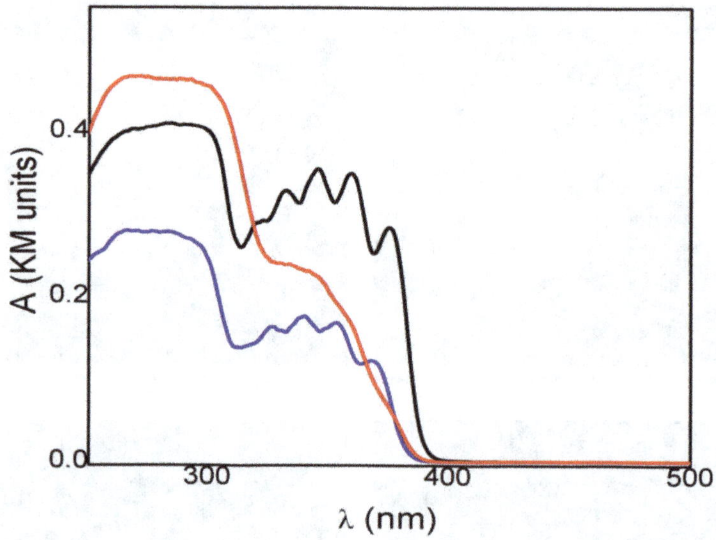

Figure 3. Absorption spectra of crystalline KET in acid form (KETH) (black line), KET-Na (blue line), and ZnAl-KET (red line).

The spectrophotometric analysis conducted on the samples under investigation before and after irradiation at 330 nm enabled us to evaluate and compare their photostability. In all cases, after 2 h of irradiation, the optical density changed (ΔOD) in the 250–400 nm range and was detected even if the relative variations were different (Figure 4). In particular, KET showed a smaller variation, compared to the other samples, in the whole spectral range investigated (black line Figure 4, Table 1). This behavior indicated that KETH had a higher photostability, in agreement with the literature data [26], where the photodecomposition of ketoprofen is reported to be pH-dependent, and a higher photodegradation is observed when the drug is in the anionic form. Therefore, KETH was not a good reference for the intercalated samples. KET-Na showed a remarkable increase in the absorption upon corresponding irradiation (blue line Figure 4, Table 1); this indicated that the deprotonated drug had a photostability lower than KETH, also when in powder form. Since the drug was intercalated in an anionic matrix, KET-Na was considered a good reference for assessing the photochemical behavior of the intercalation compound.

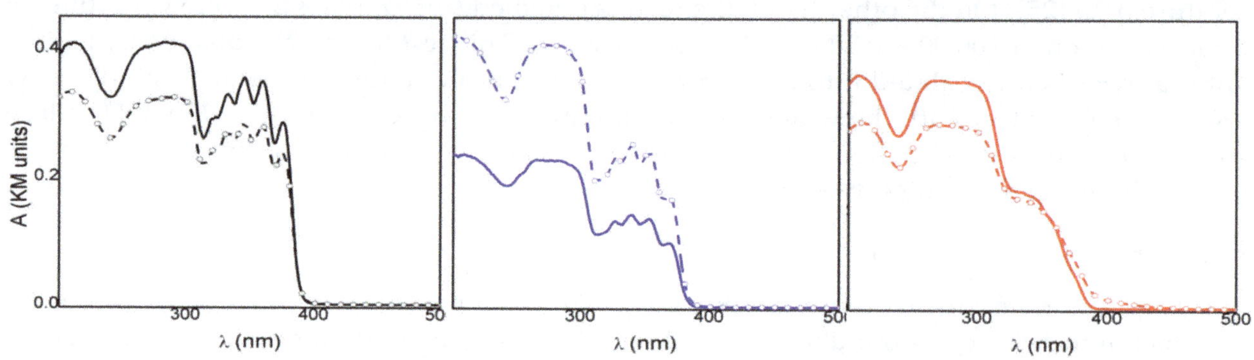

Figure 4. Absorption spectra of KETH (black line), KET-Na (blue line), and ZnAl-HTlc-KET (red line) before and after 120′ irradiation at 330 nm.

When ZnAl-KET was exposed to the 330 nm radiation (red line Figure 4) in the same experimental conditions, a decrease in the absorption at wavelengths below 360 nm was observed, while at longer wavelengths, an increase in optical density was detected. This behavior suggested that the drug underwent different photochemical processes in the inorganic matrix. However, the optical density changes of the intercalation compound were small compared to those observed for KET-Na, as shown by the data reported in Table 1.

Table 1. ΔOD measured at different λ_{obs} upon 2 h irradiation of the samples at 330 nm.

Sample	ΔOD [λ_{obs} = 280 nm]	ΔOD [λ_{obs} = 340 nm]
KETH	2%	3%
KET-Na	44%	45%
ZnAl-KET	24%	5%

ΔOD: optical density changes; λ_{obs}: observation wavelengths

The comparison of the data suggested that the hybrid ZnAl-HTlc was able to photoprotect the deprotonated form of KET. The photoprotection mechanism can be due to a physical filter effect and to a modification of the photochemical reaction paths. Indeed, it has been reported that KET carboxylate excitation produces mainly the triplet state, which undergoes a rapid and efficient photodecarboxylation reaction [27]. The intercalation in the layered solid could reduce the efficiency of the decarboxylation step due to space confinement of the species.

3.4. Patch Characterization

Previous work highlighted that patches realized starting from a hydrogel based on NaCMC (2% *wt./wt.*) as bioadhesive polymer, glycerol (10% *wt./wt.*) as a plasticizing agent, hydrotalcite ZnAl-NO_3 (1% *wt./wt.*), and water (until 100%) shows suitable mechanical properties for topical use [23]. Using this composition, a new hydrogel was prepared using ZnAl-KET 1% *wt./wt.* in place of ZnAl-NO_3. The patch was prepared to cast the hydrogel in a circular mold, obtaining a final formulation with a surface area of 10.17 cm^2, a final weight of 0.54 g ± 0.01 (0.0532 g/cm^2), and a thickness of 414 μm ± 7.42. Considering the loading percentage of ZnAl-KET (41.89% *wt./wt.*), the amount of KET/surface was measured to be 1.44 mg/cm^2.

Taking into account this datum, the patch can be prepared in different sizes to be applied on surfaces of different dimensions, as demonstrated in the pictures reported in Figure 5.

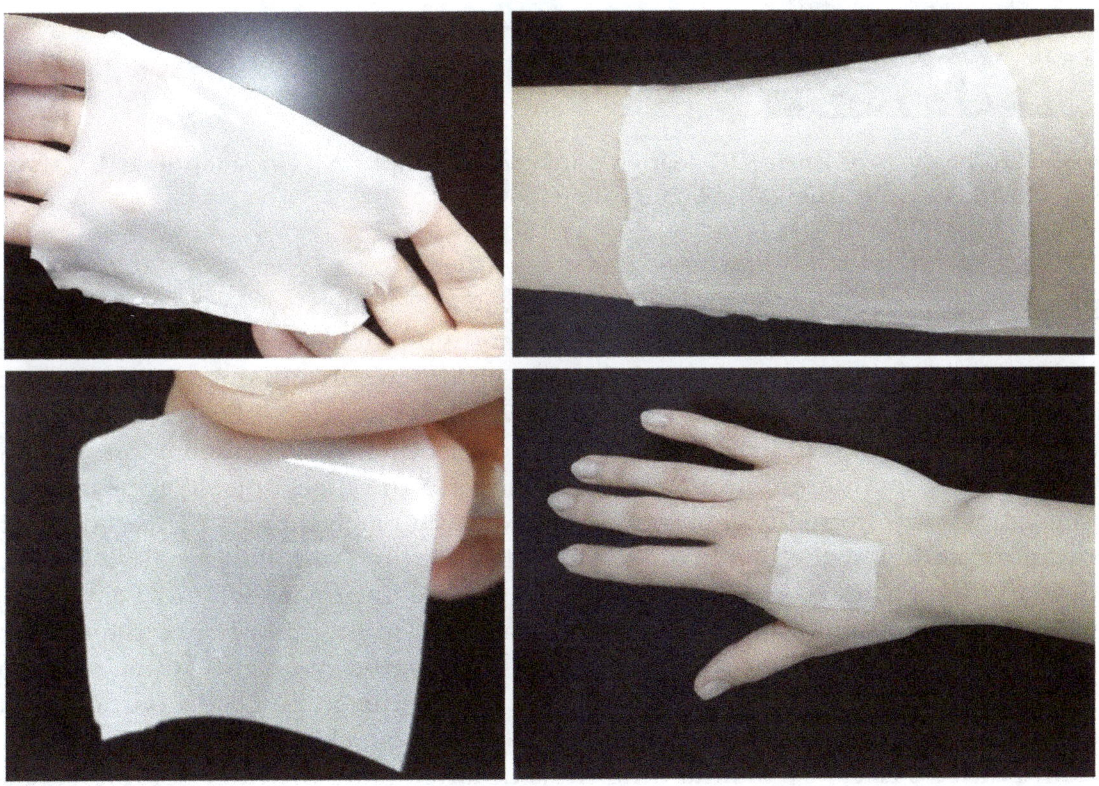

Figure 5. Examples of different sizes and shapes on which it can be applied the patch loaded with ZnAl-KET.

3.4.1. Morphological Characterization

The elemental mapping on ZnAl-KET loaded patch obtained by EDX analysis showed that the hybrid was homogeneously dispersed in the polymeric matrix (Figure 6). This result suggested that the casting method used for patch preparation allowed to obtain a homogeneous final product, and this was very important as a guarantee that the drug (KET as a hybrid) was distributed homogeneously on the whole surface. Moreover, the patch showed a wrinkled surface due to the presence of ZnAl-KET crystals.

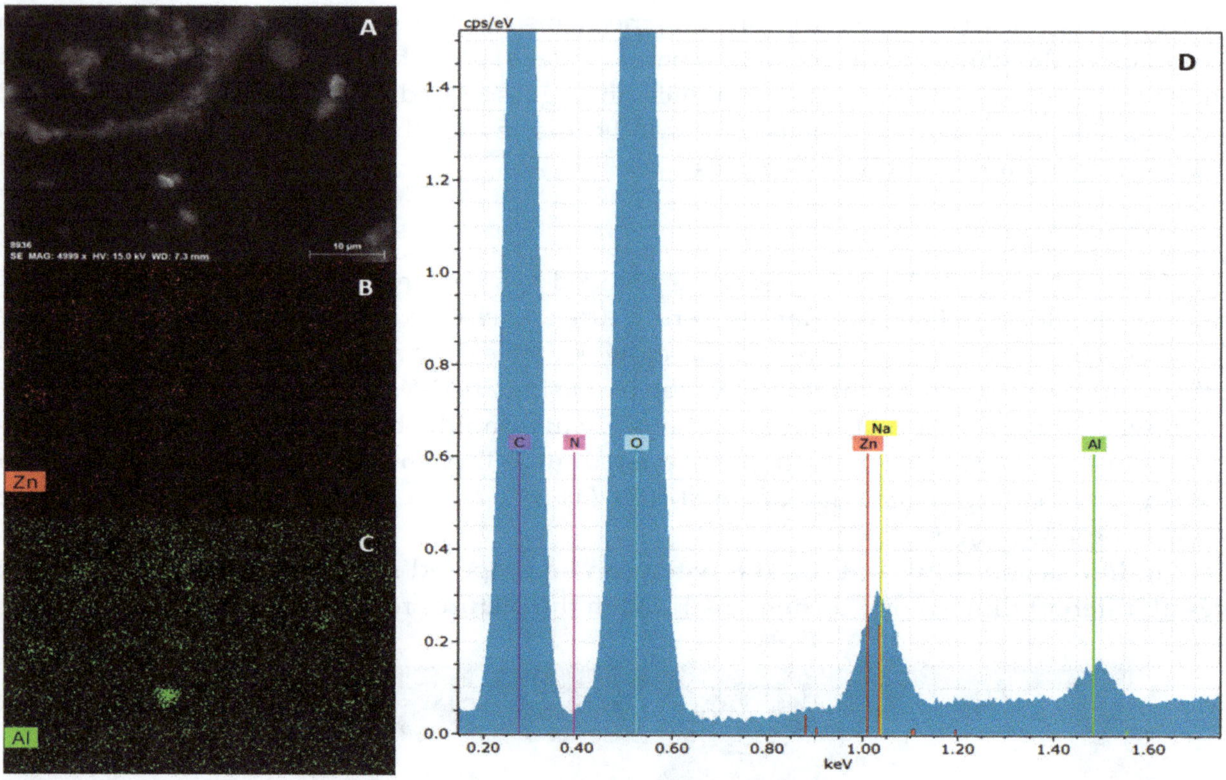

Figure 6. SEM analysis of ZnAl-KET loaded patch: micrograph (**A**), zinc mapping (**B**), aluminum mapping (**C**) and edx spectrum (**D**). Magnification 4999 X.

3.4.2. Mechanical Characterization

The presence and effect of ZnAl-KET in the NaCMC matrix were investigated in terms of mechanical properties. Mechanical parameters of the two patches, NaCMC (blank) and NaCMC loaded with ZnAl-KET, were estimated from stress-strain curves obtained by performing tensile tests at RT (Figure 7). Data are summarized in Table 2, while the stress-strain curves are reported in Figure 6. As already reported in Perioli et al. [23], the introduction of lamellar ZnAl-NO_3 at 1% *wt.* in NaCMC, even in a small amount, was able to increase the mechanical properties of reference matrix. Specifically, at low humidity conditions, the produced patch showed increased tensile strength but limited deformability at the break, as already observed by Yadollahi et al. [28]. The ductility of the NaCMC film was indeed here recovered and greatly improved when KET was intercalated in ZnAl-NO_3. The introduction of the drug into ZnAl-HTlc might enhance interfacial adhesion and compatibility between the NaCMC matrix and the layered nano clay, thus increasing tensile strength [29] and positively affecting the ductility of the produced patch. In particular, it could be considered that the presence of KET inhibited the possible restacking of the nano sheets that could appear in unmodified HTlcs, by maintaining the exfoliated state in water-soluble NaCMC before casting [30].

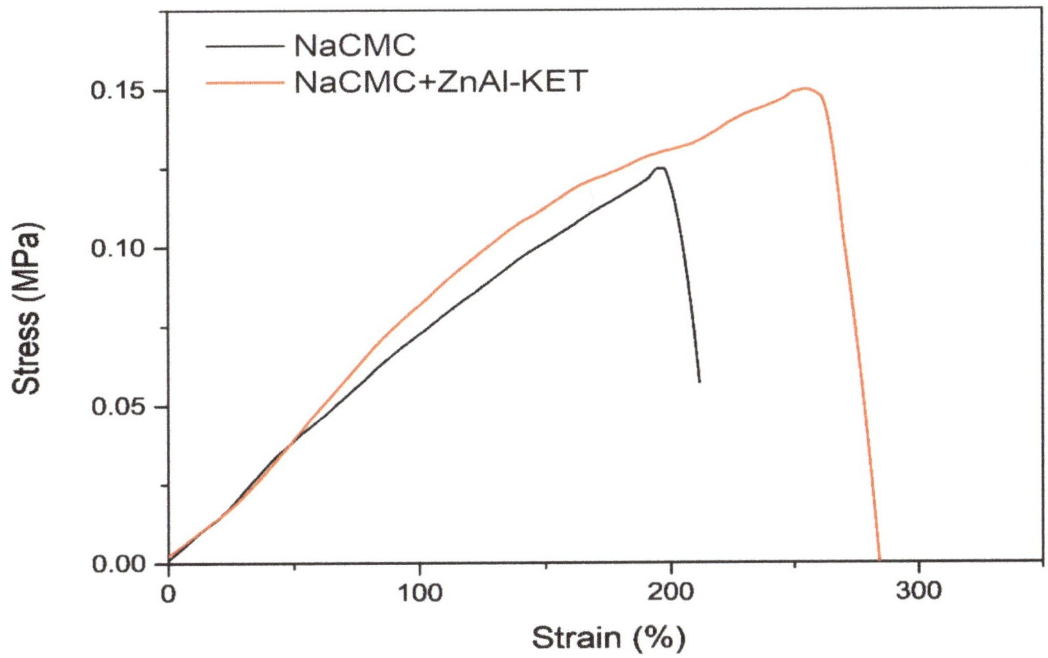

Figure 7. Stress–strain curves of NaCMC patch (NaCMC) and patch loaded with ZnAl-KET (NaCMC + ZnAl-KET).

Table 2. Mechanical properties of NaCMC patch and patch loaded with ZnAl-KET.

Formulations	σ_{max} (MPa)	$\varepsilon_{at\ \sigma max}$ (%)	E_{Young} (MPa)
NaCMC	0.134 ± 0.014	187 ± 18	0.068 ± 0.008
NaCMC + ZnAl-KET	0.149 ± 0.013	252 ± 17	0.068 ± 0.009

NaCMC: NaCMC patch; NaCMC + ZnAl-KET: patch loaded with ZnAl-KET; σ_{max}: maximum stress; $\varepsilon_{at\ \sigma max}$: deformation at the break for maximum stress; E_{Young}: elastic modulus.

3.5. *Ex Vivo Adhesion Studies*

Patch loaded with ZnAl-KET showed a bioadhesion force of 0.513 ± 0.015 N vs. 0.411 ± 0.011 N measured for the same patch without HTlc (blank). This increase was probably due to the wrinkled surface of the loaded patch, able to promote the contact and adhesion with the skin surface. Moreover, it can be hypothesized that ZnAl-KET establishes hydrophilic interactions (hydrogen bonds) with NaCMC chains involving –OH and C=O groups. This should improve the hydrophobicity of patch surface due to the exposition of NaCMC lipophilic groups (as-CH_3) freely available to bind the skin. In fact, the binding to the stratum corneum is mainly attributable to hydrophobic interactions.

3.6. *Release Studies*

The release capacity of the patch loaded with ZnAl-KET was evaluated using the in vitro method for transdermal patches, according to Ph. Eur. 10th Ed. As shown in Figure 8, a sustained release of KET was obtained from the formulation reaching 6% after 5 min, 15% after 30 min, and ~36% after 60 min. The complete release was obtained within 480 min; from this point, a steady state was observed. The same assay performed on ZnAl-KET (not formulated in the patch) showed that the amount of KET released in the first 300 min from the hybrid was higher (after 10 min 13.5% vs. ~4%; after 45 min 45% vs. 26%; after 300 min 93% vs. 89%) compared to the patch. This suggested the effect of the polymeric matrix (in the case of the patch) in controlling the drug diffusion.

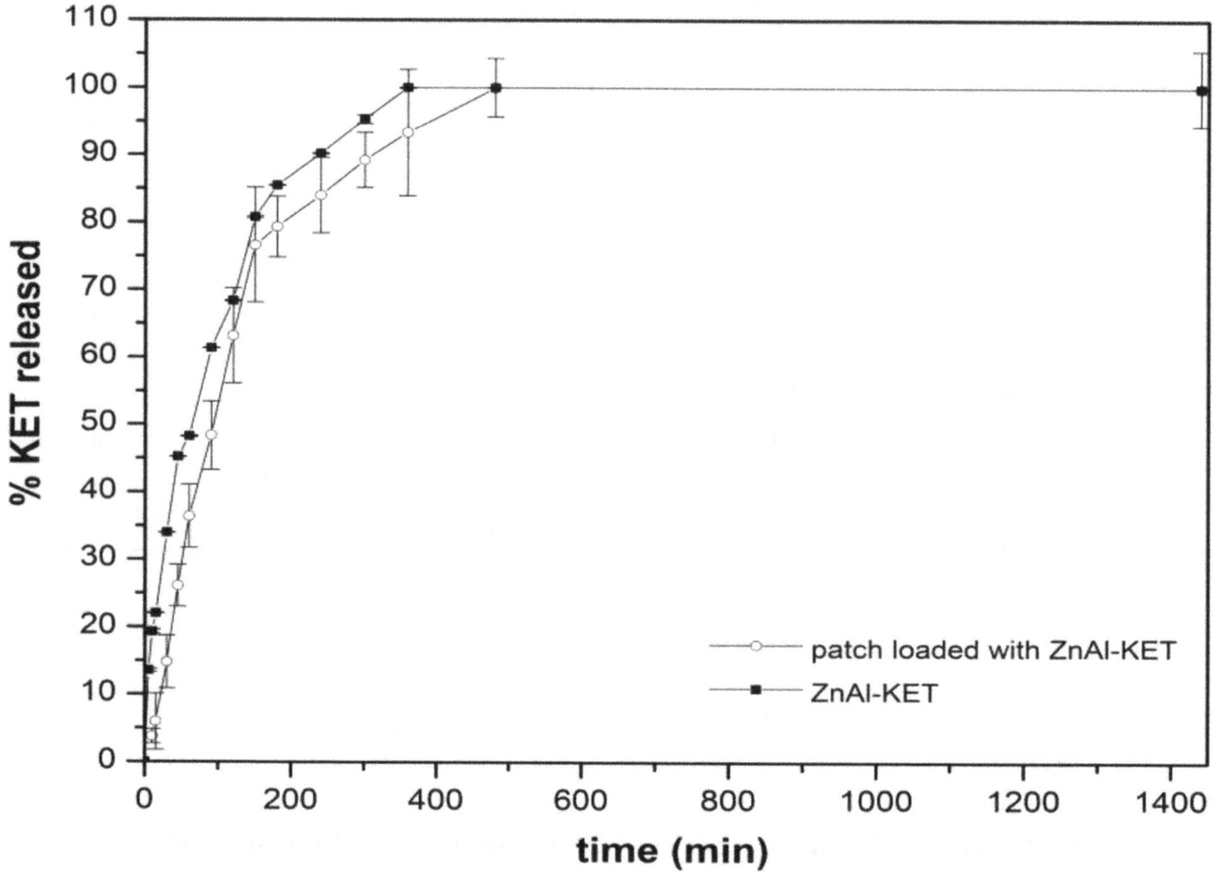

Figure 8. The release profile of KET from ZnAl-KET and from the patch loaded with ZnAl-KET ($p < 0.05$).

The kinetic of KET release from the patch can be explained considering two main mechanisms, (i) the ion exchange between KET^- stored in the HTlc interlamellar space and phosphate anions present in the dissolution medium and (ii) the effect of NaCMC polymeric network, able to modulate KET diffusion in the bulk solution.

The kinetic of KET release was deeply investigated by processing the in vitro release by the following mathematical models: zero-order, first-order, and Higuchi [31,32]. When the zero-order model describes the release rate, the latter is not dependent on the concentration; the first-order model describes the release rate concentration-dependent, and the Higuchi model explains the release based on Fickian diffusion (time-dependent). Moreover, as KET was homogeneously dispersed in the NaCMC network of the patch as intercalation product (ZnAl-KET), the influence of HTlc on the release was evaluated by the kinetic model (ion exchange resins) proposed by Bhaskar et al. [33], applied to exchangeable matrices.

The obtained results from the patch (Table 3) showed that the best fitting was obtained both for Higuchi ($R^2 = 0.98$) and Bhaskar models ($R^2 = 0.98$). This suggested that these two models were the most suitable to describe KET release from the patch. The amount of KET molecules available to cross the NaCMC polymeric network by time-dependent diffusional mechanism (Higuchi kinetic) was controlled by the ion exchange mechanism between the intercalated KET^- and phosphate ions of the dissolution medium. The good fitting obtained in the case of the Bhaskar model suggested that this process had a remarkable role in conditioning the diffusion rate.

ZnAl-KET (Table 3) showed a good fitting for the Bhaskar model ($R^2 = 0.97$), confirming that, in this case, the ion exchange between KET^- and phosphate ions was the mechanism driving the dissolution rate.

Table 3. Equations and R^2 values obtained by the application of the kinetic mathematical models (zero-order, first-order) and ion exchange resins for loaded patch and ion exchange resins for ZnAl-KET.

Sample	$M_t/M_\infty = kt$	$M_t/M_\infty = kt^{0.5}$	$M_t/M_\infty = 1 - e^{-kt}$	$M_t/M_\infty = 1 - e^{-k\,0.65}$
	Zero-order kinetic	Higuchi kinetic (release 0–60%)	First order kinetic	Ion exchange resins
ZnAl-KET	-	-	-	$y = -0.0322x + 0.1089$ $R^2 = 0.97$
patch	$y = 0.3292x + 9.8281$ $R^2 = 0.885$	$y = 6.8906x - 18.739$ $R^2 = 0.98$	$y = 0.3292x + 9.8281$ $R^2 = 0.88$	$y = -0.027x + 0.1425$ $R^2 = 0.98$

M_∞: amount of drug at the equilibrium state; M_t: amount of drug released over time t, k: release velocity constant; n: exponent of release (related to the drug release mechanism) in function of time t; e: Euler's number.

4. Conclusions

KET was intercalated into the lamellar anionic clay ZnAl-NO_3 to obtain the hybrid ZnAl-KET and then formulated in an authoadhesive patch as an alternative to conventional products (gels, foams, creams) for local treatments.

The performed studies highlighted that the intercalation is a valuable technology and advantageous to improve KET water solubilization rate and stability to UV radiations.

The hybrid ZnAl-KET was loaded in a bioadhesive polymeric patch, prepared using NaCMC, as an alternative to conventional products for local pain treatment.

It was demonstrated that the presence of ZnAl-KET crystals, homogeneously dispersed in the polymeric matrix, was able to improve the mechanical patch properties. Moreover, a sustained release was observed by in vitro method, suggesting that the planned formulation could assure prolonged KET release. The proposed patch was bioadhesive, allowing both a high residence time in the application site and easy removal by washing, avoiding the discomfort of adhesives used in conventional patches, responsible for pain during the removal.

The patch formulation is also versatile and practical to use. It can be prepared or cut, if needed, in various sizes and shapes, becoming useful to be used both for large and small surfaces.

Moreover, the production of such a formulation is easily scalable.

Author Contributions: Conceptualization, L.P. and C.P.; methodology, L.P., C.P., C.A.V.I.; formal analysis, C.P., L.L., F.L., D.P., A.D.M., C.A.V.I.; investigation, L.L., F.L., A.D.M., C.P.; resources, L.P., L.L., D.P., M.R.; data curation, C.P., L.L., A.D.M., F.L., D.P, C.A.V.I.; writing—original draft preparation, L.P., C.P., M.R., L.L., D.P.; writing—review and editing L.P., C.P., L.L., F.L., D.P.; visualization, L.P., C.P., L.L., D.P, C.A.V.I.; supervision, L.P., L.L., A.D.M., D.P., M.R.; funding acquisition, L.P., L.L., D.P. All authors have read and agreed to the published version of the manuscript.

Acknowledgments: Authors sincerely acknowledge Morena Nocchetti for X-ray patterns and registration and Marco Marani for technical assistance from the Department of Pharmaceutical Sciences. Authors wish to thank Simonetta De Angelis from ASL N. 1 (Città di Castello, Perugia, Italy), for providing pig skin samples.

References

1. Rani, S.; Savant, M.; Mahendru, R.; Bansal, P. Comparison of efficacy and safety of ketoprofen patch versus diclofenac patch as post-operative analgesic in hysterectomy patients. *Int. J. Basic Clin. Pharmacol.* **2019**, *8*, 2445–2449. [CrossRef]
2. Derry, S.; Conaghan, P.; Da Silva, J.A.P.; Wiffen, P.J.; Moore, R.A. Topical NSAIDs for chronic musculoskeletal pain in adults. *Cochrane Database Syst. Rev.* **2016**, *4*, CD007400. [CrossRef] [PubMed]
3. Shohin, I.E.; Kulinich, J.I.; Ramenskaya, G.V.; Abrahamsson, B.; Kopp, S.; Langguth, P.; Polli, J.E.; Shah, V.P.; Groot, D.W.; Barends, D.M.; et al. Biowaiver monographs for immediate-release solid oral dosage forms: Ketoprofen. *J. Pharm. Sci.* **2012**, *101*, 3593–3603. [CrossRef] [PubMed]

4. Moser, J.; Sarabia, Z.; Minter, H.; Lovell, W.W.; Beijersbergen Van Henegouwen, G.M.J. Photobinding of ketoprofen in vitro and ex vivo. *J. Photochem. Photobiol. B Biol.* **2000**, *58*, 37–45. [CrossRef]
5. Albès, B.; Marguery, M.C.; Schwarze, H.P.; Journé, F.; Loche, F.; Bazex, J. Prolonged Photosensitivity following Contact Photoallergy to Ketoprofen. *Dermatology* **2000**, *201*, 171–174. [CrossRef]
6. Kryczyk-Poprawa, A.; Kwiecień, A.; Opoka, W. Photostability of topical agents applied to the skin: A review. *Pharmaceutics* **2020**, *12*, 10. [CrossRef]
7. Nakajima, A.; Tahara, M.; Yoshimura, Y.; Nakazawa, H. Determination of free radicals generated from light exposed ketoprofen. *J. Photochem. Photobiol. A Chem.* **2005**, *174*, 89–97. [CrossRef]
8. Ray, R.S.; Mujtaba, S.F.; Dwivedi, A.; Yadav, N.; Verma, A.; Kushwaha, H.N.; Amar, S.K.; Goel, S.; Chopra, D. Singlet oxygen mediated DNA damage induced phototoxicity by ketoprofen resulting in mitochondrial depolarization and lysosomal destabilization. *Toxicology* **2013**, *314*, 229–237. [CrossRef]
9. Guy, R.H.; Kuma, H.; Nakanishi, M. Serious photocontact dermatitis induced by topical ketoprofen depends on the formulation. *Eur. J. Dermatol.* **2014**, *24*, 365–371. [CrossRef]
10. Wang, M.; Marepally, S.K.; Vemula, P.K.; Xu, C. Inorganic Nanoparticles for Transdermal Drug Delivery and Topical Application. In *Nanoscience in Dermatology*; Academic Press: Cambridge, MA, USA, 2016; ISBN 9780128029459.
11. Ioele, G.; Tavano, L.; Muzzalupo, R.; De Luca, M.; Ragno, G. Stability-Indicating Methods for NSAIDs in Topical Formulations and Photoprotection in Host-Guest Matrices. *Mini Rev. Med. Chem.* **2016**, *16*, 676–682. [CrossRef]
12. Ioele, G.; De Luca, M.; Garofalo, A.; Ragno, G. Photosensitive drugs: A review on their photoprotection by liposomes and cyclodextrins. *Drug Deliv.* **2017**, *24*, 33–44. [CrossRef]
13. Cavani, F.; Trifirò, F.; Vaccari, A. Hydrotalcite-type anionic clays: Preparation, properties and applications. *Catal. Today* **1991**, *11*, 173–301. [CrossRef]
14. Costantino, U.; Ambrogi, V.; Nocchetti, M.; Perioli, L. Hydrotalcite-like compounds: Versatile layered hosts of molecular anions with biological activity. *Micropor. Mesopor. Mater.* **2008**, *107*, 149–160. [CrossRef]
15. Ambrogi, V.; Fardella, G.; Grandolini, G.; Nocchetti, M.; Perioli, L. Effect of hydrotalcite-like compounds on the aqueous solubility of some poorly water-soluble drugs. *J. Pharm. Sci.* **2003**, *92*, 1407–1418. [CrossRef]
16. Perioli, L.; Ambrogi, V.; Nocchetti, M.; Sisani, M.; Pagano, C. Preformulation studies on host-guest composites for oral administration of BCS class IV drugs: HTlc and furosemide. *Appl. Clay Sci.* **2011**, *53*, 696–703. [CrossRef]
17. Perioli, L.; Ambrogi, V.; Bertini, B.; Ricci, M.; Nocchetti, M.; Latterini, L.; Rossi, C. Anionic clays for sunscreen agent safe use: Photoprotection, photostability and prevention of their skin penetration. *Eur. J. Pharm. Biopharm.* **2006**, *62*, 185–193. [CrossRef]
18. Schoubben, A.; Blasi, P.; Giovagnoli, S.; Nocchetti, M.; Ricci, M.; Perioli, L.; Rossi, C. Evaluation and optimization of the conditions for an improved ferulic acid intercalation into a synthetic lamellar anionic clay. *Pharm. Res.* **2006**, *23*, 604–613. [CrossRef]
19. Da Silva, T.A.; da Silva, T.A.; do Nascimento, T.G.; Yatsuzuka, R.E.; Grillo, L.A.M.; Dornelas, C.B. Recent advances in layered double hydroxides applied to photoprotection. *Einstein* **2019**, *17*, 1–6. [CrossRef]
20. Pagano, C.; Calarco, P.; Ceccarini, M.R.; Beccari, T.; Ricci, M.; Perioli, L. Development and Characterization of New Topical Hydrogels Based on Alpha Lipoic Acid—Hydrotalcite Hybrids. *Cosmetics* **2019**, *6*, 35. [CrossRef]
21. Costantino, U.; Marmottini, F.; Nocchetti, M.; Vivani, R. New Synthetic Routes to Hydrotalcite-Like Compounds−Characterisation and Properties of the Obtained Materials. *Eur. J. Inorg. Chem.* **1998**, *1998*, 1439–1446. [CrossRef]
22. Pagano, C.; Ceccarini, M.R.; Calarco, P.; Scuota, S.; Conte, C.; Primavilla, S.; Ricci, M.; Perioli, L. Bioadhesive polymeric films based on usnic acid for burn wound treatment: Antibacterial and cytotoxicity studies. *Colloids Surf. B: Biointerfaces* **2019**, *178*, 488–499. [CrossRef]
23. Perioli, L.; Dorigato, A.; Pagano, C.; Leoni, M.; Pegoretti, A. Thermo-mechanical and adhesive properties of polymeric films based on ZnAl-hydrotalcite composites for active wound dressings. *Polym. Eng. Sci.* **2019**, *59*, E112–E119. [CrossRef]
24. Pagano, C.; Perioli, L.; Latterini, L.; Nocchetti, M.; Ceccarini, M.R.; Marani, M.; Ramella, D.; Ricci, M. Folic acid-layered double hydroxides hybrids in skin formulations: Technological, photochemical and in vitro cytotoxicity on human keratinocytes and fibroblasts. *Appl. Clay Sci.* **2019**, *168*, 382–395. [CrossRef]

25. Loftsson, T.; Hreinsdóttir, D. Determination of aqueous solubility by heating and equilibration: A technical note. *AAPS Pharm. Sci. Tech.* **2006**, *7*, E29–E32. [CrossRef]
26. Cosa, G. Photodegradation and photosensitization in pharmaceutical products: Assessing drug phototoxicity. *Pure Appl. Chem.* **2004**, *76*, 263–275. [CrossRef]
27. Martínez, C.; Vilariño, S.; Fernández, M.I.; Faria, J.; Canle, M.L.; Santaballa, J.A. Mechanism of degradation of ketoprofen by heterogeneous photocatalysis in aqueous solution. *Appl. Catal. B Environ.* **2013**, *142-143*, 633–646. [CrossRef]
28. Yadollahi, M.; Namazi, H.; Barkhordari, S. Preparation and properties of carboxymethyl cellulose/layered double hydroxide bionanocomposite films. *Carbohydr. Polym.* **2014**, *108*, 83–90. [CrossRef]
29. Wang, H.; Wu, J.; Zheng, L.; Cheng, X. Preparation and Properties of ZnAl Layered Double Hydroxide/Polycaprolactone Nanocomposites for Use in Drug Delivery. *Polym. Technol. Mater.* **2019**, *58*, 1027–1035. [CrossRef]
30. Kang, H.; Huang, G.; Ma, S.; Bai, Y.; Ma, H.; Li, Y.; Yang, X. Coassembly of inorganic macromolecule of exfoliated LDH nanosheets with cellulose. *J. Phys. Chem. C* **2009**, *113*, 9157–9163. [CrossRef]
31. Ritger, P.L.; Peppas, N.A. A simple equation for description of solute release II. Fickian and anomalous release from swellable devices. *J. Control Release* **1987**, *5*, 37–42. [CrossRef]
32. Siepmann, J.; Peppas, N.A. Higuchi equation: Derivation, applications, use and misuse. *Int. J. Pharm.* **2011**, *418*, 6–12. [CrossRef] [PubMed]
33. Bhaskar, R.; Murthy, R.S.R.; Miglani, B.D.; Viswanathan, K. Novel method to evaluate diffusion controlled release of drug from resinate. *Int. J. Pharm.* **1986**, *28*, 59–66. [CrossRef]

4

New Grafted Copolymers Carrying Betaine Units Based on Gellan and N-Vinylimidazole as Precursors for Design of Drug Delivery Systems

Stefania Racovita [1], Nicolae Baranov [2,3], Ana Maria Macsim [1], Catalina Lionte [4], Corina Cheptea [5], Valeriu Sunel [3], Marcel Popa [2,6], Silvia Vasiliu [1] and Jacques Desbrieres [7,*]

1 "Petru Poni" Institute of Macromolecular Chemistry, Grigore Ghica Voda Alley, No. 41A, 700487 Iasi, Romania; stefania.racovita@icmpp.ro (S.R.); macsim.ana@icmpp.ro (A.M.M.); silvia.vasiliu@icmpp.ro (S.V.)

2 Department of Natural and Synthetic Polymers, Faculty of Chemical Engienering and Environmental Protection, "Gheorghe Asachi" Technical University of Iasi, Prof. Dr. Docent Dimitrie Mangeron Street, No. 73, 700050 Iasi, Romania; Baranov_nicolae@yahoo.com (N.B.); marpopa2001@yahoo.fr (M.P.)

3 Faculty of Chemistry, "Al. I. Cuza" University, Carol 1 Bvd., No. 11, 700506 Iasi, Romania; vsunel@uaic.ro

4 Faculty of Medicine, "Gr. T. Popa" University of Medicine and Pharmacy, Universitatii Street, No.16, 700115 Iasi, Romania; clionte@yahoo.com

5 Department of Biomedical Sciences, Faculty of Biomedical Bioengineering, "Gr. T. Popa" University of Medicine and Pharmacy, Kogalniceanu Street No. 9-13, 700454 Iasi, Romania; coricheptea@yahoo.com

6 Academy of Romanian Scientists, Splaiul Independentei Street No. 54, 050085 Bucuresti, Romania

7 Institut des Sciences Analytiques et de Physico-Chimie Pour l'Environnement et les Materiaux (IPREM), Pau and Pays de l'Adour University (UPPA), UMR CNRS 5254, Helioparc Pau Pyrenees, 2, av. President Angot, 64053 Pau CEDEX 09, France

* Correspondence: jacques.desbrieres@univ-pau.fr

Academic Editor: Sonia Trombino

Abstract: New grafted copolymers possessing structural units of 1-vinyl-3-(1-carboxymethyl) imidazolium betaine were obtained by graft copolymerization of *N*-vinylimidazole onto gellan gum followed by the polymer-analogous reactions on grafted polymer with the highest grafting percentage using sodium chloroacetate as the betainization agent. The grafted copolymers were prepared using ammonium persulfate/*N,N,N',N'* tetramethylethylenediamine in a nitrogen atmosphere. The grafting reaction conditions were optimized by changing one of the following reaction parameters: initiator concentration, monomer concentration, polymer concentration, reaction time or temperature, while the other parameters remained constant. The highest grafting yield was obtained under the following reaction conditions: $c_i = 0.08$ mol/L, $c_m = 0.8$ mol/L, $c_p = 8$ g/L, $t_r = 4$ h and T = 50 °C. The kinetics of the graft copolymerization of *N*-vinylimidazole onto gellan was discussed and a suitable reaction mechanism was proposed. The evidence of the grafting reaction was confirmed through FTIR spectroscopy, X-ray diffraction, ^{1}H-NMR spectroscopy and scanning electron microscopy. The grafted copolymer with betaine structure was obtained by a nucleophilic substitution reaction where the betainization agent was sodium chloroacetate. Preliminary results prove the ability of the grafted copolymers to bind amphoteric drugs (cefotaxime) and, therefore, the possibility of developing the new sustained drug release systems.

Keywords: graft polymerization; *N*-vinylimidazole; gellan gum; betaine structure

---

1. Introduction

In recent years, the chemical modification of natural polymers, polysaccharides in particular, by graft polymerization or by introduction of some functional groups, represents one of the most accesible and attractive method to obtain the polymeric materials with desired properties [1].

Since 1978, when gellan gum (GLL) was isolated for the first time from *Pseudomonas elodea*, this microbial polysaccharide has been used in various applications, such as in food industry as a thickening agent [2] or in biomedical and pharmaceutical fields [3,4].

This polysaccharide can be chemically modified due to the presence of many hydroxyl groups that can act as possible sites for grafting reaction. In the literature, some studies were found regarding the grafting of different vinyl monomers onto gellan gum chains using various sources of initiator radicals such as persulfate, redox systems or microwave irradiations [5,6]. Acrylic and methacrylic monomers such as, acrylamide [7], methacrylamide [8], *N,N*-dimethylacrylamide [5] or 2-(dimethylamino)ethyl methacrylate [9] were grafted onto gellan backbone in order to obtain polymeric materials with applications in industry as adsorbents/flocculants or in pharmaceutical field as sustained/controlled drug delivery systems. Verma et al. [10] combined the properties of *N*-vinyl-2-pyrrolidone and gellan gum by a grafting reaction, obtaining a new product that can be used as a coating material, superadsorbent or flocculating agent in the mining industry.

Among the vinyl monomers, *N*-vinylimidazole (NVI) has gained much attention in past years because the grafted polymers containing the imidazole ring are biocompatible, biodegradable and show antibacterial activity [11–15]. They were successfully used in medical and pharmaceutical fields. Moreover, chemical modification of imidazole-based polymers opens a huge opportunity for the development of functional polymers with complex structures [16].

The term polymers carrying betaine units (PB), or polyzwitterions, refers to polymers containing both negative (carboxylate group, sulfonate group or phosphonate/phosphate/phosphinate group) and positive (*onium* group without hydrogen atoms) charges located in the same repeat unit and separated by an alkylene group [17–20].

The grafted polymer carrying betaine units (PGB) can be obtained by one step and multistep processes [21,22].

One step process can be achieved by grafting monomers with a betaine structure onto the polymer backbone, while the multistep process consists of grafting monomers containing both nitrogen and vinyl group followed by polymer-analogous reactions onto grafted polymers in the presence of betainization agents.

The commercial interest for these polymers is determined by their possibility to be used as polymeric sorbents, oil recovery agents, fungicides, flame retardant polymers, emulsifying agents, wetting agents, cleaning agents and cryoprotectants [23–25]. Polymers having various betaine structure were synthesized in order to obtain materials sensitive to different stimuli (pH, temperature, etc.) [26].

The most interesting properties of PB are bio and hemocompatibility. Various studies have shown that polymer coatings based on poly(phosphobetaine) can improve the biocompatibility of some ocular devices by decreasing the adhesion of some microorganisms and eukaryotic cells [27,28]. Poly (methyl methacrylate) discs coated with a layer of sulfobetainic copolymer were exposed to *Staphylococcus epidermidis*, *Staphylococcus aureus* and *Pseudomonas aeruginosa* and it was found that the number of bacteria adhering to the surface of the discs coated with a layer of polybetaine decreased compared to the uncovered discs [29].

Due to the presence of vinyl groups capable of grafting polymerization and tertiary nitrogen suitable for the polymer-analogous reactions, the *N*-vinylimidazole is a very good candidate to obtain polymers carrying betaine units [30,31].

In this context, the work described in this paper follows several aspects: (1) synthesis of new grafted copolymers starting from gellan gum and *N*-vinylimidazole (PG); (2) finding the optimal conditions of the grafting reaction; (3) evidence of the grafting reaction by different methods; (4) chemical modification of new grafted copolymers containing an imidazole ring with the highest grafting yield by polymer analogous reactions in order to obtain the grafted copolymer with a betaine structure (PGB1); (5) immobilization and drug release studies of an antibiotic drug.

2. Results and Discussion

The preparation of grafted copolymers with betaine structure took place in two steps.

1. Preparation of PG and finding the optimal conditions for obtaining the grafted copolymer with maximum grafting yield.
2. Betainization reaction of PG with the highest grafting yield in the presence of sodium chloroacetate (Figure 1).

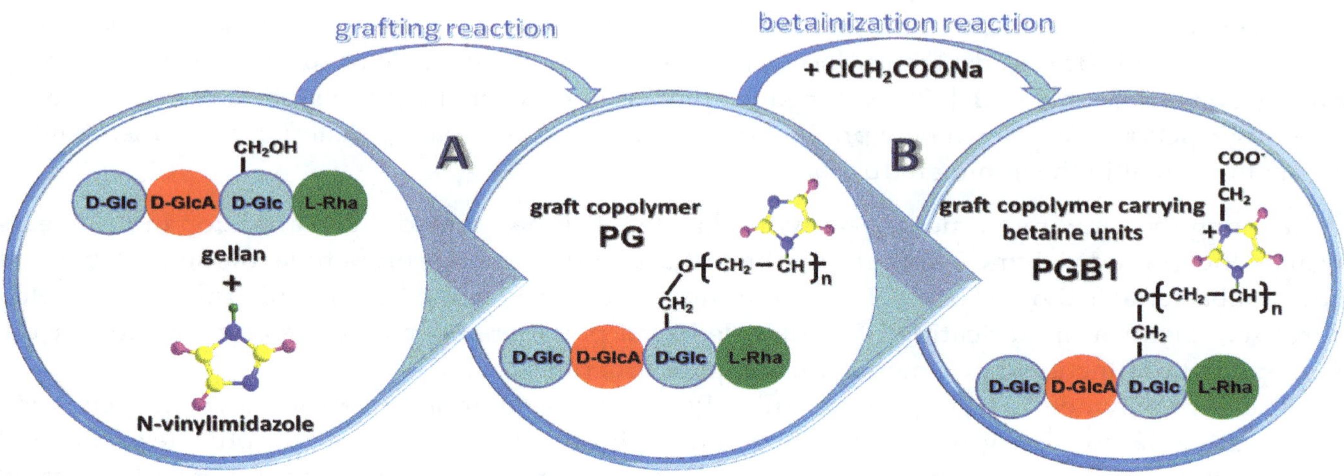

Figure 1. Graphical representation of the synthesis pathway of PG and grafted polymer carrying betaine units (PGB1) copolymers.

2.1. Optimal Conditions for the Preparation of PG

Various parameters such as monomer, initiator and polymer concentration, temperature and reaction time were investigated in order to optimize the reaction conditions in graft copolymerization of NVI onto gellan gum, as well as to improve the copolymer yield. Optimal reaction conditions were found by modifying one of the above-mentioned reaction parameters keeping the others constant, the reaction taking place under vigorous stirring and under a N_2 atmosphere.

2.1.1. Influence of Initiator Concentration

In the initiation stage, the rate of grafting can be influenced by a number of factors such as the nature and the concentration of the initiator, as well as the solubility of the initiator in the reaction medium. Among the thermal initiators, ammonium persulfate (APS) is preferred due to its high solubilization in water. In this study a redox initiator APS and *N,N,N′,N′* tetramethylethylenediamine (TEMED) (molar ratio 1:1) was used, and the influence of the initiator concentration on the grafting parameters was performed by modifying the APS/TEMED concentration in the range of 0.02–0.1 mol/L, keeping the monomer and gellan concentrations (c_m = 0.5 mol/L; c_p = 10 g/L), temperature (T = 60 °C) and reaction time (t = 4 h) constant. The graphical representation of grafting parameters versus initiator concentration is presented in Figure 2a.

As can be seen from Figure 2a grafting parameters like grafting yield (GY, %), grafting efficiency (GE, %) and conversion (C, %) increase with initiator concentration, reaching the maximal value at 0.08 mol/L APS/TEMED. After that, a slight decrease of grafting parameters is observed. This behavior could be explained in the following manner: at the beginning of the initiation reaction, the number of active sites on the gellan chain increases with the increase of initiator concentration, leading both to the formation of gellan macroradicals as well as the initiation of the grafting reaction. Then, at an initiator concentration greater than 0.08 mol/L, a decrease of grafting parameter values is observed probably because of an increase in the rate of homopolymerization compared to the grafting rate, this observation being proven by the increase in the value of homopolymer yield (H%). Another explanation of the decrease of grafting parameters can be attributed to a competition between initiation and termination reactions, the latter being achieved through chain-transfer to initiator or by a coupling reaction between initiator radicals [32]. The same behaviors were observed in the case of graft copolymerization of *N*-vinylimidazole onto various polysaccharides: xanthan [14], hyaluronic acid [11] and carboxymethyl starch [32].

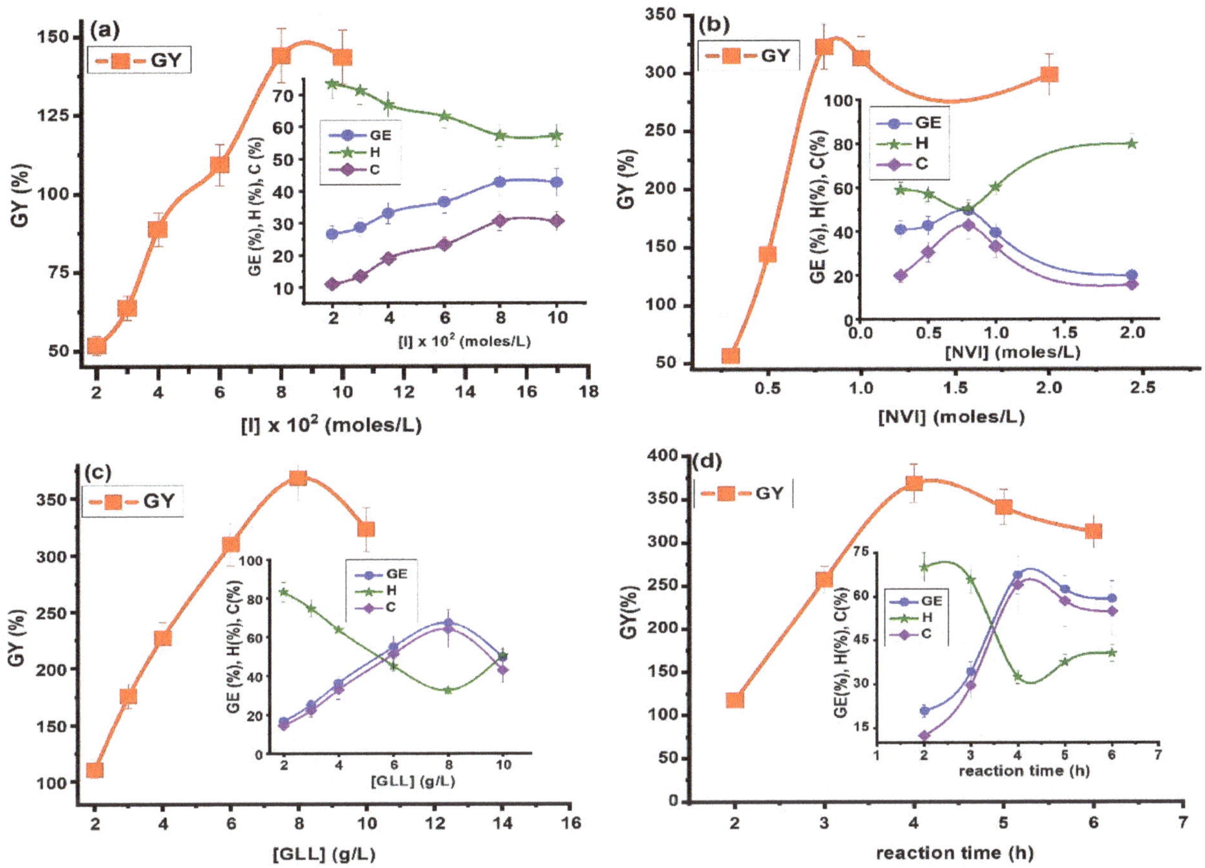

Figure 2. Influence of various factors on grafting parameters: (**a**) initiator concentration (c_m = 0.5 mol/L; c_p = 10 g/L, T = 60 °C and t = 4 h); (**b**) monomer concentration (c_i = 0.08 mol/L, c_p = 10 g/L, T = 60 °C and t_r = 4 h); (**c**) gellan concentration (c_i = 0.08 mol/L; c_m = 0.8 mol/L; T = 60 °C and t_r = 4 h); (**d**) reaction time (c_i = 0.08 mol/L; c_m = 0.8 mol/L; c_p = 8 g/L; T = 60 °C).

2.1.2. Influence of Monomer Concentration

Regarding the influence of the monomer concentration on the grafting yield, there are several factors that must be taken into account: monomer reactivity, polarity, steric hindrance, stability of the monomer radicals and concentration of monomer. In this study, the monomer concentration was varied within the range 0.3–2 mol/L, keeping the other parameters constant: c_i = 0.08 mol/L, c_p = 10 g/L, T = 60 °C and t_r = 4 h. The influence of NVI concentration on the grafting reaction is illustrated in Figure 2b. The results revealed an increase of GY%, GE% and C% with increasing NVI concentration up to 0.8 mol/L due to the greater availability of NVI molecules in the immediate vicinity of active sites located on the gellan chain, leading both to chain initiation and the formation of free radical donor that participate in the propagation reaction.

Thereafter, an increase in the monomer concentration above 0.8 mol/L caused a decrease of grafting parameter values, an exception being observed for the H% values that were found to increase. This behavior can be explained on the one hand by degradative chain-transfer to NVI as proposed in literature by Bamford and Schofield [33], and on the other hand by the poor diffusion of the monomer to the active sites situated on the polysaccharide chains leading to the homopolymer formation. A similar trend was reported in the literature for grafting of various vinyl monomers onto polysaccharides [11,32].

2.1.3. Influence of Gellan Concentration

The influence of polysaccharide concentration on grafting parameters is shown in Figure 2c. The gellan concentration was modified in the range 2–10 g/L, keeping constant the other parameters: $c_i = 0.08$ mol/L; $c_m = 0.8$ mol/L; T = 60 °C and $t_r = 4$ h. As can be seen from Figure 2c the grafting parameters (GY%, GE% and C%) increased with increasing of gellan concentration until 8 g/L and then a decrease of these parameters was observed. The increase of the grafting parameters until $c_p = 8$ g/L could be attributed to the increased number of grafting active centers situated on the polysaccharide chains leading to the formation of graft copolymers. An increase of polymer concentration above 8 g/L determines the increase of the viscosity of the reaction medium which hinders the possibility of e NVI movement toward the active sites situated on the gellan chains. The same behavior was observed in case of grafting on *N,N*-dimethylacrylamide onto gellan gum [5].

2.1.4. Influence of Reaction Time

The influence of reaction time on the grafting parameters is presented in Figure 2d and was determined by changing the time period of grafting reaction from 2 h to 6 h, keeping all the other reaction parameters constant ($c_i = 0.08$ mol/L; $c_m = 0.8$ mol/L; $c_p = 8$ g/L; T = 60 °C).

The obtained results revealed that the values of grafting parameters (GY%, GE% and C%) increased with increasing reaction time up to 4 h, due to the increase of active sites number situated on the gellan chains. After that, an increase in reaction time led to a slow decrease of the values of the grafting parameters. However, there was a slight increase in the homopolymer yield, suggesting the preference of the monomer to its own macroradical than for the one on the grafted chain, probably due to some steric hindrances. The same behavior was observed by other investigators whose results have been published in the literature [34,35].

2.1.5. Influence of Temperature

Temperature is one of the most important factors that influence the kinetics of graft copolymerization. The effect of temperature on the grafting parameters is shown in Figure 3a.

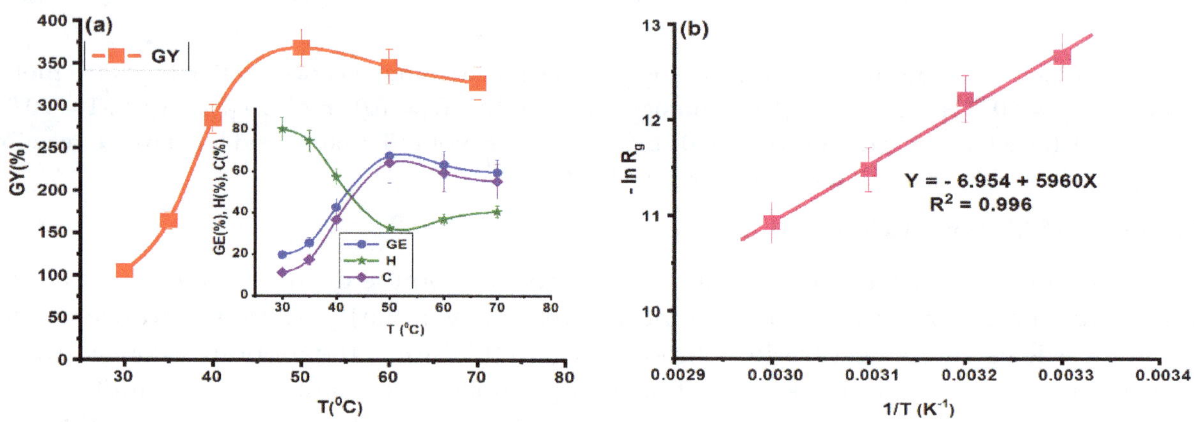

Figure 3. Influence of temperature on grafting of *N*-vinylimidazole (NVI) onto gellan gum (**a**) (c_i = 0.08 mol/L; $c_m = 0.8$ mol/L; $c_p = 8$ g/L and $t_r = 4$ h) and (**b**) the activation energy of the grafting reaction.

Temperature was varied from 30 to 80 °C, keeping constant $c_i = 0.08$ mol/L; $c_m = 0.8$ mol/L; $c_p = 8$ g/L and $t_r = 4$ h. As can be observed from Figure 3a the optimal temperature for maximum grafting yield was 50 °C and increasing temperature led to enhancement of the grafting parameters. The increase of grafting parameters until 50 °C can be attributed to:

(1) an increase in the production of free radicals resulting from thermal decomposition of initiator leading to increase in the number of the active sites on the polysaccharide chains;
(2) a decrease of reaction medium viscosity;

(3) fast diffusion of the monomer toward the active sites from the polysaccharide backbone;
(4) increase in rate of initiation and propagation steps [13,36].

Above 50 °C, the values of the grafting parameters decreased, probably due to the increase of the rate of the termination step by a combination of the monomer radicals and formation of the homopolymer. The effect may also have been due to the slower diffusion of the monomer to growing grafts due to steric hindrances, and its preference for growing homopolymer macroradicals.

The activation energy is another important parameter that can give information about the grafting process and can be determined from Arrhenius equation, as follows:

$$k = A \cdot e^{-E_a/RT} \tag{1}$$

where k is the rate constant, A is the pre-exponential factor, R is the gas constant (8.314 $J \cdot K^{-1} \cdot mol^{-1}$) and T is the absolute temperature (K).

The general rate equation of the grafting reaction can be written:

$$R_g = A \cdot [I]^a \cdot [M]^b \cdot [P]^c \cdot e^{-E_a/RT} \tag{2}$$

$$\ln R_g = \ln k' - \frac{E_a}{RT} \tag{3}$$

$$k' = A \cdot [I]^a \cdot [M]^b \cdot [P]^c \tag{4}$$

where $[I]$ = initiator concentration; $[M]$ = monomer concentration; $[P]$ = polymer concentration; a, b, and c—reaction order with respect to initiator, monomer and polymer.

The slope ($-E_a/RT$) of the ln R_g plots versus $1/T$ is used to find the E_a value (Figure 3b). The activation energy for PG was 49.5 KJ/mol. Similar results were observed in the case of grafting of various vinyl monomers (acrylamide, acrylic acid and methyl methacrylate) onto starch [37].

From the above studies it can be said that the optimized reaction conditions for grafting reaction of *N*-vinylimidazole onto gellan gum are as follows: initiator concentration = 0.08 mol/L; monomer concentration = 0.8 mol/L; polymer concentration = 8 g/L, reaction temperature = 50 °C and reaction time = 4 h.

2.2. Kinetics and Mechanism of graft Copolymerization

Generally, the rate equation of radical polymerization reaction is:

$$R_g = k \cdot [I]^{1/2} \cdot [M] \cdot [P]^{1/2} \tag{5}$$

The rate of graft copolymerization depends on several parameters such as initiator, monomer and polymer concentrations. In this study the graft copolymerization of *NVI* onto gellan was studied by modifying one of the parameters while the other parameters remained constant. In this context, the rate equations are:

$$\ln R_g = \ln k_1 + a \cdot \ln[I],\ k_1 = K \cdot [M]^b \cdot [P]^c \tag{6}$$

$$\ln R_g = \ln k_2 + b \cdot \ln[M],\ k_2 = K \cdot [I]^a \cdot [P]^c \tag{7}$$

$$\ln R_g = \ln k_3 + c \cdot \ln[P],\ k_3 = K \cdot [I]^a \cdot [M]^b \tag{8}$$

The graphical representations of ln R_g versus ln $[I]$, ln $[M]$ and ln $[P]$, respectively represent a straight line and are shown in Figure 4.

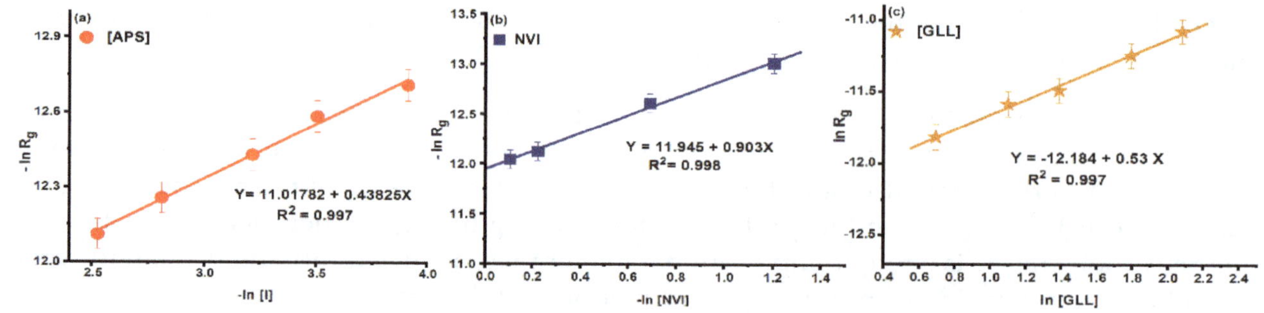

Figure 4. Plotting ln R_g versus (**a**) ln $[I]$; (**b**) ln $[NVI]$; and (**c**) ln $[GLL]$.

From Figure 4 the values of the slopes of the plots suggest that the reaction order with respect to initiator, monomer and polymer are 0.44, 0.90 and 0.53, respectively. Thus, the rate equation of grafting reaction of *N*-vinylimidazole onto gellan gum is:

$$R_g = k{\cdot}[APS/TEMED]^{0.44}{\cdot}[NVI]^{0.903}{\cdot}[GLL]^{0.53} \tag{9}$$

Equation (13) is very similar to Equation (9) and, for this reason, the mechanism of the grafting reaction of NVI onto gellan involves the same elementary reactions encountered in the free radical polymerization, namely, initiation, chain growth or chain propagation, chain transfer and termination of polymer chains [38].

The first step of the radical polymerization reaction corresponds to the formation of active species (radicals) followed by their addition to the monomer molecule (Figure 5).

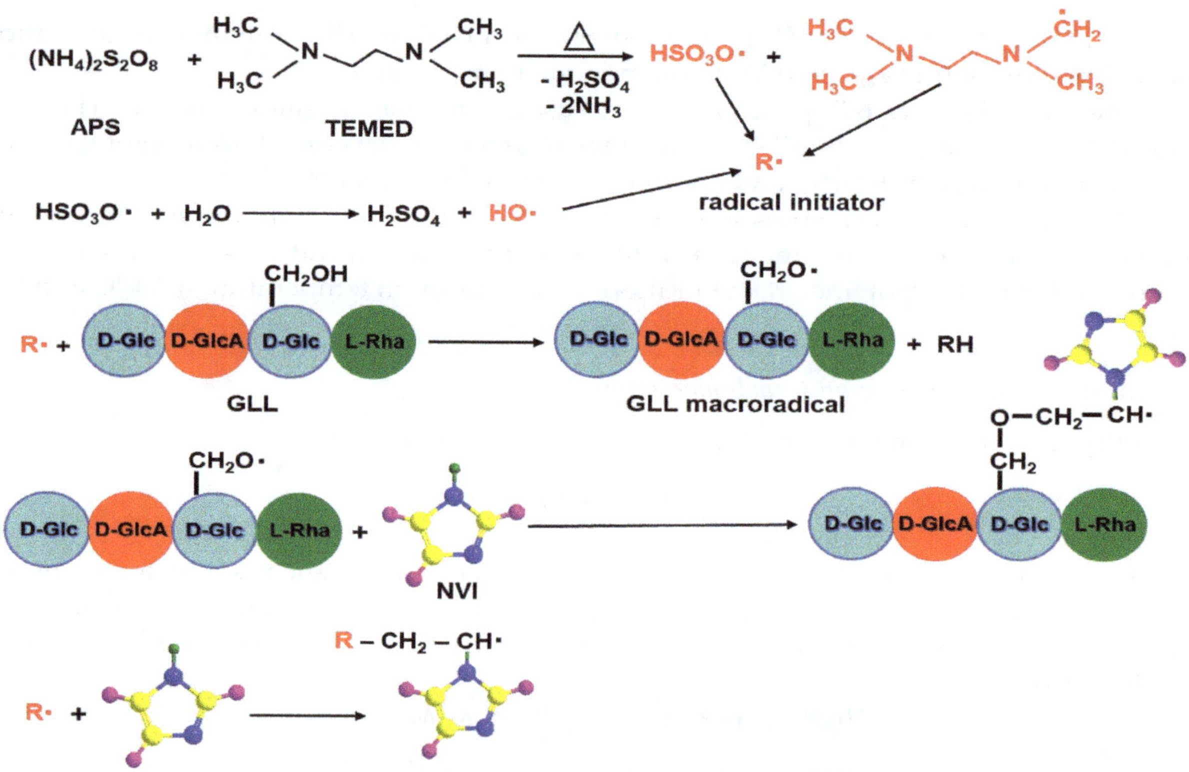

Figure 5. Initiation step of grafting copolymerization.

When the initiation system is heated, it decomposes in radical species that are able to initiate the polymerization reaction. In the case of the APS and TEMED system, two types of radicals (alkylaminoethyl radical derived from TEMED and sulfate radical from APS) [39] are formed and are able to initiate the graft copolymerization of *N*-vinylimidazole onto the gellan backbone. The propagation step consists of successive addition of a large number of monomer molecule to the promoter generated in the initial step (Figure 6).

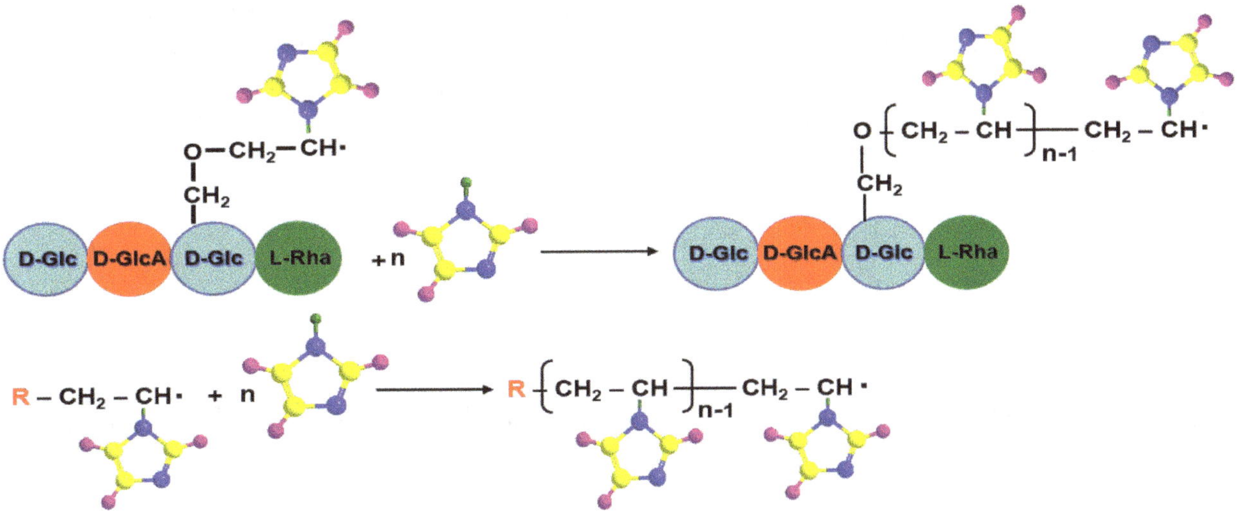

Figure 6. Propagation step of grafting copolymerization.

The termination reactions depend on the size, activity and structure of the macroradical, the viscosity of the medium, the temperature and the composition of the reaction mixture (Figure 7). Depending on these factors, the mechanism of the termination reaction is different and occurs as follows: (a) reaction with the initiator; (b) coupling/combination and disproportionation reaction; (c) inactivation of the growth radicals by inhibitors.

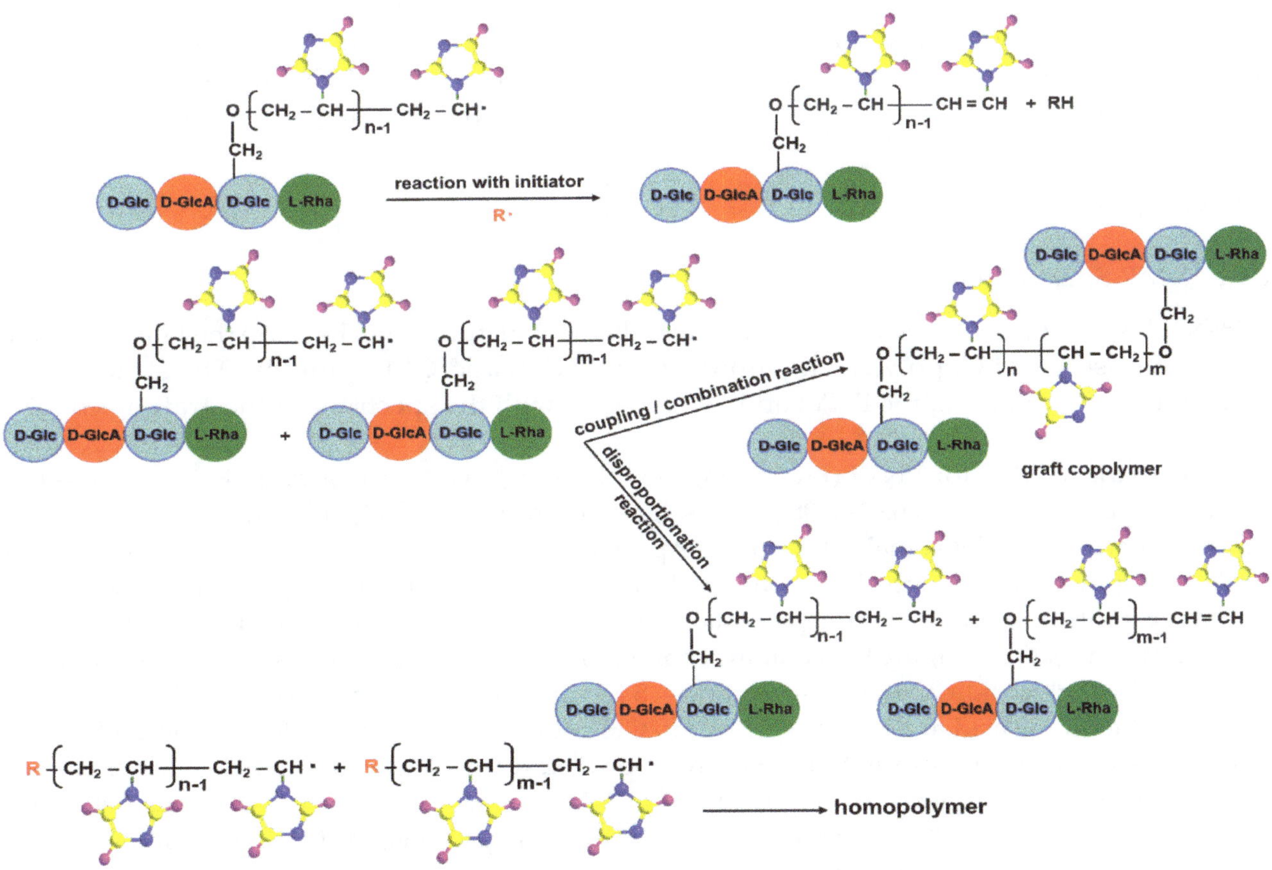

Figure 7. Termination steps of graft copolymerization.

2.3. Synthesis of Copolymer Carrying Betaine Structure

The second stage for preparation of grafted copolymer carrying structural units of 1-vinyl-3(1-carboxymethyl) imidazolium betaine consists in polymer-analogous reactions on grafted copolymer with the highest grafting yield in the presence of sodium chloroacetate as a betainization agent. From the reaction mechanism point of view, the grafted betaine copolymer with one methylene group between the opposite charges is achieved by the nucleophilic substitution reaction. The chemical structure of PGB1 is presented in Figure 8.

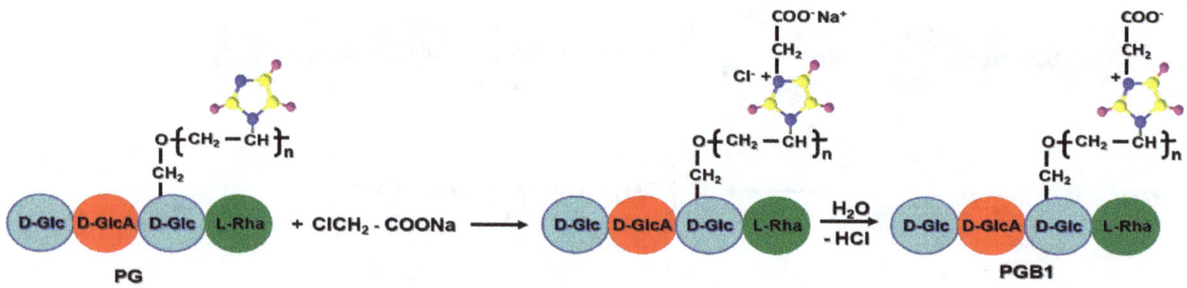

Figure 8. Betainization reaction of PG copolymer with sodium chloroacetate.

Different reaction parameters (temperature, reaction time, concentration of betainization agent) were modified in order to find the optimal value of betainization degree. It was found that the increase of all parameters mentioned above, up to a certain value, led to an increase of betainization degree. The optimal conditions for synthesis of graft copolymers carrying betaine structure was found to be: concentration of betainization degree = 20%, T = 60 °C and the reaction time = 72 h.

The degree of betainization was obtained by FTIR spectroscopy using the relative ratio between integrated area of betainized (1637 cm^{-1}) and chemically unmodified imidazole ring (1500 cm^{-1}). The curve fitting of the FTIR spectrum of PGB1 in the region 1700–1420 cm^{-1} was realized using OPUS Software on the basis of a linear regression Levenberg-Marquardt model, the method being similar to that mentioned in our previous paper [40]. In this case, the betainization degree was found to be 89.97%.

2.4. Characterization of PG and PGB1

2.4.1. ^{1}H-NMR Spectroscopy

^{1}H-NMR spectroscopy was used to elucidate only the structure of PG because the PGB1 is insoluble in the solvent used for PG, poly(*N*-vinylimidazole) (PNVI) and GLL samples. The structure of PG was elucidated by comparing the PNVI and GLL spectra with the spectrum of the grafting copolymer (Figure 9).

It is well known that for PNVI (Figure 9b) the following characteristic signals can be observed:

(1) multiplet signals at δ = 6.61–7.08 ppm assigned to the protons (H_2, H_4 and H_5) belonging to the imidazole ring; (2) multiplet signals at δ = 3.7–3.9 ppm due to the methine protons; (3) doublet signal at δ = 2.07–2.13 ppm assigned to the backbone methylene protons; (4) triplet signal at δ = 2.58–2.87 ppm related to the splitting chain -CH group (isotactic, heterotactic and syndiotactic triads) [41].

The spectrum of GLL (Figure 9a) contains characteristic peaks of the tetrasaccharide repeating units as follows: -CH of glycosidic bonds in sugar at δ = 5.83 ppm; -CH of rhamnose at δ = 5.15 ppm; -CH of glucose and glucuronic acid at δ = 3.36–4.61 ppm; -CH_3 of rhamnose at δ = 1.29–1.31 ppm [42,43].

The ^{1}H-NMR spectrum presented in Figure 9c proved the synthesis of the PG copolymer because in this spectrum the characteristic signals of both PNVI (δ = 6.72–7.13 ppm—protons belonging to the imidazole ring; δ = 2.14–2.35 ppm—backbone methylene protons) and GLL (δ = 3.37–4.61 ppm—protons of the tetrasaccharide repeating units; δ = 1.29–1.31—CH_3 of rhamnose) polymers are found.

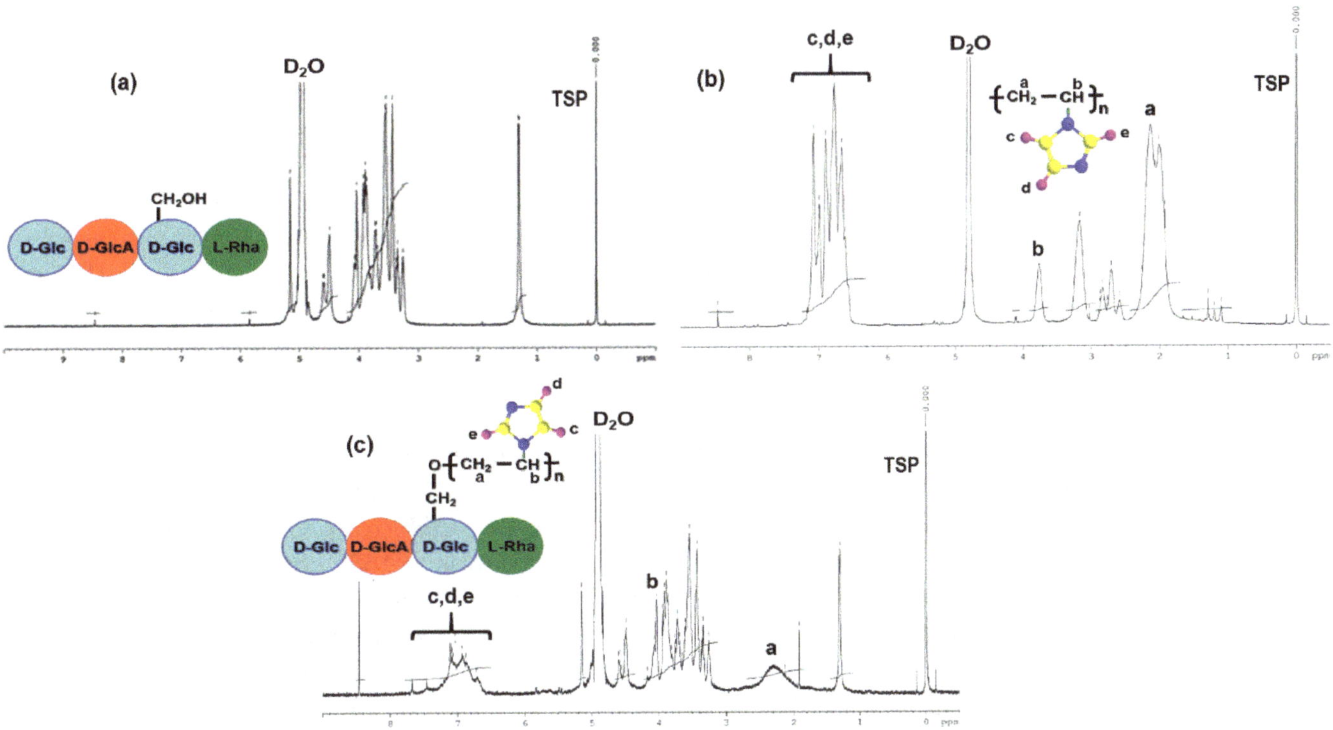

Figure 9. ^{1}H-NMR spectra of GLL (**a**); PNVI (**b**) and PG samples (**c**).

2.4.2. FTIR Spectroscopy

The infrared spectra of PNVI, GLL PG and PGB1 samples are presented in Figure 10.

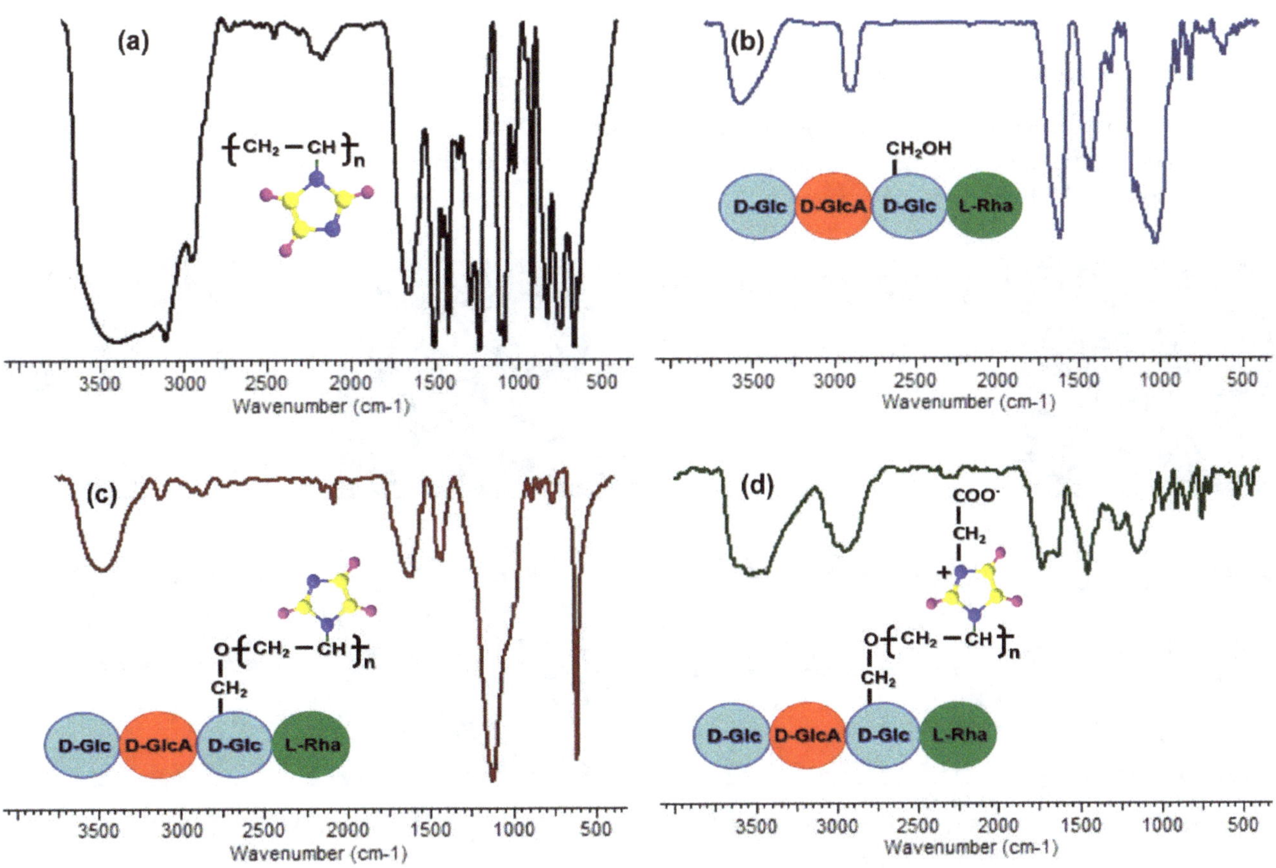

Figure 10. The infrared spectra of PNVI (**a**); GLL (**b**); PG (**c**) and PGB1 samples (**d**).

The infrared spectrum analysis of gellan gum (Figure 10b) showed the following adsorption bands: 3566 cm^{-1} attributed to the O-H stretching of hydroxyl groups of glucopyranose ring; 2892 cm^{-1} characteristic of the aliphatic-CH; 1611 and 1420 cm^{-1} assigned to the asymmetric and symmetric vibrations of the carboxylate group and 1027 cm^{-1} attributed to the C-O-C bonds.

In the PNVI spectrum (Figure 10a) the following characteristic absorption bands are observed: 3100 cm^{-1} assigned to C-H stretching vibration; 2957 cm^{-1} attributed to the C-H and CH_2 stretching vibrations of the backbone chain. A strong and broad band is observed at 1655 cm^{-1} that is characteristic of the C=C ring stretching vibrations. The bands observed at 1500, 1285, 1230, 1083 and 914 cm^{-1} are assigned to C-C, C=N ring stretching vibrations, C-H bending vibration, the ring C-H bending and C-C-C bending vibration of the backbone of the aliphatic chain. Two characteristic bands for the imidazole ring were observed at 1500 and 665 cm^{-1}, the last being attributed to the puckering vibration of imidazole ring [41].

In the FT-IR spectrum of the PG copolymer (Figure 10c) a shifting of -OH stretching vibration from about 3400 cm^{-1} (3392 cm^{-1} for PNVI and 3415 cm^{-1} for GLL) to 3479 cm^{-1} is observed, as well as a decrease of intensity of the absorption bands corresponding to the -OH group vibration, indicating the participation of hydroxyl groups in the grafting reaction. The bands at 1630 cm^{-1} (>C=C< stretching vibrations in imidazole ring), 1545 cm^{-1} (>C=N$^-$ stretching vibration) and 1124 cm^{-1} (in-plane bending vibration of the C-H bond inside imidazole ring) indicate the presence of PNVI in the structure of the grafted copolymer, and also the confirmation of grafting of the vinyl monomer onto the gellan backbone.

If the FT-IR spectra of PG and PGB1 copolymers are compared (Figure 10d) the appearance of new absorption bands specific to the betaine structure can be observed as follows: the band at 3439 cm^{-1} appears due to the >C=N$^+$ group, and the shift of the adsorption band from 1630 cm^{-1} to 1637 cm^{-1} is due to the overlap the vibration band of >C=N$^-$ group from PNVI with the absorption band corresponding to the asymmetric COO$^-$ group. The absorption bands at 1340 and 1266 cm^{-1} may be attributed to the stretching vibration of carboxylate group.

2.4.3. Surface Morphology Analysis

Surface morphology images at high magnification (2000×) of PNVI, GLL, PG and PGB1 samples were analyzed using a scanning electron microscope coupled with an energy dispersive X-ray system and are presented in Figure 11.

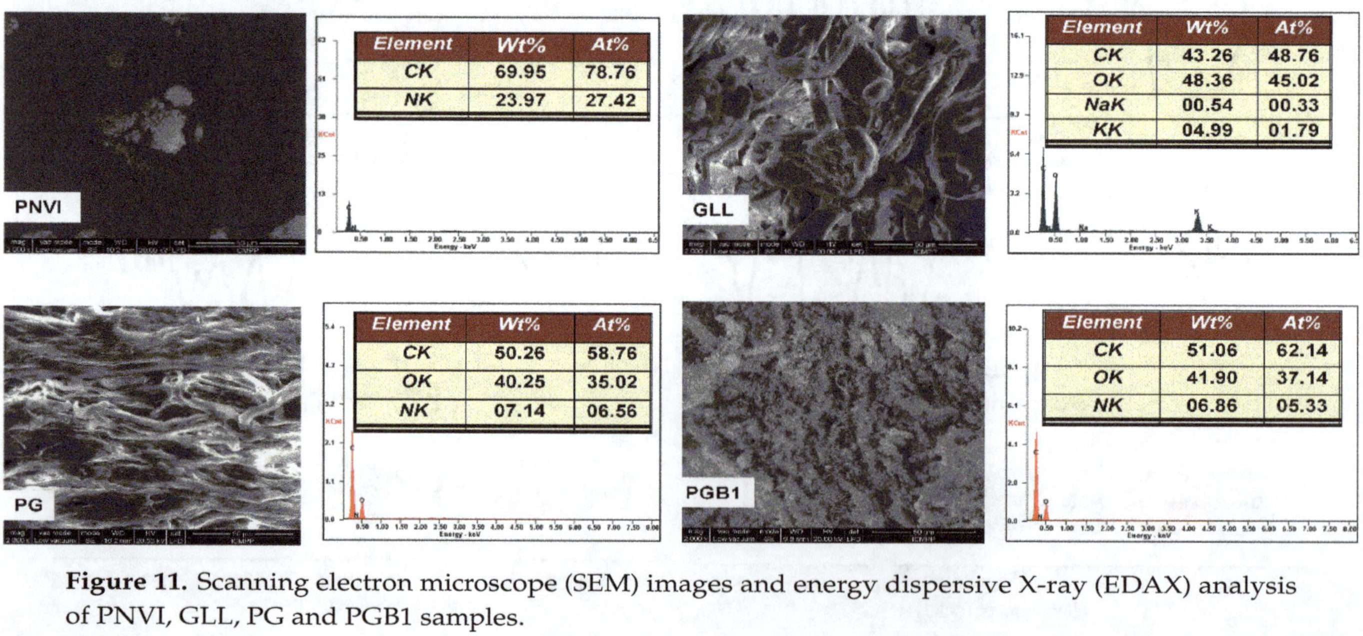

Figure 11. Scanning electron microscope (SEM) images and energy dispersive X-ray (EDAX) analysis of PNVI, GLL, PG and PGB1 samples.

The PNVI sample showed a compact porous structure while GLL and PG samples seemed to have a fibrous structure. When NVI was grafted onto the GLL backbone, microstructural changes were observed, the PG copolymer having a more ordered structure compared to that of the gellan. The reaction between PG copolymer and sodium chloroacetate led to the preparation of the grafting copolymer with betaine structure having a porous structure.

The EDAX analysis confirmed both grafting of *N*-vinylimidazole onto gellan gum and the formation of graft copolymer carrying betaine units as follows:

(1) the presence of nitrogen belonging only to NVI on the surface of PG and PGB1 copolymers;
(2) increase of C% value of the PG molecule compared to that from GLL indicating the presence of PNVI in the PG structure;
(3) increase of C% and O% values, as well as the decrease of N% values, of the PGB1 copolymer compared those from the PG copolymer due to the formation of betaine units.

2.4.4. X-Ray Diffractions Analysis (XRD)

XRD patterns of GLL, PNVI, PG and PGB1 samples are illustrated in Figure 12.

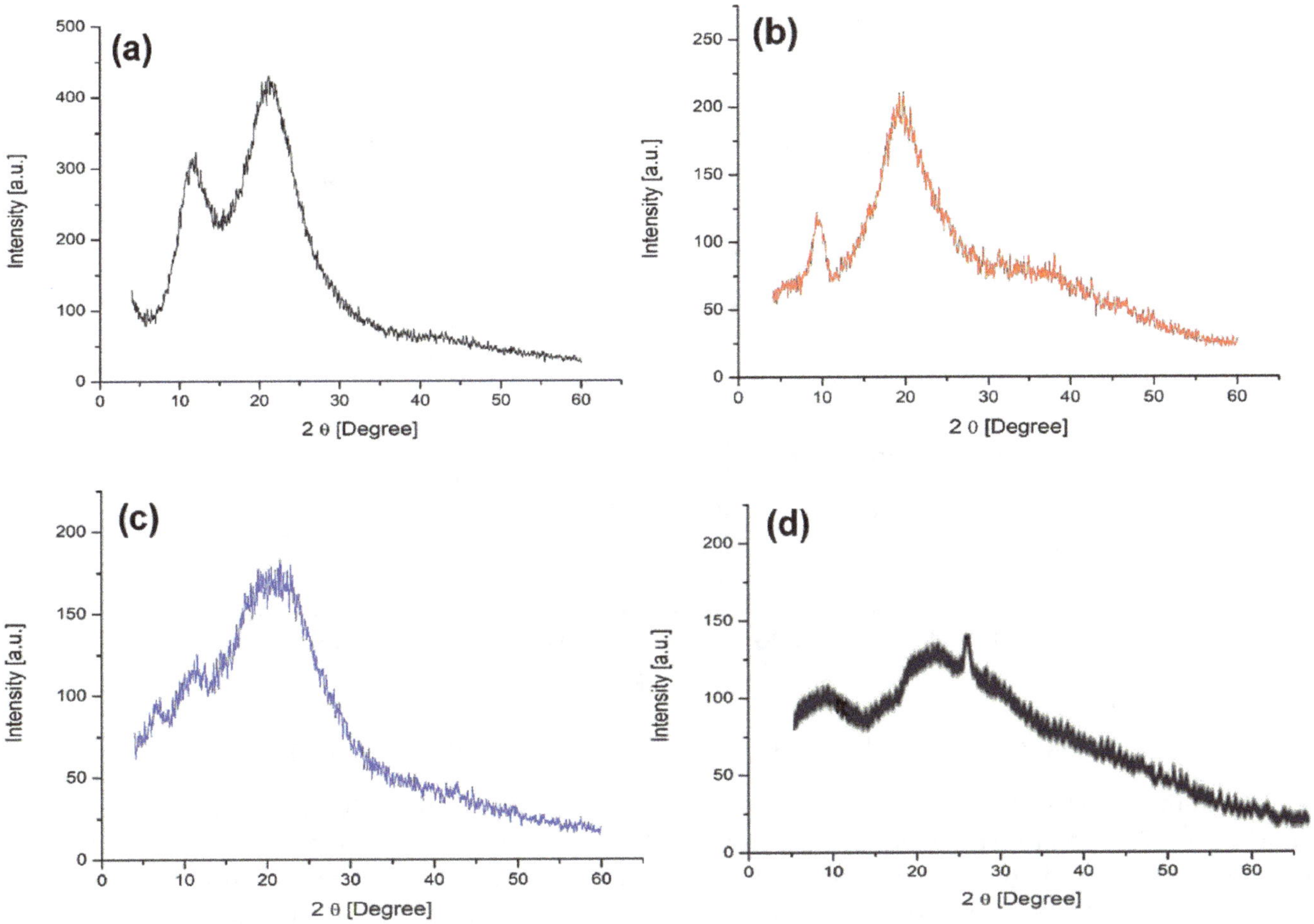

Figure 12. XRD patterns of PNVI (**a**); GLL (**b**); PG (**c**) and PGB1 samples (**d**).

X-ray diffraction spectra of PNVI and GLL show two broad diffraction peaks at lower diffraction angle values (2θ = 20° and 10°) indicating the amorphous structure of both polymers. The XRD pattern of PG copolymer presents the combined signals of started polymers leading to the conclusion that the grafting of PNVI onto gellan gum was successfully completed. The PGB1 copolymers presented an amorphous structure.

2.4.5. Thermogravimetric Studies

Thermogravimetric studies were realized to prove the preparation of both grafted copolymers and grafted copolymers carrying betaine units. The thermal stability of PNVI, GLL, PG and PGB1 samples was discussed according to the temperature at which intensive degradation took place and the results are presented in Table 1.

Table 1. Thermogravimetric analysis data for main stage of decomposition.

Sample Codes	Decomposition Temperature			Weight Loss (%)	Residual Mass (%)
	T_i (°C)	T_m (°C)	T_f (°C)		
PNVI	406	433	519	47.3	3.9
GLL	241	250	322	45.0	16.1
PG	429	454	548	15.9	53.3
PGB1	256	278	410	40.9	31.2

Thermogravimetric (TG) and derivative thermogravimetric (DTG) curves of PNVI, GLL, PG and PGB1 samples (Figure 13) showed that thermal degradation was characterized by four (PNVI), three (GLL), five (PG) and three (PGB1) stages of degradation.

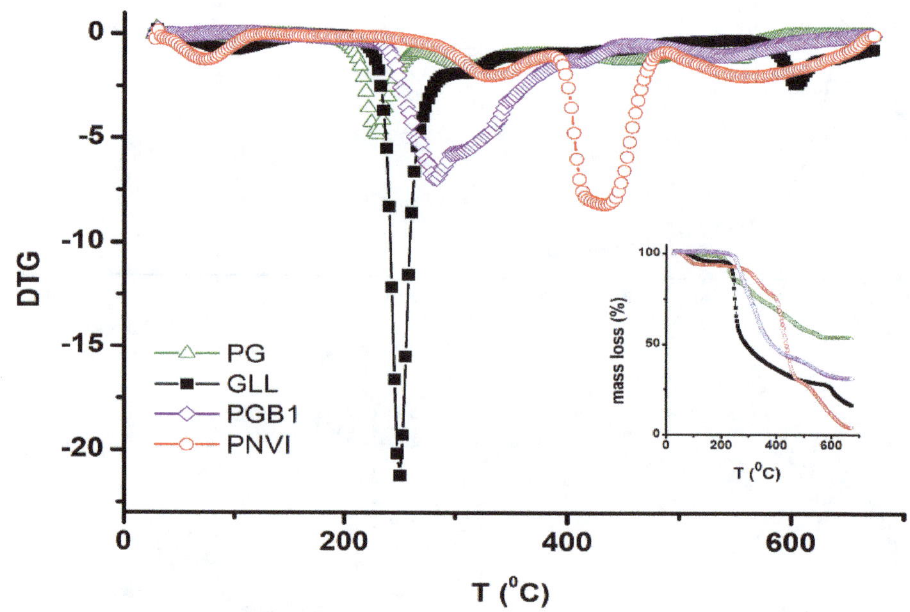

Figure 13. TG and DTG curves of PNVI, GLL, PG and PGB1 samples.

The main stages of degradation for PNVI and gellan occurred in the temperature ranges 406–519 °C and 241–322 °C, respectively being characterized by an important weight loss of 47.30% and 44.96%, probably due to the degradation of the polymer backbone. The degradation results of PG showed that the grafting of NVI onto gellan gum increased the thermal stability of the copolymer, the main stage of decomposition occurring in the range 429–548 °C with a weight loss of 15.85%. This behavior can be explained by the presence of an imidazole ring belonging to PNVI which is thermally stable. The same observations were reported by other authors for grafting of poly(*N*-vinylimidazole) onto carboxymethyl chitosan [32]. The introduction of betaine units led to decrease of thermal stability of PGB1, the main stage of decomposition taking place in the range 256–410 °C with a weight loss of 40.92%. After thermal treatment up to 700 °C the remaining residual masses were 3.92% (PNVI), 16.14% (GLL), 53.29% (PG) and 31.18% (PGB1), respectively. Taking into account the results previously presented, it can be said that the grafting reaction was realized and the grafting of NVI onto gellan gum led to an increase in thermal stability of the PG copolymers, whereas the introduction of betaine units induced a slight decrease in the thermal stability of PGB1 copolymers.

2.5. Immobilization and Drug Release

The synthesis of grafted copolymers with *N*-vinyl imidazole (PG), and subsequently functionalized with betaine structure (PGB1), was made in order to obtain precursors capable of binding amphoteric drugs through ionic interactions. Consequently, a preliminary study was performed on the immobilization; respectively the release of an amphoteric model drug (cefotaxime sodium salt) to verify our hypothesis. The ionic interaction of the drug is possible both with the copolymer PG, which contains carboxylic groups belonging to gellan, and especially with the copolymer PGB1, which contains carboxylic groups belonging to both the gellan and the betaine structure.

Cefotaxime sodium salt (CF) is a semisynthetic third generation cephalosporin with bactericidal activity, being more active against gram-negative bacteria than gram-positive bacteria [44].

Cefotaxime sodium salt was immobilized onto PG and PGB1 samples in a bach system. The maximum immobilization capacities of CF onto PG and PGB1 samples were found to be 420 mg/g and 473.2 mg/g, repectively. Obviously, the higher CF binding capacity was higher for the PGB1 copolymer which contains a higher number of carboxylic groups compared to the PG copolymer.

The release profiles of CF as a function of time are presented in Figure 14.

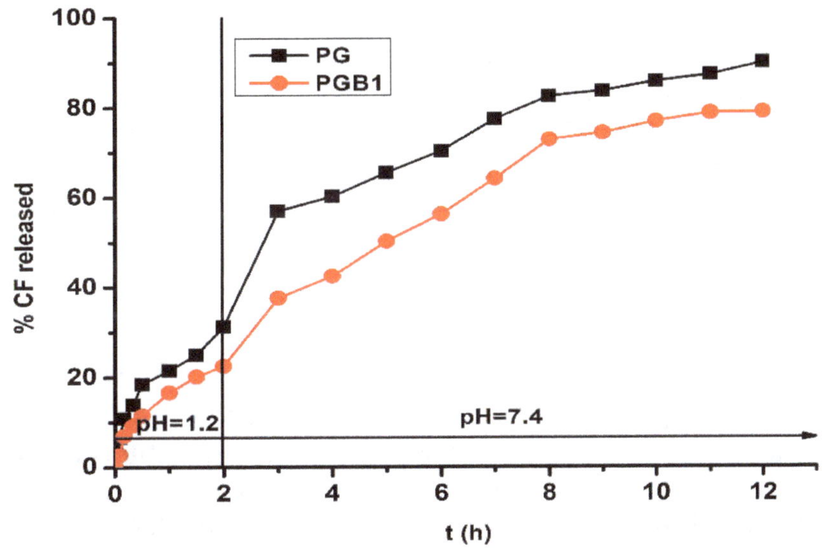

Figure 14. Release profile of cefotaxime sodium salt from PG and PGB1 samples.

From Figure 14, it can be observed that the amount of CF released from PG and PGB1 was higher at pH = 7.4 than pH = 1.2. In acidic pH values, the carboxylate groups of gellan became protonated, the repulsions between polymer chains being much diminished resulting in a decrease of swelling degree and finally in a decrease of the amount of drug released. At higher pH values, the carboxylate groups were ionized and the electrostatic repulsive forces between COO^- groups located on the copolymer backbone caused an increase of the swelling capacity leading to an increase of amount of drug released.

To analyze the type of release mechanism, the drug release data were fitted using two release kinetic models: the Higuchi and Korsmeyer-Peppas models.

The Higuchi model is based on the Fick's law and is used to describe the release of a water soluble drug from solid matrices [45]. The mathematical equation of Higuchi model is:

$$Q_t = k_H \cdot t^{\frac{1}{2}} \tag{10}$$

where k_H is Higuchi dissolution constant.

The Korsmeyer-Peppas model describes the mechanism of drug release from polymeric systems [46]:

$$\frac{M_t}{M_\infty} = k_r \cdot t^n \tag{11}$$

where Mt/M_∞ = fraction of drug released at time t; k_r = release rate constant that is characteristic to polymer-drug interactions; n = the diffusion exponent is characteristic to the different release mechanisms.

Depending on the values of n, the release can take place through several mechanisms such as: $n = 0.5$, Case I diffusion or Higuchi kinetic (diffusion/controlled drug release); $0.5 < n < 1$, anomalous diffusion; $n = 1$, Case II transport (swelling-controlled drug release); $n > 1$, super Case II transport.

The values of the release parameters of CF from PG and PGB1 are presented in Table 2.

Table 2. Kinetic parameters of CF release from PG and PGB1.

Sample Codes	Higuchi Model		Korsmeyer-Peppas Model		
	k_H ($h^{-1/2}$)	R^2	k_r (min^{-n})	n	R^2
PG	0.249	0.993	0.053	0.377	0.992
PGB1	0.236	0.990	0.023	0.550	0.991

Based on the release exponent n from the Korsmeyer-Peppas equation, the release mechanism of CF from the PG sample is controlled by a diffusion process while the release mechanism of CF from the PGB1 sample is more complex, being controlled by both swelling and diffusion processes.

The results presented in this study attest the ability of the two types of copolymers to bind amphoteric drugs through electrostatic interactions. An in-depth study on the immobilization of biologically active principles with cationic or anionic characteristics on grafted copolymers carrying betaine units is the subject of further work.

3. Materials and Methods

3.1. Materials

Gellan gum ($M_w = 1 \times 10^6$ g/mol), ammonium persulfate, *N,N,N′,N′*-tetramethylethylenediamine, acetone, ethanol, sodium chloroacetate, hydrochloric acid, potassium chloride, monobasic and dibasic sodium phosphate and cefotaxime sodium salt were supplied from Sigma-Aldrich, Germany and were used as received. *N*-vinylimidazole was purchased from Sigma Aldrich, Germany and was distilled under vacuum. Ultrapure grade water ($\Omega < 10^{-6}$ s/cm) was prepared by purifying deionized water with Millipore Simplicity-UV apparatus.

3.2. Synthesis of Grafted Polymers (PG)

The PG copolymers were prepared by using the free radical polymerization technique in presence of redox initiator (APS + TEMED) in nitrogen atmosphere.

60 mL of (2–10 g/L) gellan solution in ultrapure distilled water was added into a 250 mL three-necked round-bottom flask equipped with a magnetic stirrer and a thermostater water bath. To gellan solution various amounts of NVI (c_m = 0.3–2 mol/L) were added followed by the addition of different amounts of initiator solutions (c_i = 0.02–0.1 mol/L). The molar ratio between APS and TEMED was 1:1, which has been reported in literature to be the optimal value for obtaining free radicals as well as the polymer with highest grafting yield [47]. The grafting reactions were carried out at different reaction temperatures (30–80 °C) and at various periods of time (2–6 h). Finally, the grafting mixture was precipitated under vigourous stirring in cold acetone and then the grafted copolymers were separated by filtration under vacuum using borosilicate glass filter crucibles, porosity 4. Thereafter, the grafted copolymers were purified by extraction with ethanol in a Soxhlet apparatus in order to remove the homopolymer, and were dried in vacuum oven at 50 °C for 48 h.

3.3. Estimation of Grafting Parameters

The grafting parameters were calculated as follows [48,49].

$$GY\ (\%) = \frac{weight\ of\ grafted\ PNVI}{weight\ of\ gellan} \cdot 100 \tag{12}$$

$$GE\ (\%) = \frac{weight\ of\ grafted\ PNVI}{weight\ of\ polymer\ formed} \cdot 100 \tag{13}$$

$$C\ (\%) = \frac{weight\ of\ polymer\ formed}{weight\ of\ monomer\ fed} \cdot 100 \tag{14}$$

$$H\ (\%) = 100 - GE\ (\%) \tag{15}$$

3.4. Synthesis of Grafted Polymer Carrying Betaine Units

Grafted polymer carrying betaine units was prepared by the betainization reaction of PG with maximum grafting yield in the presence of sodium chloroacetate. Thus, 5 g of PG were swollen in water for 24 h at room temperature then centrifuged at 78 RCF for 10 min after which an aqueous solution of sodium chloroacetate (100 mL, c = 20%, *w*/*v*) was added. To calculate the amount of betainization agent required for the polymer-analogous reaction, the molar ratio between nitrogen and sodium chloroacetate was considered to be 1:1.5. The reaction mixture was gently stirred at T = 60 °C for 72 h. The final product was removed from the reaction medium by precipitation in acetone and then the precipitate was extracted with water in a Soxhlet apparatus. The final product was insoluble in water.

3.5. Infrared Spectroscopy

FTIR spectra were recorded on a Bruker Vertex 70 FTIR spectrometer (Wien, Austria) at a resolution of 2 cm^{-1} in the frequency range of 400–4000 cm^{-1}, by the KBr pellet technique (pellets obtained at a pressure of 2 tons for 1 min).

3.6. ^{1}H-NMR Analysis

^{1}H-NMR measurements of PNVI, gellan and PG were performed on a high-resolution liquid NMR 400 MHz spectrometer Bruker Neo-1 (Rheinsteitten, Germany) for direct detection probe, with 5 mm Quadra nuclei probes, QNP (four nuclei, $^1H/^{13}C/^{19}F/^{29}Si$). Sample solutions were prepared with deuterated water and 1N NaOH as solvent. TSP (trimethylsilylpropanoic acid) (δ = 0.0 ppm) was used as an internal standard. Detection temperature was set at 25 °C and the sample was scanned 64 times.

3.7. Scanning Electron Microscopy (SEM)

The surface morphologies of gellan, PNVI, PG and PGB1 in powder form were analyzed with an environmental scanning electron microscope type Quanta 200 at 25 kV with secondary electrons in low vacuum. The microscope was coupled with an energy dispersive X-ray system for qualitative and quantitative analysis.

3.8. X-Ray Diffraction Analysis (XRD)

The XRD patterns of PNVI, GLL, PG and PGB1 samples were recorded employing a D8 Advance Bruker AXS device using a CuKα radiation at a current/voltage of 36 mA/30 kV.

3.9. Thermogravimetric Analysis (TG/DTG)

The thermal stability of the crosslinked epoxy resins were thermogravimetrically analyzed using a STA 449 F1 Jupiter apparatus (Netzsch, Selb, Germany) coupled to a Vertex 70 spectrophotometer for FT-IR analysis and Aeölos QMS 403C mass spectrometer (Netzsch-Germany) for the mass spectroscopic analysis of the evolved gases. Samples of about 10 mg placed in Al_2O_3 crucibles were thermally degraded at a heating rate of 10 °C min^{-1}, under air atmosphere in the temperature range between 25 °C and 700 °C.

3.10. Immobilization and Drug Release

CF immobilization was realized as follows: 0.2 g of PG and PGB1 copolymers were weighed into 50 mL conical flasks and then 20 mL of CF ($c_{CF} = 3 \cdot 10^{-3}$ g/mL) were added. The samples were placed in a thermostatic shaker bath (Memmert MOO/M01, Schwabach, Germany) and shaken at 180 strokes/minute until equilibrium was reached. The flasks were removed from the shaker and the copolymers were centrifuged at 78 RCF for 10 min. The amount of CFR immobilized onto PG and PGB1 copolymers was determined by UV-VIS spectrophotometry (SPEKOL 1300 Spectrophotometer, Analytik Jena, Jena, Germany) at a wavelength of 236 nm, based on a calibration curve.

The amount of drug immobilized was obtained using the following equation:

$$q_e = \frac{(C_0 - C_e) \cdot V}{W} \quad (16)$$

where q_e is the amount of CF immobilized onto PG and PGB1 copolymers (mg/g), C_0 is the initial concentration of drug (mg/mL), C_e is the drug concentration at equilibrium (mg/mL), V is the volume of drug solution (mL) and W is the weight of the copolymers.

In vitro release studies of cefotaxime sodium salt were performed by immersing the PG and PGB1 samples (0.1 g) in 10 mL of simulated gastric fluid (pH = 1.2) for 2 h and phosphate buffer solution (pH = 7.4) for 10 h at 37 °C. The buffer solutions were prepared according to protocols well known in the literature [50,51]. The samples were placed in a thermostated shaker bath (Memmert M00/M01, Germany) under gentle shaking (50 strokes/minute). Withdrawal of a small volume (1 µL) of release solution was done and the CF solutions collected at different intervals of time were measured spectrophotometrically at a wavelength of 236 nm using a UN-VIS spectrophotometer (Nanodrop ND 100, Wilmington, DE, USA). The amount of CF released was calculated using a calibration curve.

4. Conclusions

Grafted polymers carrying betaine units were obtained by grafting *N*-vinylimidazole onto a gellan gum backbone followed by a betainization reaction of the grafted copolymer with maximum grafting yield in the presence of sodium chloroacetate. The grafted copolymers were successfully obtained by a free radical polymerization technique in the presence of redox initiator (APS + TEMED) and a nitrogen atmosphere. From the point of view of the reaction mechanism, the betainization reaction is a nucleophilic reaction and the betainization degree estimated by FTIR spectroscopy was found to be about 90%. The grafting parameter (GY%, GE%, H% and C%) could be adjusted by changing one of the reaction parameters. The optimized reaction conditions for the grafting reaction of NVI onto GLL were as follows: initiator concentration = 0.08 mol/L; monomer concentration = 0.8 mol/L; polymer concentration = 8 g/L; reaction temperature = 50 °C and the reaction time = 4 h. The mechanism of grafting reaction is similar with that of free radical polymerization.

FTIR spectroscopy, ^{1}HNMR spectroscopy, X-ray diffraction, thermogravimetric analysis and scanning electron microscopy confirmed the grafting reaction of NVI onto gellan, as well as the synthesis of grafted polymers having betaine structure.

In vitro release studies of CF proved the capacity of the new grafted copolymers to immobilize amphoteric drugs and highlighted the fact that the release mechanism of CF from PG and PGB1 samples is controlled by diffusion process or by a combination between diffusion and swelling processes. These results demonstrated that the grafted copolymer with betaine structure can be a potential candidate for developing sustained/controlled drug delivery systems.

Author Contributions: Conceptualization, S.R. and S.V.; methodology, S.R., N.B. and S.V.; validation, V.S., M.P. and J.D.; formal analysis, N.B., A.M.M. and C.C.; investigation, C.L. and V.S.; data curation, S.R., N.B. and S.V.; writing—original draft preparation, S.R. and S.V.; writing—review & editing, M.P. and J.D., visualization and supervision, S.V., M.P. and J.D. All authors have read and agreed to the published version of the manuscript.

References

1. Garcia-Valdez, O.; Champagne, P.; Cunningham, M.F. Graft modification of natural polysaccharides via reversible deactivation radical polymerization. *Prog. Polym. Sci.* **2018**, *76*, 151–173. [CrossRef]
2. Cassanelli, M.; Prosapio, V.; Norton, I.; Mills, T. Acidified/basified gellan gum gels: The role of the structure in drying/rehydration mechanisms. *Food Hydrocoll.* **2018**, *82*, 346–354. [CrossRef]
3. Osmałek, T.; Froelich, A.; Tasarek, S. Application of gellan gum in pharmacy and medicine. *Int. J. Pharm.* **2014**, *466*, 328–340. [CrossRef]
4. Chang, S.J.; Huang, Y.-T.; Yang, S.-C.; Kuo, S.M.; Lee, M.-W. In vitro properties of gellan gum sponge as the dental filling to maintain alveolar space. *Carbohydr. Polym.* **2012**, *88*, 684–689. [CrossRef]
5. Pandey, V.S.; Verma, S.K.; Yadav, M.; Behari, K. Studies on graft copolymerization of gellan gum with *N,N*-dimethylacrylamide by the redox system. *Int. J. Biol. Macromol.* **2014**, *70*, 108–115. [CrossRef]
6. Giri, T.K.; Verma, P.; Tripathi, D.K. Grafting of vinyl monomer onto gellan gum using microwave: Synthesis and characterization of grafted copolymer. *Adv. Compos. Mater.* **2014**, *24*, 531–543. [CrossRef]
7. Vijan, V.; Kaity, S.; Biswas, S.; Isaac, J.; Ghosh, A. Microwave assisted synthesis and characterization of acrylamide grafted gellan, application in drug delivery. *Carbohydr. Polym.* **2012**, *90*, 496–506. [CrossRef]
8. Nandi, G.; Patra, P.; Priyadarshini, R.; Kaity, S.; Ghosh, L.K. Synthesis, characterization and evaluation of methacrylamide grafted gellan as sustained release tablet matrix. *Int. J. Biol. Macromol.* **2015**, *72*, 965–974. [CrossRef]
9. Karthika, J.S.; Vishalakshi, B. Microwave-Assisted Synthesis and Characterization of Poly(2-(dimethylamino)ethyl methacrylate) Grafted Gellan Gum. *Int. J. Polym. Anal. Charact.* **2014**, *19*, 709–720. [CrossRef]
10. Verma, S.K.; Pandey, V.S.; Behari, K. Gellan gum-g-*N*-vinyl-2-pyrrolidone: Synthesis, swelling, metal ion uptake and flocculation behavior. *Int. J. Biol. Macromol.* **2015**, *72*, 1292–1300. [CrossRef]
11. Abu Elella, M.H.; Mohamed, R.R.; Sabaa, M.W. Synthesis of novel grafted hyaluronic acid with antitumor activity. *Carbohydr. Polym.* **2018**, *189*, 107–114. [CrossRef]
12. Caner, H.; Yilmaz, E.; Yilmaz, O. Synthesis, characterization and antibacterial activity of poly(N-vinylimidazole) grafted chitosan. *Carbohydr. Polym.* **2007**, *69*, 318–325. [CrossRef]
13. Unal, H.I.; Inegollu, C.; Sanli, O. Graft copolymerization of N-vinylimidazole on poly(ethylene tetephthalate) fibers in a swelling solvent using azobisisobutyronitrile as initiator. *Turk. J. Chem.* **2003**, *27*, 403–415.
14. Abu Elella, M.H.; Mohamed, R.R.; Elhafeez, E.A.; Sabaa, M.W. Synthesis of novel biodegradable antibacterial grafted xanthan gum. *Carbohydr. Polym.* **2017**, *173*, 305–311. [CrossRef]
15. El-Hamshary, H.; Fouda, M.M.; Moydeen, M.; El-Newehy, M.H.; Al-Deyab, S.S.; Abdel-Megeed, A. Synthesis and antibacterial of carboxymethyl starch-grafted poly(vinyl imidazole) against some plant pathogens. *Int. J. Biol. Macromol.* **2015**, *72*, 1466–1472. [CrossRef]
16. Anderson, E.B.; Long, T.E. Imidazole- and imidazolium-containing polymers for biology and material science applications. *Polymer* **2010**, *51*, 2447–2454. [CrossRef]
17. Pineda-Contreras, A.; Hernández-Madrigal, J.V.; Vázquez-Vuelvas, O.F.; Fomine, S. Synthesis and ROMP of new sulfobetaine and carboxybetaine norbornene. *e-Polymers* **2016**, *16*, 181–188. [CrossRef]
18. Vasiliu, S.; Neagu, V.; Popa, M.; Luca, C. Materials with special properties based on polybetaines. *Mater. Plast.* **2008**, *45*, 177–183.
19. Barboiu, V.; Holerca, M.N.; Streba, E.; Luca, C. Reactions on polymers with amine groups. 3. Description of the addition reaction of pyridine and imidazole compounds with alpha, beta-unsaturated monocarboxylic acids. *J. Polym. Sci. Part A Polym. Chem.* **1996**, *34*, 261–270. [CrossRef]
20. Gonsior, N.; Mohr, F.; Ritter, H. Synthesis of mesomeric betaine compounds with imidazolium-enolate structure. *Beilstein J. Org. Chem.* **2012**, *8*, 390–397. [CrossRef]
21. Laschewsky, A. Structures and Synthesis of Zwitterionic Polymers. *Polymer* **2014**, *6*, 1544–1601. [CrossRef]
22. Liu, D.; Zhu, J.; Qiu, M.; He, C. Antifouling PVDF membrane grafted with zwitterionic poly(lysine methacrylamide) brushes. *RSC Adv.* **2016**, *6*, 61434–61442. [CrossRef]
23. Li, M.; Zhuang, B.; Yu, J. Functional Zwitterionic Polymers on Surface: Structures and Applications. *Chem. Asian J.* **2020**, *15*, 2060–2075. [CrossRef]

24. Blackman, L.D.; Gunatillake, P.A.; Cass, P.; Locock, K.E.S. An introduction to zwitterionic polymer behavior and applications in solution and at surfaces. *Chem. Soc. Rev.* **2019**, *48*, 757–770. [CrossRef]
25. Tarannum, N.; Singh, M. Advances in Synthesis and Applications of Sulfo and Carbo Analogues of Polybetaines: A Review. *Rev. Adv. Sci. Eng.* **2013**, *2*, 90–111. [CrossRef]
26. Didukh, A.G.; Koizhaiganova, R.B.; Khamitzhanova, G.; Bimendina, L.A.; Kudaibergenov, S.E. Stimuli-sensitive behaviour of novel betaine-type polyampholytes. *Polym. Int.* **2003**, *52*, 883–891. [CrossRef]
27. Tada, S.; Inaba, C.; Mizukami, K.; Fujishita, S.; Gemmei-Ide, M.; Kitano, H.; Mochizuki, A.; Tanaka, M.; Matsunaga, T. Anti-Biofouling Properties of Polymers with a Carboxybetaine Moiety. *Macromol. Biosci.* **2008**, *9*, 63–70. [CrossRef]
28. Lewis, A.L. Phosphorylcholine-based polymers and their use in the prevention of biofouling. *Colloids Surf. B Biointerfaces* **2000**, *18*, 261–275. [CrossRef]
29. West, S.L.; Salvage, J.P.; Lobb, E.J.; Armes, S.P.; Billingham, N.C.; Lewis, A.L.; Hanlon, G.W.; Lloyd, A.W. The biocompatibility of crosslinkable copolymer coatings containing sulfobetaines and phosphobetaines. *Biomaterials* **2004**, *25*, 1195–1204. [CrossRef]
30. Luca, C.; Mihailescu, S.; Popa, M. Polymers containing quaternary ammonium groups based on poly(N-vinylimidazole). *Eur. Polym. J.* **2002**, *38*, 1501–1507. [CrossRef]
31. Racovita, S.; Vasiliu, S.; Neagu, V. Solution properties of three polyzwitterions based on poly (N-vinylimidazole). *Iran. Polym. J.* **2010**, *19*, 333–341.
32. Sabaa, M.W.; Mohamed, N.A.; Mohamed, R.R.; Khalil, N.M.; El Latif, S.M.A. Synthesis, characterization and antimicrobial activity of poly (N-vinyl imidazole) grafted carboxymethyl chitosan. *Carbohydr. Polym.* **2010**, *79*, 998–1005. [CrossRef]
33. Bamford, C.; Schofield, E. Non-classical free-radical polymerization: Degradative addition to monomer in the polymerization of 1-vinylimidazole. *Polymer* **1981**, *22*, 1227–1235. [CrossRef]
34. Behari, K.; Pandey, P.; Kumar, R.; Taunk, K. Graft copolymerization of acrylamide onto xanthan gum. *Carbohydr. Polym.* **2001**, *46*, 185–189. [CrossRef]
35. Badwaik, H.; Sakure, K.; Alexander, A.; Ajazuddin Dhongade, H.; Tripathi, D.K. Synthesis and characterisation of poly(acryalamide) grafted carboxymethyl xanthan gum copolymer. *Int. J. Biol. Macromol.* **2016**, *85*, 361–369. [CrossRef]
36. Bhattacharyya, S.; Maldas, D. Graft copolymerization onto cellulosics. *Prog. Polym. Sci.* **1984**, *10*, 171–270. [CrossRef]
37. Taghizadeh, M.T.; Khosravy, M. Kinetics and mechanism of graft copolymerization of vinyl monomers (acrylamide, acrylic acid and methacrylate) onto starch by potassium dichromate as redox initiator. *Iran. Polym. J.* **2003**, *12*, 497–505.
38. Sirirat, T.; Vatanatham, T.; Hansupalak, N.; Rempel, G.L.; Arayapranee, W. Kinetics and modeling of methyl methacrylate graft copolymerization in the presence of natural rubber latex. *Korean J. Chem. Eng.* **2015**, *32*, 980–992. [CrossRef]
39. Mostafa, K.; Samarkandy, A.R.; El-Sanabary, A. Grafting onto carbohydrate polymer using novel potassium persulfate/tetramethylethylene diamine redox system for initiating grafting. *Adv. Polym. Technol.* **2011**, *30*, 138–149. [CrossRef]
40. Neagu, V.; Vasiliu, S.; Racovita, S. Adsorption studies of some inorganic and organic salts on new zwitterionic ion exchangers with carboxybetaine moieties. *Chem. Eng. J.* **2010**, *162*, 965–973. [CrossRef]
41. Talu, M.; Demiroğlu, E.U.; Yurdakul, Ş.; Badoğlu, S. FTIR, Raman and NMR spectroscopic and DFT theoretical studies on poly(*N*-vinylimidazole). *Spectrochim. Acta Part. A Mol. Biomol. Spectrosc.* **2015**, *134*, 267–275. [CrossRef]
42. Coutinho, D.F.; Sant, S.V.; Shin, H.; Oliveira, J.T.; Gomes, M.E.; Neves, N.M.; Khademhosseini, A.; Reis, R.L. Modified Gellan Gum hydrogels with tunable physical and mechanical properties. *Biomaterials* **2010**, *31*, 7494–7502. [CrossRef]
43. Lu, Y.; Zhao, X.; Fang, S. Characterization, Antimicrobial Properties and Coatings Application of Gellan Gum Oxidized with Hydrogen Peroxide. *Foods* **2019**, *8*, 31. [CrossRef]
44. Vasiliu, S.; Bunia, I.; Racovita, S.; Neagu, V. Adsorption of cefotaxime sodium salt on polymer coated ion exchange resin microparticles: Kinetics, equilibrium and thermodynamic studies. *Carbohydr. Polym.* **2011**, *85*, 376–387. [CrossRef]
45. Higuchi, W.I. Diffusional Models Useful in Biopharmaceutics. *J. Pharm. Sci.* **1967**, *56*, 315–324. [CrossRef]

46. Korsmeyer, R.W.; Gurny, R.; Doelker, E.; Buri, P.; Peppas, N.A. Mechanisms of solute release from porous hydrophilic polymers. *Int. J. Pharm.* **1983**, *15*, 25–35. [CrossRef]
47. Sepulveda, P.; Binner, J.G.P. Persulfate–Amine Initiation Systems for Gelcasting of Ceramic Foams. *Chem. Mater.* **2001**, *13*, 4065–4070. [CrossRef]
48. Constantin, M.; Mihalcea, I.; Oanea, I.; Harabagiu, V.; Fundueanu, G. Studies on graft copolymerization of 3-acrylamidopropyl trimethylammonium chloride on pullulan. *Carbohydr. Polym.* **2011**, *84*, 926–932. [CrossRef]
49. Srivastava, A.; Behari, K. Studies on Graft Copolymerization of *N*-Vinyl-2-pyrrolidone on to Carboxymethylcellulose (Sodium Salt) and Metal Ion Sorption Behavior. *J. Macromol. Sci. Part A* **2006**, *43*, 1065–1081. [CrossRef]
50. Clark, W.M.; Lubs, H.A. The Colorimetric Determination of Hydrogen ion Concentration and its Applications in Bacteriology PART I1. *J. Bacteriol.* **1917**, *2*, 1–34. [CrossRef]
51. Sorensen, S.P.L. Enzyme studies II. On the measurement and the importance of hydrogen ion concentrationduring enzymatic processes. *Biochem. Z.* **1909**, *21*, 131–200.

5

Tablets of "Hydrochlorothiazide in Cyclodextrin in Nanoclay": A New Nanohybrid System with Enhanced Dissolution Properties

Francesca Maestrelli [1], Marzia Cirri [1,*], Fátima García-Villén [2], Ana Borrego-Sánchez [3], César Viseras Iborra [2,3] and Paola Mura [1]

1 Department of Chemistry, University of Florence, via Schiff 6, Sesto Fiorentino, 50019 Florence, Italy; francesca.maestrelli@unifi.it (F.M.); paola.mura@unifi.it (P.M.)

2 Department of Pharmacy and Pharmaceutical Technology, University of Granada, Campus de Cartuja, s/n 18071 Granada, Spain; fgarvillen@ugr.es (F.G.-V.); cviseras@ugr.es (C.V.I.)

3 Andalusian Institute of Earth Sciences, CSIC-University of Granada, Avda. de Las Palmeras 4, 18100 Armilla (Granada), Spain; anaborrego@iact.ugr-csic.es

* Correspondence: marzia.cirri@unifi.it

Abstract: Hydrochlorothiazide (HCT), a Biopharmaceutical Classification System (BCS) class IV drug, is characterized by low solubility and permeability, that negatively affect its oral bioavailability, reducing its therapeutic efficacy. The combined use of cyclodextrins (CDs) and nanoclays (NCs) recently proved to be a successful strategy in developing delivery systems able to merge the potential benefits of both carriers. In this work, several binary systems of CDs or NCs with the drug were obtained, using different drug:carrier ratios and preparation techniques, and characterized in solution and in solid state, to properly select the most effective system and preparation method. Then, the best CD (RAMEB) and NC (sepiolite), at the best drug:carrier ratio, was selected for preparation of the ternary system by co-evaporation and emerged as the most effective preparation method. The combined presence of RAMEB and sepiolite gave rise to a synergistic improvement of drug dissolution properties, with a two-fold increase in the amount of drug dissolved as compared with the corresponding HCT-RAMEB system, resulting in an approximately 12-fold increase in drug solubility as compared with the drug alone. The ternary system that was co-evaporated was then selected for a tablet formulation. The obtained tablets were fully characterized for technological properties and clearly revealed a better drug dissolution performance than the commercial reference tablet (Esidrex®).

Keywords: hydrochlorothiazide; cyclodextrins; sepiolite; nanoclay; dissolution rate; tablet

1. Introduction

Hydrochlorothiazide (HCT) is a thiazide diuretic drug widely used in the treatment of heart failure, hypertension, hypovolemic shock, or edema [1]. HCT is a class IV drug, according to the Biopharmaceutical Classification System (BCS), characterized by low aqueous solubility and low permeability [2]. Due to these factors, this drug is poorly absorbed in the gastrointestinal tract, thus, resulting in a variable and low bioavailability after oral administration [3]. Moreover, HCT can be easily hydrolyzed in an aqueous environment, which also poses stability problems [4].

Cyclodextrins (CDs) are a family of cyclic oligosaccharides with a hydrophilic outer surface and a lipophilic central cavity used as complexing agents to increase aqueous solubility of poorly soluble drugs and to increase their bioavailability and stability. The natural CDs, named $\alpha-$, $\beta-$, and γCD consist of six, seven, or eight glucopyranose units and among them, βCD usually demonstrates the higher complexing ability toward drugs [5]. Cyclodextrins (CDs) have been successfully used as carriers to improve the solubility and bioavailability of antihypertensive agents such as HCT [6]. CD complexation can provide additional advantages, including taste masking, increased drug stability, and drug permeation, thus, leading to dose lowering and reduction of side effects [7]. Mendes et al., 2016 showed the capacity of βCD to increase HCT solubility, protect the drug from hydrolysis and enhance the in vivo effect [8]. Moreover, the effectiveness of βCD in increasing drug permeability across the small intestine of rats was recently demonstrated by Altamimi et al., 2018 [9]. However, βCD has relatively low solubility and often cannot be used at concentrations suitable for pharmaceutical applications. For these reasons several modified βCDs have been prepared, and now its hydroxypropyl, methyl, and sulfobutylether derivatives have been commercially used as new pharmaceutical excipients.

Clay minerals can be used as excipients in several medicinal products and can be effectively used in the development of new formulations. Nanoclays (NCs) are fibrous inorganic matrices that are able to entrap little molecules and release them in particular conditions and have aroused particular interest as drug carriers due to their biocompatibility, high drug loading power, low cost, and very poor toxicity [10,11]. Moreover, their ability to enhance the dissolution properties and, then, the bioavailability of poorly soluble drugs has been reported [12,13].

Tablets are still the most used solid dosage form in the market due to their manufacturing efficiency, good stability, and good patient acceptance [14]; and CD and fibrous clays used as excipients for tablet formulation is well recognized and consolidated [13,15]. Recently, "drug-in-CD-in-NC" hybrid systems have been developed and used to prepare tablets of oxaprozin, a poorly water-soluble NSAID, with improved dissolution properties and enhanced therapeutic effect on rats [16,17]. Taking these considerations into account, the aim of this work was to assess the effectiveness of such a particular approach, based on the combined use of CDs and NCs as drug carriers, for the development of a powerful tablet formulation for oral delivery of HCT. With this purpose, the solubilizing effect of different CDs and NCs towards the drug was first investigated, in order to select the best carriers. In fact, it is not possible to determine in advance which kind of CD or NC better improves the drug dissolution properties, as well as it is not possible to predict the effect of drug-CD complexation on the nanoclay interaction and entrapment. Moreover, in order to evaluate the influence of the preparation technique in establishing effective drug-carrier interactions, binary and ternary combinations of the drug with CDs and NCs were prepared by different methods and characterized for solid-state (by differential scanning calorimetry and X-ray powder diffractometry) and dissolution properties. The best CD and NC carriers and the most effective preparation method were then selected to obtain the hybrid ternary system, which was used for the development of tablets. These were suitably evaluated for technological properties and tested for dissolution behavior and compared with a marketed tablet formulation.

2. Materials and Methods

2.1. Materials

Hydrochlorothiazide (HCT) was a gift from Menarini (L'Aquila, Italy). β-Cyclodextrin (βCD) and hydroxypropyl-β-cyclodextrin (Kleptose HP, HPβCd) were kindly donated by Roquette (Lestrem, France). Amorphous randomly methylated-β-cyclodextrin (RAMEB, average MS 1.8) and hydroxyethyl-β-cyclodextrin (HEβCD, average MS 1.0) were a gift from Wacker-Chemie GmbH (Munchen, Germany). Sulfobutylether-β-cyclodextrin (SBEβCD) Dexolve® was gifted from CycloLab (Budapest, Ungary). Sepiolite was from Vicalvaro (Spain) (SV); attapulgite (Pharmasorb colloidal, PHC) was from BASF, and bentonite (or smectite) (VeegumHS, VHS) was kindly gifted by Vanderbilt Minerals (USA). Magnesium stearate and polyvinylpyrrolidone (PVP K 30) were obtained from Sigma-Aldrich Chemie GmbH (Steinhelm, Germany). Sodium starch glycolate (Explotab®) was from JRS Pharma (Rosenberg, Germany). Tablets of HCT commercially available in Italy (Esidrex®) containing 25 mg of drug were from Novartis Farma Spa (Varese, Italy). Other chemicals and solvents were of reagent grade and used without further purification.

2.2. *Phase Solubility Studies*

Phase-solubility studies of HCT with different cyclodextrins were performed by adding an excess of drug to phosphate buffer solutions (pH 5.5) containing increasing concentrations of CD, i.e., 0 to 12.5 mM for βCD and 0 to 25 mM for the other CD derivatives. The vials were sealed, and the suspensions were electromagnetically stirred (500 rpm) at a constant temperature (25 °C) until equilibrium (3 days). Then, an aliquot of solution was withdrawn with a filter-syringe (pore size 0.45 μm), and the drug concentration was spectrometrically determined (UV/Vis 1601 Shimadzu, Tokyo, Japan) at λ_{max} 272.2 nm. The linearity was determined on five concentration levels (from 3 to 20 mg/L). The calibration curve was $y = 0.0623x + 0.003$, $r^2 = 0.999$. LOQ = 1 mg/L and LOD = 0.33 mg/L. The presence of CD did not interfere with the drug spectrophotometric assay. Each experiment was performed in triplicate (C.V. < 2.5%). The apparent stability constants of the drug–CD complexes were calculated from the slope of the linear portion of the phase-solubility diagrams and the drug solubility (S_o) in the dissolution medium according to Equation (1) [18]:

$$Ks = slope/S_o{*}(1 - slope) \tag{1}$$

The complexation efficiency (CE) was calculated from the slope of the phase-solubility diagrams according to Equation (2) [19]:

$$CE = slope/(1 - slope) \tag{2}$$

The solubilizing efficiency (SE) of CDs towards the drug was calculated as the ratio of drug solubility in the presence of the maximum concentration of CD used with respect to that of the drug alone.

2.3. *Preparation of Drug–CD and Drug–NC Binary Systems*

Physical mixtures (PM) were prepared by mixing equimolar amounts of drug and CD with the same granulometric size (75 to 150 μm). By submitting the PM to grinding, using a high-energy vibrational micro-mill for 30 min at 24 Hz (Mixer Mill MM 200, Retsch GmbH, Dusseldorf, Germany), co-ground binary systems were obtained. Kneaded products (KN) were prepared starting from the corresponding PM. Briefly, the PM were placed in a mortar and 0.2 mL of a water/ethanol 50:50 *v/v* solution were added until a dough was obtained. The mixture was then manually ground with a pestle until a powder was obtained. A complete drying was achieved putting the powder in an oven at 40 °C for 24 h.

HCT binary systems with NCs (PHC, VHS, and SV) were prepared at different w/w ratios (1:1; 1:2; 1:4) by physical mixing (i.e., PM), as described above for HCT-CD systems. Binary systems with the selected NC (SV) at the selected *w/w* ratio (1:4 *w/w*) were prepared by different techniques. Co-evaporated products (COE) were prepared by dissolving HCT in the minimum amount of ethanol and suspending SV in water, mixing and removing the solvent by rotary evaporation; the solid product was collected and left to dry in an oven for 24 h at 40 °C. Cofused products (COF) were realized by heating the PM under magnetic stirring at 300 °C for 10 min. Co-ground systems (GR) were obtained by ball-milling the PM in a high-energy vibrational micro-mill (Mixer Mill MM 200, Retsch GmbH, Dusseldorf, Germany) at 24 Hz for 30 min [10,16]. Solvent-heated products (SH) were obtained by adding 5 mL of ethanol to the PM under magnetic stirring for 5 min and heating at 300 °C for 5 min until the solvent evaporation [20,21]. Solvent-sonicated products (SS) were prepared by a partial modification of the method of Yendluri et al., 2017 [22,23]. Briefly, 20 mg of drug were dissolved in 1 mL of ethanol to obtain a saturated solution where SV was added. The mixture was sonicated with a Sonopuls HD2200 ultrasound homogenizer (Bandelin Electronic GmbH, Berlin, Germany) equipped with a KE76 probe at 50% of power for 10 min and left to dry overnight to ensure maximum loading. The day after, the sample was washed with fresh ethanol and filtered in order to remove aggregates. The sample was dried in a vacuum desiccator overnight and powdered. The solvent magnetic stirring technique (SMS) is a partial variation of the method used by Lun et al., 2014 [24].

Briefly, the saturated solution of drug in ethanol containing SV was kept under stirring overnight; then, the solid in suspension was separated by centrifugation, filtered and dried overnight at 60 °C.

2.4. Preparation of Drug-CD-Sepiolite (SV) Ternary Systems

Ternary physical mixtures (PM) were prepared by 15 min tumble mixing the drug with the selected CD (HCT:RAMEB 1:1 mol/mol) and SV (HCT:SV 1:4 *w/w* ratio). Co-evaporated ternary products (COE) were prepared by dissolving equimolar amounts of HCT and RAMEB in the minimum amount of ethanol and water, respectively, mixing the solutions, suspending SV (HCT:SV 1:4 *w/w* ratio) under mixing and removing the solvent by rotary evaporation; the solid product was collected and left to dry in an oven for 24 h at 40 °C.

2.5. Solid-State Characterization

Thermal analysis of pure components, drug–CD and drug-SV binary systems obtained with the different techniques was performed by a Mettler TA 4000 Star^e system (Mettler Toledo, Greifensee, Switzerland). About 5 to 10 mg of each sample were accurately weighed by a MX5 Microbalance (Mettler-Toledo, Greifensee, Switzerland), placed in sealed aluminum pans with pierced lid, and scanned at a heating rate of 10 °C min^{-1} under static air atmosphere, at a temperature in the range 30–300 °C. The instrument was calibrated using Indium as a standard (99.98% purity, melting point 156.61 °C, and fusion enthalpy 28.71 J/g).

The relative degree of drug crystallinity (RDC) in the samples was calculated according to Equation (3) [17]:

$$RDC = \frac{\Delta Hsample}{\Delta Hdrug} \times 100\% \qquad (3)$$

where ΔH *sample* and ΔH *drug* are, respectively, the heat of fusion of the drug in the sample (normalized to the drug content) and of the pure drug. Measurements were performed in triplicate and the relative standard deviation of crystallinity data was about ±4% to 5%.

The X-ray powder diffraction analysis (XRPD) was conducted at room temperature (2θ = 5 to 30° and scan rate = 0.05°/s) with Bruker D8-advance apparatus (Silberstreifen, Germany) at a 40 mV voltage and 55 mA current using a Cu Kα radiation and a graphite monochromator.

2.6. Dissolution Rate Studies

Dissolution rate studies of HCT as such and from its different binary and ternary systems as well as from the final tablets were performed according to the dispersed amount method.

Powder samples, containing a fixed amount of drug, were sieved and the selected granulometric fraction (75 to 150 μm) was placed into a 150 mL beaker containing 75 mL of pH 5.5 phosphate buffer solution. In the beaker, thermostated at 37 ± 0.5 °C, a three-blade paddle (1.5 cm radius) was centrally placed and rotated at 100 rpm. Drug content was determined as described above (Section 2.1) in samples (3 mL) periodically withdrawn and filtered with a syringe-filter (pore size 0.45 μm). Fresh medium was added to replace the sampling and a correction was made for the cumulative dilution.

Each test was repeated four times (C.V. < 5%). All data were analyzed by ANOVA (one-way analysis of variance) (GraphPad Prism version 4.0 program, Inc. San Diego, CA, USA). Differences were considered statistically significant when p values were <0.05.

2.7. Tablet Formulation and Characterization

Flat tablets containing 25 mg of drug were prepared with the selected ternary system (COE HCT-RAMEB-SV). In order to obtain mixtures with proper flowability, disintegration, and compactability properties, 4% sodium starch glycolate (Explotab®) as superdisintegrant, 10% of polyvinylpirrolidone (PVP K30) as binder, and 1% of Mg stearate as lubricant were combined to the drug or drug-carrier systems. After a mixing of 15 min in a turbula mixer, the powders were compressed at 2.5 tons for 3 min using a hydraulic press. Uniformity of content, weight, diameter, thickness, hardness, friability, and disintegration tests were performed according to European Pharmacopoeia (Ph. Eur.) 9th Edition. In order to obtain results comparable with the powders, dissolution studies were instead performed according to the method described above (Section 2.5).

The same test was also performed on Esidrex®, an HCT tablet formulation present on the market.

3. Results and Discussion

3.1. Phase Solubility Studies

The phase solubility studies evidenced a linear increase of drug solubility with increasing CDs concentration (A_L type), as reported in Figure 1. The results indicate, in all cases, the formation of soluble complexes of probable 1:1 mol:mol stoichiometry [18]. The parameters, reported in Table 1, evidenced the difference in the solubilizing and complexing power towards HCT among the different CDs.

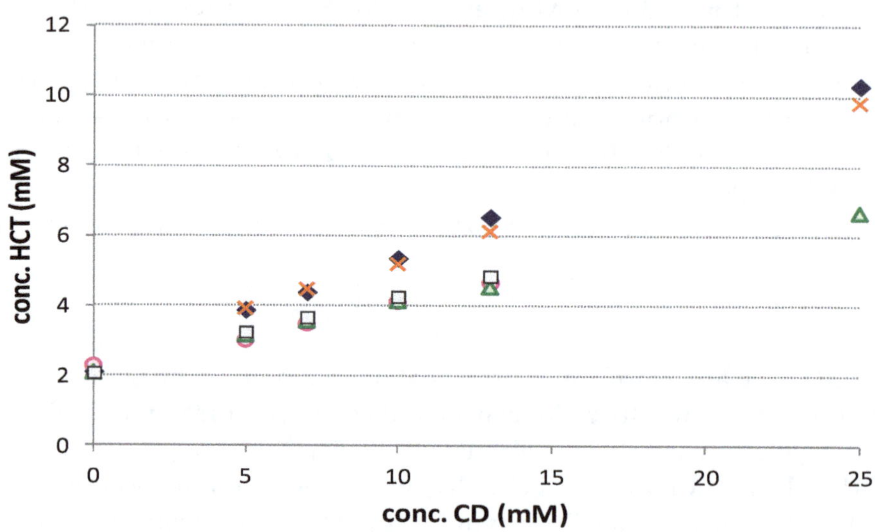

Figure 1. Phase solubility diagrams of HCT with βCD(□), HPβCD (Δ), HEβCD (○), SBEβCD (X), and RAMEB (♦). Each value represents the mean of 9 measurements.

Table 1. Stability constant ($K_{1:1}$), complexation efficiency (CE), and solubilizing efficiency (SE) of complexes of the different examined cyclodextrins (CDs) with hydrochlorothiazide in pH 5.5 phosphate buffer at 25 °C.

CD Type	$K_{1:1}$ M^{-1} ± s.d.	CE	SE [a]
βCD	131 ± 2	0.27	2.3
HPβCD	106 ± 3	0.28	3.1
HEβCD	114 ± 1	0.23	3.3
SBEβCD	213 ± 4	0.44	4.7
RAMEB	234 ± 2	0.48	4.8

[a] ratio between drug water solubility in presence of the highest CD concentration used (12.5 mM for βCD and 25 mM for other CDs) and alone.

Our results were in full agreement with those of Onnainty et al., 2013 [25], who reported the same type of phase-solubility diagrams for HCT complexation with βCD. The highest values of complex apparent stability constant ($K_{1:1}$), complexation efficiency (CE), and solubilizing efficiency (SE) were obtained with RAMEB and SBEβCD that gave rise to an approximately five-fold increase in drug solubility as compared with the drug alone (Table 1). The better performance of these derivatives can be attributed to the presence of methyl and sulfobutylether substituents which extended the CD hydrophobic region and improved substrate binding via a hydrophobic effect, as just observed for other lipophilic drugs [16,26].

3.2. *Characterization of the Drug–CD Binary Systems*

DSC curves of pure HCT and CDs and of their binary systems obtained with the different techniques were recorded in order to investigate the effect of the CD type and preparation technique towards drug amorphization and complexation (Figure 2A). Thermograms of pure drug submitted to the different treatments used for the preparation of the binary systems were also recorded, in order to evidence any effect of the preparation technique on drug solid-state properties.

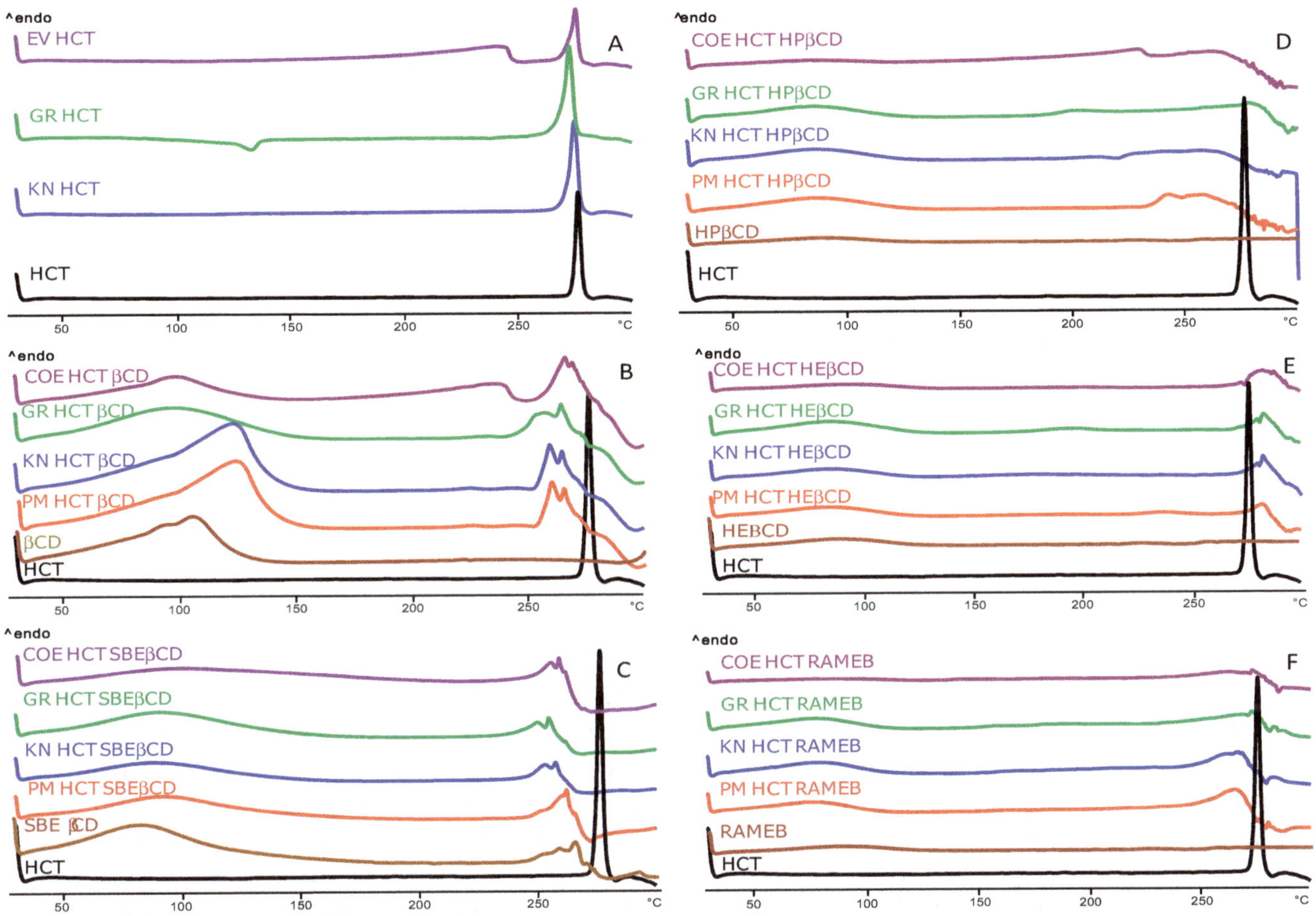

Figure 2. DSC curves of pure HCT (**A**) untreated or submitted to kneading (KN), grinding (GR) or dissolution-solvent evaporation (EV) and its binary systems with βCD (**B**), HPβCD (**C**), HEβCD (**D**), SBEβCD (**E**), and RAMEB (**F**), obtained by physical mixing (i.e., PM), co-grinding (GR), kneading (KN), and co-evaporation (COE).

The drug alone thermogram showed a sharp melting peak (T_{peak} = 274.4 °C and ΔH = 152.8 $J \cdot g^{-1}$), as expected for an anhydrous crystalline compound. The kneading does not seem to affect the thermal behavior, causing just a slight decrease in T_{peak} (272.2 °C) and RDC (98.96%).

The thermal curve of the drug submitted to the grinding process showed an exothermic phenomenon at 134.5 °C which is attributed to the recrystallization of the drug fraction amorphized during the grinding procedure; it was followed by the melting peak at 271.2 °C, whose reduced intensity (ΔH_{fus}128.1 Jg^{-1}) indicated some loss of crystallinity (RDC 83.23%). In the evaporated product, the drug melting peak at 274.1 °C was characterized by a sensible reduction of fusion enthalpy

(72.1 Jg^{-1}). The calculated RDC of 46% suggested an appreciable drug amorphization, as a consequence of its dissolution in the water-ethanol mixture and the following solvent evaporation.

In Figure 2B, the thermal profiles of HCT binary systems with βCD are reported. The DSC curve of βCD in the examined temperature range was characterized by an intense and broad endothermic effect that ranged between 50 to 130 °C, due to its dehydration. The PM showed the CD dehydration band, followed at higher temperatures by an endothermic event characterized by the presence of two peaks at 265 °C and 269 °C. These can be attributed to the partial superimposition of the drug melting and the CD thermal decomposition, both shifted at lower temperature than the corresponding pure components, due to their co-presence, as observed also by other authors [27,28]. In fact, CD alone started to decompose usually over 300 °C [29]. A thermal behavior substantially similar to that of PM was found for GR, KN, or COE products, suggesting poor host–guest interactions. A rather similar behavior (Figure 2C) was observed for the series of products with SBEβCD. As previously observed by Cirri et al., 2017, the thermal profile of this CD showed a broad endothermic effect between 60 to 110 °C due to its dehydration, and another endothermic band between 250 and 280 °C, due to degradation phenomena [30]. All binary systems prepared with the different techniques showed the superimposition of HCT melting and CD decomposition phenomena, similar to that observed in the simple PM. As for the thermal profiles of binary systems with HPβCD, HEβCD and RAMEB (Figure 2D–F, respectively) after the initial broad endothermic effect, due to the amorphous CD dehydration, the drug and CD endothermic decomposition phenomena in the range 250–260 °C was still barely detectable only for the PM with HPβCD, while the drug melting peak completely disappeared in all other systems, where only the CD decomposition band was observed.

In order to better elucidate the DSC findings and, in particular, to evidence any possible artifact of the technique, due to a heating-induced interaction between the components as a consequence of the thermal energy supplied to the sample during the DSC scans [31], XRPD analysis was conducted. As shown in Figure 3A, the patterns of pure drug and βCD presented several sharp peaks, characteristic of crystalline substances, whereas all βCD derivatives, as shown, as example, for HPβCD, presented an almost flat pattern typical of amorphous substances. Representative drug peaks were clearly detectable in the patterns of all PMs (Figure 3B), even if reduced in intensity, particularly, in combinations with the amorphous partners, indicating that any solid-state interaction occurred during the simple mixing of drug and CDs. However analogous results to those of PMs were also obtained for all binary systems with βCD and different CD derivatives, with the only exception for COE products obtained with RAMEB and SBEβCD (Figure S1, Supplementary Material). Thus, the disappearance of the drug melting peak, observed in the other cases can be attributed to heating-induced interactions due to the thermal energy supplied to the sample during the scan. However, the completely amorphous pattern exhibited by the COE products with RAMEB and SBEβCD proved that the actual drug amorphization and complexation was achieved only by this preparation technique with these CDs (Figure 3C).

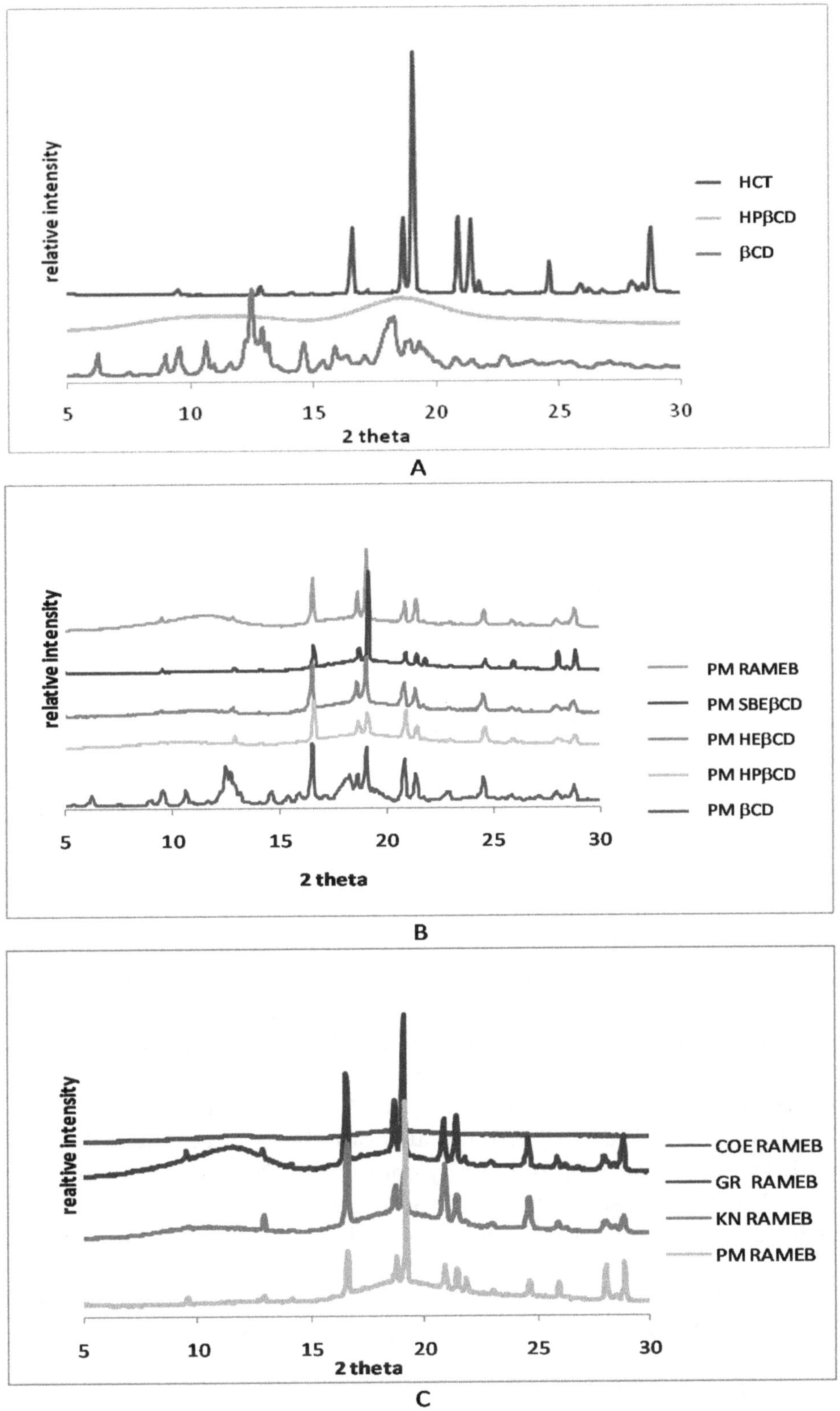

Figure 3. XRPD patterns of pure HCT and CDs (**A**) and of equimolar physical mixtures (PM) (**B**) with all CDs and the co-ground (GR), kneaded (KN), and co-evaporated (COE) products with RAMEB (**C**).

The results of dissolution rate studies performed on pure drug, both untreated and submitted to the different techniques and on the different binary systems with all the CDs, are presented in Figure 4.

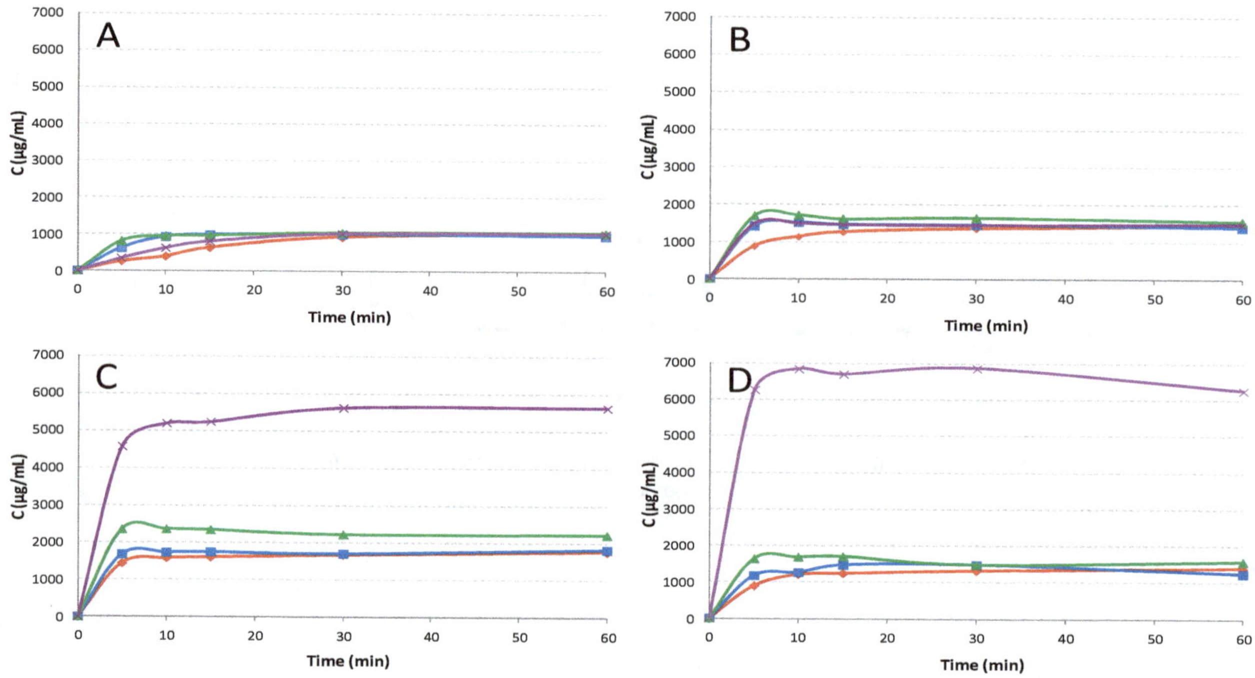

Figure 4. Dissolution profiles of pure HCT (**A**) untreated (♦ red line) or submitted to kneading (■ blue line), grinding (▲ green line), or dissolution-solvent evaporation (x violet line) and from its binary systems with βCD (**B**), SBEβCD(**C**), and RAMEB (**D**), obtained by physical mixing (PM) (♦ red line), kneading (KN) (■ blue line), co-grinding (GR) (▲ green line), and co-evaporation (COE) (x violet line). Each value represents the mean of 3 experiments.

As shown, HCT alone (Figure 4A) always reached a solubility of 1 mg/mL, even if the treatments, especially the grinding one, initially allowed a more rapid release, probably due to a particle size reduction of the powder. In binary systems with βCD (Figure 4B) a better profile was also observed for the simple PM that reached a plateau level of 1.45 ± 0.5 mg/mL, due to the improved drug wettability and possible in situ complexation phenomena. A little more favorable effect on the drug dissolution rate, particularly in the first minutes, was observed for all treated products, in virtue of the more intimate contact between the components brought about by the sample preparation method. Similar results were obtained for drug systems with HEβCD and HPβCD (data not shown), regardless of the sample preparation technique. Instead, significant differences were observed for the series of products with SBEβCD and RAMEB (Figure 4C,D) especially for COE systems, which achieved plateau levels around 5.5 ± 0.3 and 6.8 ± 0.2 mg/mL, respectively. It should be pointed out that the COE systems with SBEβCD and RAMEB were the only ones actually containing the drug in an amorphous/complexed status, as revealed by XRPD analysis. Moreover, the results were in accordance with phase solubility studies, where SBEβCD and RAMEB showed the higher complexing and solubilizing efficiency towards HCT.

Taking into account these results, co-evaporation was selected as the most effective preparation technique and RAMEB as CD that lead to the best drug dissolution profile.

3.3. *Characterization of Drug–NC Binary Systems*

DSC analyses were then performed on HCT binary systems with three different nanoclays (SV, PHC, and VHS) at three different drug:NC *w/w* ratios (1:1, 1:2, and 1:4) in order to find the nanoclay that more strongly interacts with the drug and the most suitable weight ratio between the components. The results, as summarized in Table 2, show evidence that no interaction occurred between HCT and VHS, as indicated by the absence of variations in drug melting peak or enthalpy. Evidently, on the one hand, the typical lamellar stratified structure of VHS, despite having proven to effectively entrap molecules by cation, exchange with the hydrated cations present in its interlayers [10] showed limited interaction with a lipophilic molecule as HCT. On the other hand, the typical fibrous structure of SV and PHC, consisting in hollow nanotubes, seemed to be more suitable to entrap lipophilic drugs. SV proved to have a greater interaction ability towards HCT, raising to the highest reduction in drug crystallinity at the 1:4 *w*/*w* ratio (RDC 37%) as a consequence of its better dispersion into the nanoclay structure. The higher interaction ability of SV than PHC towards HCT probably could be related to the different dimensions of their channels (0.37 × 1.06 nm for SV and 0.37 × 0.64 nm for PHC) [32]. Moreover, these findings were in accordance with those previously obtained with another lipophilic drug, oxaprozin, where SV provided the best results in terms of NC–drug interactions [16].

Table 2. Thermal parameters and % residual drug crystallinity (% RDC) of hydrochlorothiazide (HCT) alone or in the presence of the different examined nanoclays (NCs).

NC Type	HCT:NC Ratio (*w*/*w*)	HCT Melting Peak (°C)	HCT ΔH_{fus}(J/g)	% RDC
- - - -	/	274.4	152.8	100.0
PHC	1:1	274.3	92.0	60.2
PHC	1:2	274.3	77.9	51.0
PHC	1:4	274.1	64.4	42.2
VHS	1:1	274.4	152.6	100.0
VHS	1:2	274.3	152.5	100.0
VHS	1:4	274.2	152.2	100.0
SV	1:1	274.4	84.2	55.1
SV	1:2	270.4	71.9	47.1
SV	1:4	269.2	56.5	37.0

SV was then selected in order to test the effect of different preparation methods and experimental conditions (such as use of solvent, stirring rate, temperature, etc.) on the performance of drug-nanoclay systems. Binary systems at 1:4 *w*/*w* drug:SV ratio were prepared by co-evaporation (COE), co-fusion (COF), co-grinding (GR), solvent-heating (SH), solvent-sonication (SS), and solvent magnetic stirring (SMS) techniques. The products obtained were submitted to DSC analyses and the results are summarized in Table 3 in terms of drug melting temperature and enthalpy and percent of residual drug crystallinity (RDC %).

Table 3. Thermal parameters and % residual drug crystallinity (% RDC) of hydrochlorothiazide (HCT) alone or in the different 1:4 *w*/*w* systems with sepiolite prepared by physical mixing (PM), solvent-sonication (SS), solvent magnetic stirring (SMS), co-grinding (GR), co-fusion (COF), solvent-heating (SH), and co-evaporation (COE).

Batch	Drug Melting Peak (°C)	H_{fus} (J/g)	% RDC
HCT	274.4	152.8	100.0
PM	269.2	56.5	37.0
SS	263.9	28.3	18.5
SMS	262.8	28.2	18.3
GR	260.4	15.4	10.1
COF	274.1	9.9	6.5
SH	274.0	8.2	5.4
COE	/	/	/

Even if all the used techniques gave rise to a marked reduction of intensity of the drug melting peak, with the trend PM < SS = SMS < GR < COF < SH, its complete disappearance was obtained just with the COE.

The XRPD patterns of pure components, PM and COE product are reported in Figure 5. SV showed a typical crystalline pattern clearly recognizable in the PM and still detectable in the COE product with the drug. However, the crystallinity peaks of HCT were well visible in the PM and in the other binary systems (data are reported just for PM as example) while they completely disappeared in the COE product.

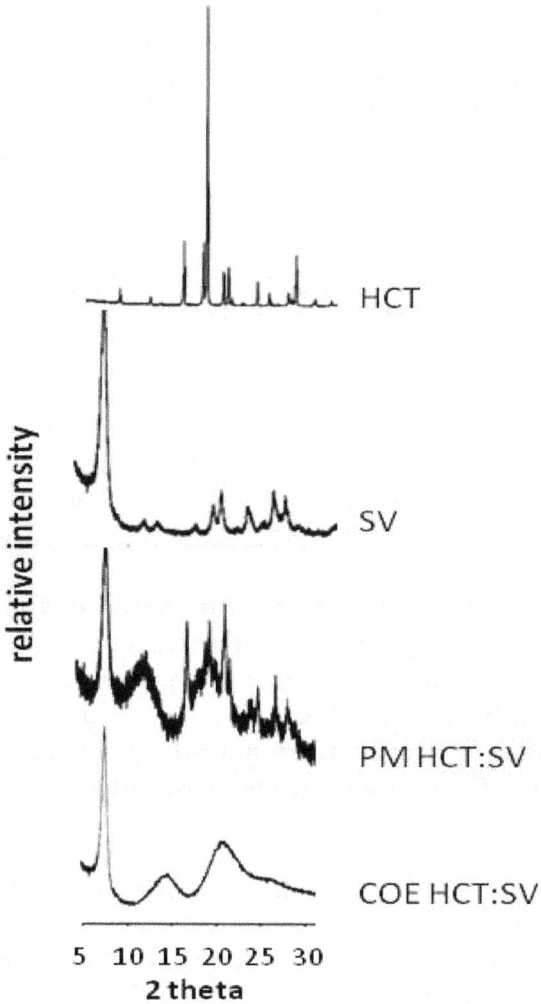

Figure 5. Patterns of HCT, SV, and their 1:4 *w/w* binary systems obtained by physical mixing (PM) and co-evaporation (COE).

On the basis of these results, ternary systems were prepared by physical mixture and co-evaporation with RAMEB (HCT-RAMEB 1:1 molar ratio) and SV (HCT-SV 1:4 *w/w* ratio) and compared with the corresponding binary systems. X-ray diffractograms, performed on ternary PM and COE products confirmed the complete drug amorphization in the COE product, thus, confirming the DSC results.

3.4. Dissolution Rate Studies

The dissolution profiles of binary and ternary PM and COE products with RAMEB and SV are shown in Figure 6.

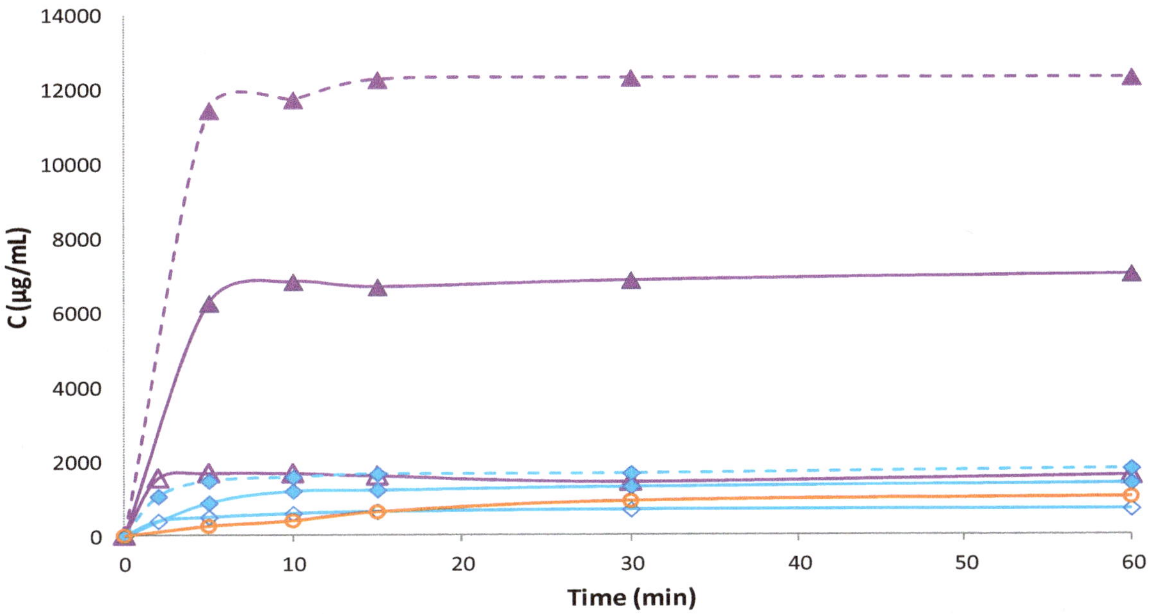

Figure 6. Dissolution profiles of HCT alone (o) and from its binary and ternary systems with RAMEB and SV: Physical mixtures (PM) (blue lines) with RAMEB (♦), SV (◊), and both (♦ dotted line) and co-evaporated (COE) products (violet lines) with RAMEB (▲), SV (Δ), and both (▲ dotted line). Each value represents the mean of 3 experiments.

Binary HCT-SV systems obtained by co-evaporation revealed an increase in drug dissolution rate with respect to pure drug, more evident as compared with the simple PM, probably, due to the complete drug amorphization and its closer dispersion within the NC matrix. However, the dissolution performance of drug-SV systems was considerably worse than the corresponding binary systems with RAMEB, indicating that drug complexation with RAMEB was far more effective than NC entrapment. The simultaneous presence of both carriers in the ternary systems gave rise to a synergistic effect in improving HCT dissolution properties. This was particularly evident in the ternary COE product, which showed about a two-fold increase of the dissolved drug amount after 5 min, with respect to the binary HCT-RAMEB COE system and reached a plateau level of 12.3 ± 0.9 mg/mL. Analogous results have been previously obtained for oxaprozin [16]. However, it is necessary to evidence that, in the case of oxaprozin, the grinding technique with CDs and the cofusion technique with nanoclay resulted in the best technique to improve the drug solubility, whereas in the case of HCT, the best results were obtained with co-evaporation. These findings confirm that the combined use of cyclodextrins and nanoclays, joined with the most appropriate sample preparation technique, can be a successful strategy to strengthen the benefits related to their potential to enhane solubility and dissolution rate of lipophilic drugs. Nevertheless, it is evident that preformulation studies are important in order to find the most appropriate preparation technique.

On the basis of these findings, the HCT-SV-RAMEB COE product was selected for the development of a new tablet formulation.

3.5. Tablet Formulation and Characterization

Compatibility studies performed by DSC analysis demonstrated the complete compatibility between the drug and the selected tablet excipients, as shown in Figure S2 of Supplementary materials. Preliminary studies conducted on the excipients allowed the obtainment of the selected tablet composition. Particularly, it was necessary to bring the binder percentage up to 10% because tablets prepared with a lower content did not pass the friability test. Tablets prepared with COE HCT SV RAMEB were fully characterized according to Ph. Eur. 9th Edition and compared with the marketed product, Esidrex®and the tablet properties in terms of hardness, friability, and disintegration time are summarized in Table 4. The batches demonstrated a good uniformity passing the tests of content (RDS < 1%), diameter (RSD < 0.3%), thickness (RSD < 1%) and weight (RSD < 3%), and uniformity. As reported, the new tablets showed higher hardness and higher disintegration time than the commercial ones, but they were within the limits of the values imposed by the Ph. Eur. 9th Edition for uncoated tablets (15 min). The SV presence was fundamental to the improvement of the powder compactability and the obtainment of tablets with acceptable hardness and low friability properties, thus, demonstrating its suitability for direct compression.

Table 4. Technological properties of the new tablet formulation and of the commercial reference tablet.

Tablet	Drug Content (%)	Diameter (cm)	Thickness (cm)	Weight (mg)	Hardness (N)	Friability (%)	Disintegration Time (min)
Esidrex®	98.5 ± 0.5	0.7 ± 0.0	0.25 ± 0.02	139.3 ± 1.9	4.0 ± 0.2	0.00 ± 0.00	6.0 ± 0.1
New tablet	99.2 ± 0.8	1.3 ± 0.0	0.20 ± 0.01	384.6 ± 0.5	6.6 ± 0.3	0.63 ± 0.01	13.0 ± 0.5

Dissolution studies were performed using the dispersed amount method with an excess drug amount in order to evidence the effectiveness of our formulation. As shown in Figure 7, the results clearly demonstrated the better dissolution profile of the new tablet that reached the 100% of dissolved drug within 60 min vs. about the 40% obtained with the commercial tablet.

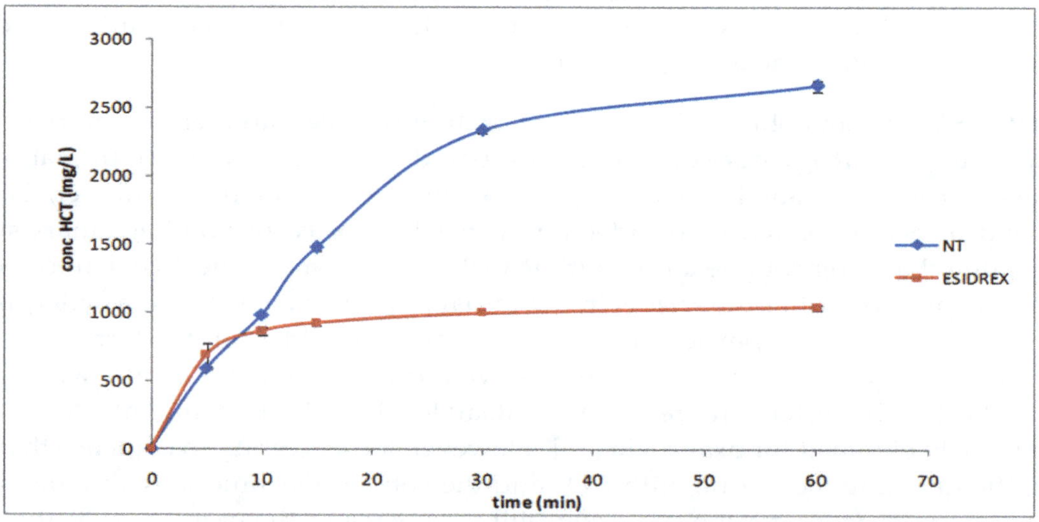

Figure 7. Dissolution profiles of HCT from the new tablet formulation and from the marketed tablet. The results proved the maintenance of the synergistic effect of NC and CD in improving the dissolution behavior also in the tablet formulation. Each value represents the mean of 3 measurements.

An improved drug bioavailability can be reasonably expected as a consequence of the increased drug solubility and dissolution rate. Moreover, the permeation enhancer properties of cyclodextrins, included methyl βCD derivatives, are well documented [33–35]. In particular, other authors observed an increased HCT permeability in the presence of βCD, by performing experiments on non-everted intestinal sac model [9]. Further in vivo studies have been planned in order to demonstrate the actual improvement of therapeutic efficacy of the new tablet formulation.

4. Conclusions

An exhaustive study of the interactions between HCT and several kinds of cyclodextrins, in combination with different preparation methods for binary systems resulted in the selection of the COE product with RAMEB as the most appropriate to improve drug dissolution properties, as a result of the best complexing-solubilizing ability of such CD and the complete drug amorphization achieved by co-evaporation in its presence. Solid-state studies of HCT in mixtures with three types of NCs at different w/w ratios led to the choice of SV at the 1:4 *w/w* ratio as the best for establishing effective interactions with the drug. Among the different techniques used for HCT:SV binary systems preparation, the co-evaporation showed the greater ability to improve drug amorphization and dissolution.

Ternary systems prepared by co-evaporation with both selected carriers, evidenced a synergistic effect of CD and NC in enhancing drug dissolution properties, giving a two-fold and a 12-fold increase in drug solubility as compared with the binary HCT-RAMEB COE product and the pure drug, respectively, thus confirming the great potential of such a combined approach.

Tablets prepared with the selected ternary systems clearly showed a better dissolution profile as compared with a marketed formulation, with an approximate 60% increase of the drug amount dissolved at 60 min. Therefore, the new tablets give proof of their ability to strongly improve the HCT dissolution properties, thus, increasing the amount of drug available for oral absorption.

Author Contributions: Conceptualization, P.M.; methodology, F.G.-V.; software, A.B.-S.; validation, F.G.-V. and A.B.-S.; formal analysis, M.C. and A.B.-S.; investigation, F.M. and A.B.-S.; resources, P.M., C.V.I.; data curation, F.M., M.C. and F.G.-V.; writing—original draft preparation, F.M. and M.C.; writing—review and editing, P.M.; visualization, M.C., F.M.; supervision, C.V.I.; project administration, C.V.I. All authors have read and agreed to the published version of the manuscript.

References

1. Musini, V.M.; Nazer, M.; Bassett, K.; Wright, J.M. Blood pressure-lowering efficacy of monotherapy with thiazide diuretics for primary hypertension. *Cochrane Database Syst. Rev.* **2014**, *29*, 003824. [CrossRef] [PubMed]
2. Amidon, G.L.; Lennernas, H.; Shah, V.P.; Crison, J.R. A theoretical basis for a biopharmaceutic drug classification: The correlation of in vitro drug product dissolution and in vivo bioavailability. *Pharm. Res.* **1995**, *12*, 413–420. [CrossRef] [PubMed]
3. Sanphui, P.; Devi, V.K.; Clara, D.; Malviya, N.; Ganguly, S.; Desiraju, G.R. Cocrystals of hydrochlorothiazide: Solubility and diffusion/permeability enhancements through drug–coformer interactions. *Mol. Pharm.* **2015**, *12*, 1615–1622. [CrossRef] [PubMed]
4. Mahajan, A.A.; Thaker, A.K.; Mohanraj, K. LC, LC-MS/MS studies for the identification and characterization of degradation products of hydrochlorothiazide and establishment of mechanistic approach towards degradation. *J. Braz. Chem. Soc.* **2012**, *23*, 445–452. [CrossRef]
5. Uekama, K.; Hirayama, F.; Tetsumi, I. Cyclodextrin drug carrier systems. *Chem. Rev.* **1998**, *98*, 2045–2076. [CrossRef]
6. Lovatti Alves, Q.; Barbosa Camargo, S.; Leonne Cruz de Jesus, R.; Flávia Silva, D. Drugs–β-Cyclodextrin inclusion complex: Would be a new strategy to improve Antihypertensive Therapy? *Clin. Res. Trials* **2019**, *5*, 1–3. [CrossRef]
7. Loftsson, T.; Duchêne, D. Cyclodextrins and their therapeutic applications. *Int. J. Pharm.* **1998**, *329*, 1–11. [CrossRef]
8. Mendes, C.; Buttchevitz, A.; Kruger, J.H.; Kratz, J.M.; Simões, C.M.; de Oliveira Benedet, P.; Oliveira, P.R.; Silva, M.A. "Inclusion complexes of hydrochlorothiazide and β-cyclodextrin: Physicochemical characteristics, in vitro and in vivo studies. *Eur. J. Pharm. Sci.* **2016**, *83*, 71–78. [CrossRef]
9. Altamimi, M.A.; Elzayat, E.M.; Alhowyan, A.A.; Alshehri, S.; Shakeel, F. Effect of β-cyclodextrin and different surfactants on solubility, stability, and permeability of hydrochlorothiazide. *J. Mol. Liquids* **2018**, *250*, 323–328. [CrossRef]
10. Aguzzi, C.; Cerezo, P.; Viseras, C.; Caramella, C. Use of clays as drug delivery systems: Possibilities and limitations. *Appl. Clay Sci.* **2007**, *36*, 22–36. [CrossRef]

11. Viseras, C.; Cerezo, P.; Sanchez, R.; Salcedo, I.; Aguzzi, C. Current challenges in clay minerals for drug delivery. *Appl. Clay Sci.* **2010**, *48*, 291–295. [CrossRef]
12. Kinnari, P.; Mäkiläb, E.; Heikkiläb, T.; Salonen, J.; Hirvonen, J.; Santos, H.A. Comparison of mesoporous silicon and non-ordered mesoporous silica materials as drug carriers for itraconazole. *Int. J. Pharm.* **2011**, *414*, 148–156. [CrossRef] [PubMed]
13. Mura, P.; Valleri, M.; Fabianelli, E.; Maestrelli, F.; Cirri, M. Characterization and evaluation of different mesoporous silica kinds as carriers for the development of effective oral dosage forms of glibenclamide. *Int. J. Pharm.* **2019**, *563*, 43–52. [CrossRef] [PubMed]
14. Leane, M.; Pitt, K.; Reynolds, G. The Manufacturing Classification System (MCS) Working Group. A proposal for a drug product Manufacturing Classification System (MCS) for oral solid dosage forms. *Pharm. Dev. Technol.* **2015**, *20*, 12–21. [CrossRef]
15. Conceição, J.; Adeoye, O.; Cabral-Marques, H.M.; Sousa Lobo, J.M. Cyclodextrins as excipients in tablet formulations. *Drug Discov. Today* **2018**, *23*, 1274–1284. [CrossRef]
16. Mura, P.; Maestrelli, F.; Aguzzi, C.; Viseras, C. Hybrid systems based on "drug—in cyclodextrin—in nanoclays" for improving oxaprozin dissolution properties. *Int. J. Pharm.* **2016**, *509*, 8–15. [CrossRef]
17. Maestrelli, F.; Mura, P.; Cirri, M.; Mennini, N.; Ghelardini, C.; Di Cesare Mannelli, L. Development and characterization of fast dissolving tablets of oxaprozin based on hybrid systems of the drug with cyclodextrins and nanoclays. *Int. J. Pharm.* **2017**, *531*, 640–649. [CrossRef]
18. Higuchi, T.; Connors, K.A. Phase-solubility techniques. *Adv. Anal. Chem. Instr.* **1965**, *4*, 117–212.
19. Saokham, P.; Muankaew, C.; Jansook, P.; Loftsson, T. Solubility of Cyclodextrins and Drug/Cyclodextrin Complexes. *Molecules* **2018**, *23*. [CrossRef]
20. Sareen, S.; Mathew, G.; Joseph, L. Improvement in solubility of poor water-soluble drugs by solid dispersion. *Int. J. Pharm. Investig.* **2012**, *2*, 2–17. [CrossRef]
21. Sridhar, I.; Doshi, A.; Joshi, B.; Wankhede, V.; Doshi, J. Solid Dispersions: An approach to enhance solubility of poorly water soluble drug. *Int. J. Sci. Innov. Res.* **2013**, *2*, 685–694.
22. Yendluri, R.; Otto, D.P.; De Villiers, M.M.; Vinokurovc, V.; Lvova, Y.M. Application of halloysite clay nanotubes as a pharmaceutical excipient. *Int. J. Pharm.* **2017**, *521*, 267–273. [CrossRef]
23. Yendluri, R.; Lvov, Y.; De Villiers, M.M.; Vinokurov, V.; Naumenko, E.; Tarasova, E.; Fakhrullin, R. Paclitaxel Encapsulated in Halloysite Clay Nanotubes for Intestinal and Intracellular Delivery. *J. Pharm. Sci.* **2017**, *106*, 3131–3139. [CrossRef] [PubMed]
24. Lun, H.; Ouyang, J.; Yang, H. Natural halloysite nanotubes modified as aspirin carrier. *RSC Adv.* **2014**, *83*, 83. [CrossRef]
25. Onnainty, R.; Shenfeld, E.M.; Quevedo, M.A.; Fernández, M.A.; Longhi, M.R.; Granero, G.E. Characterization of the Hydrochlorothiazide: β-cyclodextrin inclusion complex. Experimental and theoretical methods. *J. Phys. Chem. B* **2013**, *117*, 206–217. [CrossRef]
26. Mennini, N.; Bragagni, M.; Maestrelli, F.; Mura, P. Physico-chemical characterization in solution and in the solid state of clonazepam complexes with native and chemically-modified cyclodextrins. *J. Pharm. Biom. Anal.* **2014**, *89*, 142–149. [CrossRef]
27. Pires, M.A.; Souza dos Santos, R.A.S.; Sinisterra, R.D. Pharmaceutical Composition of Hydrochlorothiazide: β-Cyclodextrin: Preparation by Three Different Methods, Physico-Chemical Characterization and In Vivo Diuretic Activity Evaluation. *Molecules* **2011**, *16*, 4482–4499. [CrossRef]
28. Hădărugă, D.I.; Birău (Mitroi), C.L.; Gruia, A.T.; Păunescu, V.; Geza, N.B.; Hădărugă, N.G. Moisture evaluation of β-cyclodextrin/fish oils complexes by thermal analyses: A data review on common barbel (Barbus barbus L.), Pontic shad (Alosa immaculata Bennett), European wels catfish (Silurus glanis L.), and common bleak (Alburnusalb L.) living in Danube river. *Food Chem.* **2017**, *236*, 49–58.
29. Boldescu, V.; Bratu, I.; Borodi, G.; Kacso, I.; Bende, A.; Duca, G.; Macaev, F.; Pogrebnoi, S.; Ribkovskaia, Z. Study of binary systems of β -cyclodextrin with a highly potential anti-mycobacterial drug. *J. Incl. Phenom. Macrocycl. Chem.* **2012**, *74*, 129–135. [CrossRef]
30. Cirri, M.; Mennini, N.; Maestrelli, F.; Mura, P.; Ghelardini, C.; Di Cesare Mannelli, L. Development and in vivo evaluation of an innovative "Hydrochlorothiazide-in Cyclodextrins-in Solid Lipid Nanoparticles" formulation with sustained release and enhanced oral bioavailability for potential hypertension treatment in pediatrics. *Int. J. Pharm.* **2017**, *521*, 73–83. [CrossRef]

31. Mura, P. Analytical techniques for characterization of cyclodextrin complexes in the solid state: A review. *J. Pharm. Biomed. Anal.* **2015**, *113*, 226–238. [CrossRef] [PubMed]
32. Viseras, C.; Aguzzi, C.; Cerezo, P. Medical and health applications of natural mineral nanotubes. In *Natural Mineral Nanotubes*; Apple Academic Press, Inc.: Palm Bay, FL, USA, 2015.
33. Schipper, N.G.M.; Romeijn, S.G.; Verhoef, J.C.; Merkus, F.W.H.M. Nasal insulin delivery with dimethyl-β-cyclodextrin as an absorption enhancer in rabbits: Powder more effective than liquid formulations. *Pharm. Res.* **1993**, *5*, 682–686. [CrossRef] [PubMed]
34. Schoch, C.; Bizec, J.C.; Kis, G. Cyclodextrin derivatives and cyclofructan as ocular permeation enhancers. *J. Incl. Phenom. Macrocycl. Chem.* **2007**, *57*, 391–394. [CrossRef]
35. Kurkov, S.V.; Loftsson, T. Cyclodextrins. *Int. J. Pharm.* **2013**, *453*, 167–180. [CrossRef] [PubMed]

6

Praziquantel–Clays as Accelerated Release Systems to Enhance the Low Solubility of the Drug

Ana Borrego-Sánchez [1,2,*], Rita Sánchez-Espejo [1], Fátima García-Villén [2], César Viseras [2] and C. Ignacio Sainz-Díaz [1]

1 Instituto Andaluz de Ciencias de la Tierra, CSIC-University of Granada, Av. de las Palmeras 4, 18100 Granada, Spain; ritase@correo.ugr.es (R.S.-E.); ignacio.sainz@iact.ugr-csic.es (C.I.S.-D.)

2 Department of Pharmacy and Pharmaceutical Technology, Faculty of Pharmacy, University of Granada, Campus de Cartuja s/n, 18071 Granada, Spain; fgarvillen@ugr.es (F.G.-V.); cviseras@ugr.es (C.V.)

* Correspondence: anaborrego@iact.ugr-csic.es

Abstract: Praziquantel is an antiparasitic drug indicated for the treatment of the schistosomiasis disease. This drug has very low aqueous solubility, requiring high oral doses for its administration which gives rise to side effects, therapeutic noncompliance and the appearance of resistant forms of the parasite. Clay minerals, like sepiolite and montmorillonite, are innocuous, non-toxic, biocompatible and low-cost excipients. Additionally, clays have high adsorbent properties that allow them to encapsulate drugs in nanometric spaces present in the channels in the case of the sepiolite or between the layers in the case of the montmorillonite. The interactions between the drug and clay minerals are studied experimentally with the strategy for preparing interactions products in organic solvents (ethanol, acetonitrile and dichloromethane) so that the interaction will be more effective and will be enhanced the aqueous solubility of praziquantel. The results showed that in the interaction products, the drug interacted with both clay minerals, which produced the loss of the crystallinity of the drug demonstrated by different techniques. This led to a significant increase in the dissolution rate of the praziquantel in all the interaction products in the simulated gastrointestinal tract media, except for the praziquantel–montmorillonite product prepared in dichloromethane that presented a controlled release in acid medium. Moreover, in vitro cytotoxicity and cell cycle studies were performed in the interaction products prepared with ethanol. The interaction product with sepiolite was biocompatible with the HTC116 line cells, and it did not produce alterations in the cell cycle. However, interaction products with montmorillonite did not produce cell death, but they showed affectation and damage of cells in the cell cycle study at the highest concentration tested (20–100 μM). Therefore, the different organic solvents used are adequate for the improvement of the biopharmaceutical profile of praziquantel. Drug–clay interaction products, specifically with sepiolite, showed very promising results in which new accelerated oral release systems of the praziquantel were obtained.

Keywords: praziquantel; drug; montmorillonite; sepiolite; organic solvents; in vitro dissolution tests; cytotoxicity

---

1. Introduction

Neglected tropical diseases are infectious diseases that affect a sixth of the world population, more than a billion people, mainly in poor populations of tropical countries in Africa, Latin America, Asia and the Middle East. Their prevalence increases with the absence of salubrious water and adequate sanitation conditions and the most vulnerable population are children in contact with contaminated water [1].

Schistosomiasis is the second neglected tropical disease with the highest prevalence, widespread mainly in tropical Africa. Therefore, the improvement of the existing treatment with the praziquantel

(PZQ) drug is very important for saving lives. Since schistosomiasis is in the expansion phase and currently affects 240 million people in the world, of which only 88 million receive adequate treatment, it is estimated that it produces more than 200,000 deaths annually, and it is extended in 78 countries around the world, mainly in the tropical and subtropical region, being in Africa the second most prevalent disease in children. This disease is acquired by contact with fresh water infested with larvae of the parasite [2–5].

PZQ is the recommended treatment against all forms of schistosomiasis. It has high efficacy, low toxicity and is administered orally. In addition, the cost of production and sale of PZQ is low [2,6]. However, it has a few disadvantages. First, it is a racemic compound, with only one of its enantiomers being pharmacologically active [7,8]. In addition, it is a Class II drug of the Biopharmaceutical Classification System (BCS) and has very low aqueous solubility and high permeability, so that the dissolution is the factor limiting the rate of absorption [9–11]. Its low solubility in water makes it necessary to administer high oral doses, which gives rise to secondary effects that increase the therapeutic noncompliance and favor the appearance of resistant forms of the parasite. For these reasons, the use of low-cost natural inorganic excipients was proposed as a starting hypothesis to improve the aqueous solution profile of the PZQ, maintaining the final cost of the drug, which is very important given the population to which it is subject destined.

Montmorillonite and sepiolite are innocuous, non-toxic, biocompatible and low-cost clay minerals. Additionally, clays have high adsorbent properties that allow them to encapsulate drugs in nanometric spaces present between the layers in the case of the montmorillonite or in the channels in the case of the sepiolite [12–17].

The interaction between PZQ and other excipients was also studied in order to improve the low solubility of the drug, for example, with calcium carbonate [18–20], β-cyclodextrins [21–23], polyvinyl-pyrrolidone [24,25], polyethylene glycols [26–28], sodium starch glycolate [29], phosphatidylcholine–containing liposomes [30], layered double hydroxides [31], among others. Specifically, the interaction between PZQ and montmorillonite in aqueous medium was previously studied, although no improvements of in vitro dissolution and absorption rates were observed [32]. The lack of relevant biopharmaceutical improvements was explained by the absence of PZQ in the interlayer space of montmorillonite. Water molecules present in the clay interlayer space would be blocking the entrance of the drug, thus PZQ would be solely absorbed in the external surface of montmorillonite. Therefore, in our previous studies [33,34], the interactions between PZQ and montmorillonite and sepiolite in absence of water were studied as a strategy for enhancing the aqueous solubility of the drug. To do this, ethanol 99% (*v*/*v*) was used as a solvent increasing the interaction between the drug and the excipient. The results showed a great increase in the dissolution rate of the drug and the total amount of drug dissolved in vitro in the interaction products, due to the high interaction between both components. Therefore, this new procedure was found to be an effective strategy to improve the biopharmaceutical profile of the PZQ.

Hence, in this work, the preparation of interaction products is studied following the previously described procedure [33,34] comparing the use of different organic solvents, like ethanol, acetonitrile and dichloromethane. The aim is to prepare and characterize these systems and, by these means, to determine the potential influence of the organic solvent on the release and solubility of the drug. In particular, the results were compared with those obtained with ethanol in which a significant improvement in the biopharmaceutical profile was described. As well as this, in vitro cytotoxicity and cell cycle studies are carried out for checking if these systems are biocompatible and suitable for human use.

2. Materials and Methods

2.1. Materials

Pristine racemic PZQ drug was purchased from Sigma Aldrich (St. Louis, MO, USA). Purified pharmaceutical degree. Montmorillonite (Veegum HS®, VHS, Norwalk, CT, USA) was purchased from Vanderbilt Company (Norwalk, CT, USA). The Sepiolite samples from Vicálvaro (Madrid) (SEP) were kindly gifted by TOLSA (Madrid, Spain). Ethanol of 99% (*v*/*v*) of purity, acetonitrile, and dichloromethane were used as solvents.

2.2. Methods

2.2.1. Preparation of Praziquantel–Clay Minerals Interaction Products

PZQ was put in contact with montmorillonite and sepiolite clay powders in 100 mL of different solvents: ethanol 99% (*v*/*v*), acetonitrile, and dichloromethane, in such way that the clay/drug ratio was 5:1 *w*/*w*. The dispersion was put into magnetic stirring for 24 h at room temperature. After 24 h, the solvent was evaporated at 40 °C using a rotary evaporator (Buchi® R II, Flawil, Switzerland). The solid residue was stored in a desiccator at room temperature with freshly activated silica-gel grafted with a moisture indicator of Co salt.

The interaction products obtained were: PZQ–VHSet prepared with VHS and dispersed in ethanol, PZQ–VHSac prepared with VHS and dispersed in acetonitrile, PZQ–VHSdic prepared with VHS and dispersed in dichloromethane, PZQ–SEPet prepared with SEP and dispersed in ethanol, PZQ–SEPac prepared with SEP and dispersed in acetonitrile and PZQ–SEPdic prepared with SEP and dispersed in dichloromethane.

2.2.2. X-ray Diffraction

Powder X-ray diffraction was performed with equipment of Panalytical X'Pert Pro (Marvel Panalytical, Madrid, Spain) model, which is managed by a fully computerized system. It also has an automatic charger system and uses the X'Celerator detector (Marvel Panalytical) (linear type, detects the RX along a line) with the Cu Kα wavelength that allows a quick and accurate study. The information of diffraction was analyzed using X'Pert HighScore® software (Version 2.2., Marvel Panalytical, Madrid, Spain).

2.2.3. Thermal Analysis

Differential Scanning Calorimetric analysis (DSC) and Thermogravimetric Analysis (TGA) were performed with a Mettler Toledo mod. TGA/DSC1 calorimeter (Mettler Toledo, Barcelona, Spain). The TGA equipment sensor is a thermostatic microbalance with an accuracy of 0.1 µg, which is the limit established for weighing precision. On the other hand, the TGA/DSC1 has sensors that obtain the DSC signal directly and in real-time.

The TGA was performed in air using a heating rate of 10 °C/min in the 30–400 °C temperature range and the DSC runs were performed with a heating rate of 2 °C/min and nitrogen was used as a purge gas in DSC under the flow of 15 mL/min.

2.2.4. Fourier Transform Infrared (FTIR) Spectroscopy

FTIR spectra were performed with the JASCO 6200 spectrophotometer (JASCO, Pfungstadt, Germany) which has an attenuated total reflectance (ATR) accessory. Measurements were performed in the range 4000–600 cm^{-1} with a 0.5 cm^{-1} resolution and a well-plate sampler. The results were analyzed using the Spectra Manager II software (Version 2, JASCO).

2.2.5. In Vitro Release Studies

In vitro dissolution tests were performed according to the European Pharmacopoeia procedures dealing with solid oral dosage forms. In particular, the paddle apparatus (apparatus 2, Sotax AT7, Teknokroma®, Barcelona, Spain) with sinkers was set at 150 rpm and 37 °C, filled with 1 L of dissolution medium and working at sink conditions. Stomach physiological fluid was simulated by using a dissolution medium composed of HCl 0.001 M, while simulated intestinal fluid (SIF) was used with a phosphate buffer (pH = 6.8) without enzymes.

Hard gelatin capsules were subjected to the in vitro dissolution test. The capsules were prepared with 210 mg of each PZQ–VHS and PZQ–SEP interaction product, in which 35 mg corresponds to PZQ. Each of these interaction products (PZQ–VHS and PZQ–SEP) were prepared with the different solvents previously explained. Similarly, hard gelatin capsules containing 35 mg of PZQ were elaborated as reference.

During the in vitro dissolution tests, at predetermined time intervals, 5 mL of samples were withdrawn, the volume immediately replenished with fresh dissolution medium. The drug amount was quantified by High-Performance Liquid Chromatography (HPLC) after being filtered through 0.45 μm nitrocellulose membranes (Merck-Millipore®, Darmstadt, Germany). HPLC was performed in a 1260 Infinity II HPLC (Agilent Technologies Inc., Santa Clara, CA, USA) equipped with a quaternary pump, autosampler, column oven and UV-VIS diode-array spectrophotometer. The stationary phase was a Lichrospher® (100 RP-18, C18, 5 μm, 15 cm × 3.2 mm) column (Merck Millipore®, Darmstadt, Germany). Isocratic conditions were used, the mobile phase formed by a mixture of H_2O and CH_3CN (35:65 *v*/*v*). The flow rate was set at 0.8 mL/min with a sample injection volume of 10 μL. PZQ was detected at 225 nm during the 5 min of the run time of the HPLC analysis. The software LC Open LAB HPLC 1260 (Agilent Technologies Inc.) was used to record and treat the chromatograms. The linear analytical method was obtained in the concentration range of 5 to 100 mg/L of PZQ in both dissolution media (correlation coefficients of 1 in both HCl 0.001 M and in SIF).

Subsequently, release data fitting was performed using kinetic models intended to describe the drug release from immediate or modified dosage forms [35–37]. These models, such as zero order, first order, cube root, Higuchi, Peppas, and Weibull, were used to fit experimental data obtained from in vitro dissolution studies. The fitting was carried out linearizing the equations. The choice of the best model to describe the dissolution/release process of the drug was based on the correlation coefficient (R^2) criterium. A second evaluation criterium that is frequently used is called the Akaike Information Criterion (AIC) [38,39]. Herein, it is also considered.

2.2.6. Solubility Studies

The solubility of PZQ, PZQ–VHSet and PZQ–SEPet, which was used as a reference for the rest of the interaction products, were obtained in both HCl 0.001 M and SIF (phosphate buffer at pH = 6.8, without enzymes). PZQ solubility was obtained by placing 30 mg of drug in 10 mL of HCl and SIF (supersaturated conditions). The solution was stirred at 37 °C for 24 h (thermostatic bath). Then, the solution was centrifuged, the supernatant filtered (nitrocellulose membranes, 0.45 μm, Merck Millipore®) and quantified by HPLC (Agilent Techonologies Inc.). The amount of dissolved drug, determined by the chromatography, corresponds to PZQ solubility in the corresponding medium. In order to demonstrate the solubility improvement of PZQ in the composites (PZQ–VHSet and PZQ–SEPet), drug solubility was determined with the very same procedure. Triplicate experiments were performed in all samples.

2.2.7. Cell Culture

Cellular viability and cell cycle profiles were studied over a human colorectal carcinoma cell line HCT 116 (ATCC® CCL-247™, Manassas, VA, USA). HCT 116 cells were cultured in Dulbecco's Modified Eagle's Medium (DMEM, Gibco™, Dublin, Ireland) supplemented with 10% *w*/*w* of Fetal

Bovine Serum (FBS, Gibco™, Dublin, Ireland), 1% of Glutamax (BioWhittaker®, Cologne, Germany) and 1% of penicillin/streptomycin (BioWhittaker®). Cells were cultured in an incubator set at 37 °C and 5% of CO_2.

2.2.8. Cytotoxicity Studies

Cytotoxicity studies of PZQ, VHS and SEP were performed by using PZQ veterinary antiparasitic doses. Consequently, the amount of mineral (VHS and SEP) that should be subjected to study was five times higher than that of PZQ. To do so, intermediate dilutions of 100 mM and 10 mM were prepared in dimethyl sulfoxide (DMSO). The same procedure and concentrations were used for cytotoxicity studies of PZQ–VHSet and PZQ–SEPet.

AlamarBlue™ bioassay (Thermo Fisher Scientific, Carlsbad, CA, USA) was used to study cell proliferation. To do so, HCT 116 cells were seeded in 96-well plates (density of 3–6 × 10^4 cells/cm^2) in a final DMEM volume of 200 μL. The corresponding solid samples were subsequently added (PZQ, VHS, SEP, IP PZQ–VHSet, or IP PZQ–SEPet). All samples were tested in a wide range of concentrations (100 μM, 20 μM, 4 μM, 800 nM, 160 nM, 32 nM, and 6.4 nM) and three replicates were used for each experience. Then, the well plates were incubated at 37 °C, 5% CO_2 for 48 h. At the end of contact time, 10 μL of cell viability reagent (PrestoBlue™, Thermo Fisher Scientific) was added to each well. The PrestoBlue™ reagent is a resazurin compound that works as a cellular viability indicator since its color changes from blue to pink when reduced by living cells. After 15 min of incubation in presence of PrestoBlue™ reagent, fluorescence was quantified at 535–90 nm in a microplate reader (Tecan, Zürich, Switzerland).

2.2.9. Cell Cycle Studies

HCT 116 cells were cultured in 24 well-plates (250,000 cells/well) in a final DMEM volume of 500 μL. In these conditions, cells were subjected to PZQ, VHS, SEP, IP PZQ–VHSet, and IP PZQ–SEPet samples for 48 h. Increasing concentrations of each sample (0.8 μM, 4 μM, 20 μM, and 100 μM) were used. Cells entering the apoptotic or necrotic cycle were detected with a propidium iodide staining procedure, as explained in a previous protocol [40]. Briefly, once the cells were in contact with each sample, they were collected and washed with 2 mL of phosphate-buffered saline (PBS) at 4 °C and subsequently fixed with ethanol 70° (V_f = 1 mL, diluted 1:9 in PBS) for 5 min, while maintained on ice. Ethanol was withdrawn and fixed cells were washed with PBS. Then, they were resuspended in a solution consisting of 250 μL of PBS and 250 μL of a DNA extraction solution (0.2 M Na_2HPO_4, 0.1 M $C_6H_8O_7$, pH 7.8) for 10 min at 37 °C. Then, the supernatant removed and 200 μL of the staining solution were added (8 μL propidium iodide (1 mg/mL) and 2 μL RNAse 100 (μg/mL)), the cells further incubated in the dark at 37 °C for 10 min. A FACScalibur cytometer (Becton Dickinson and Co., Franklin Lakes, NJ, USA) was used to measure the fluorescence (FL2 detector). Sub-G1 cells (dead cells, that is, cells that entered either necrotic or apoptotic phases) were detected by the Cell Quest software (Version 1.0.2, BD, Biosciences, Franklin Lakes, NJ, USA).

3. Results

3.1. X-ray Diffraction

The interaction products were prepared following the methodology described above in drug–clay. These materials and raw materials were characterized by powder XRD, showing the results in Figure 1. PZQ drug revealed the most intense reflection at around 16.5° (2θ units) and other intense reflections at approximately 8.0°, 19.1° and 23.3° (2θ units) in accordance with that previously reported [41].

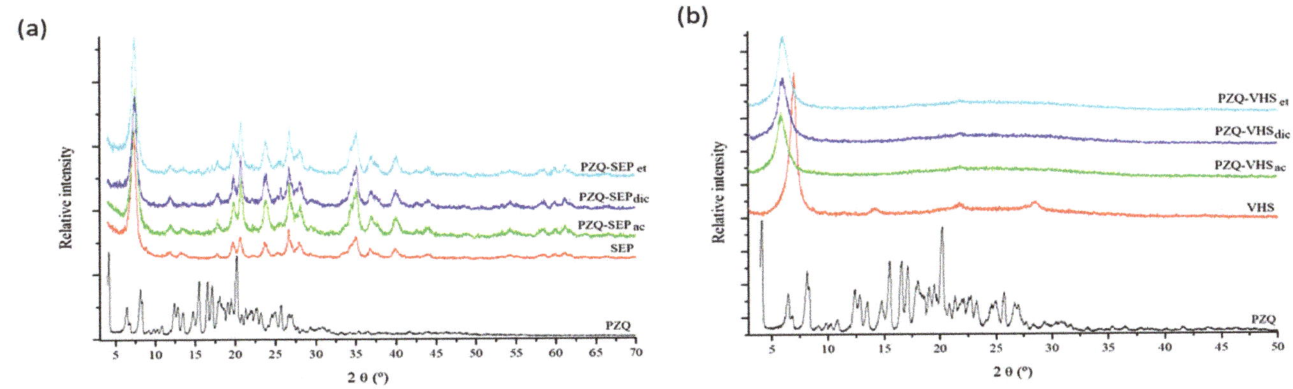

Figure 1. XRPD patterns of the studied samples with sepiolite (**a**) and montmorillonite (**b**).

After interaction with the clay minerals, a practically complete absence of drug reflection was observed, probably due to a loss of crystallinity of PZQ (Figure 1). In previous works, similar behavior of PZQ was observed in the formation of a solid dispersion with polyvinylpyrrolidone [24], with sodium starch glycolate [29], and with glycyrrhizic acid–forming micelles [42].

The interaction product of PZQ with sepiolite using different solvents in the preparation method (Figure 1a) showed an XRD pattern similar in all the cases. In the profiles, clear peaks of the PZQ drug were not observed; only the peaks of sepiolite were observed. Therefore, after the interaction, a loss of drug crystallinity was found.

In the oriented aggregate powder X–ray diffraction pattern of the interaction products of PZQ with montmorillonite (Figure 1b), the peaks of PZQ were not observed either in any of the products. However, the (001) reflection peak of the VHS increased in the interaction products, confirming the intercalation and the presence of PZQ in the interlayer space of the clay.

The interaction product PZQ–VHSet showed an increase in the interlayer space of montmorillonite from 1.26 nm to $d(001)$ = 1.50–1.61 nm in accordance with that reported previously [33,43]. The interaction product PZQ–VHSdic increased to $d(001)$ = 1.47 nm; and the spacing of PZQ–VHSac increased to $d(001)$ = 1.51 nm (Figure 1b). These results corroborated that the PZQ is present in the interaction products and the peaks of PZQ were not observed probably due to the complete intercalation of the drug in the interlayer space of the clay and the loss of crystallinity of the drug. The PZQ molecules intercalate in the confined space of montmorillonite as individual molecules where no recrystallization is possible. Nevertheless, the $d(001)$ reflection peaks are wider in the interaction products than in the pristine VHS. This indicates than a range of different $d(001)$ spacings can be produced, especially in PZQ–VHSdic, where two peaks can be distinguished. In previous modeling studies, we observed the formation of a monolayer of PZQ in the interlayer space of VHS, where different densities of the drug can be found and several conformations of the adsorbate molecule can happen [44]. These differences can be responsible for the variation of $d(001)$ spacing widening this (001) peak, maintaining the monolayer configuration.

3.2. Thermal Analysis

The DSC profiles of the pristine PZQ showed a strong endothermic peak at 144 °C, according to previous work [18] (Figure 2). The DSC profile of SEP and VHS indicated broad endothermic peaks in the range 50–90 °C due to the evaporation of water (Figure 2).

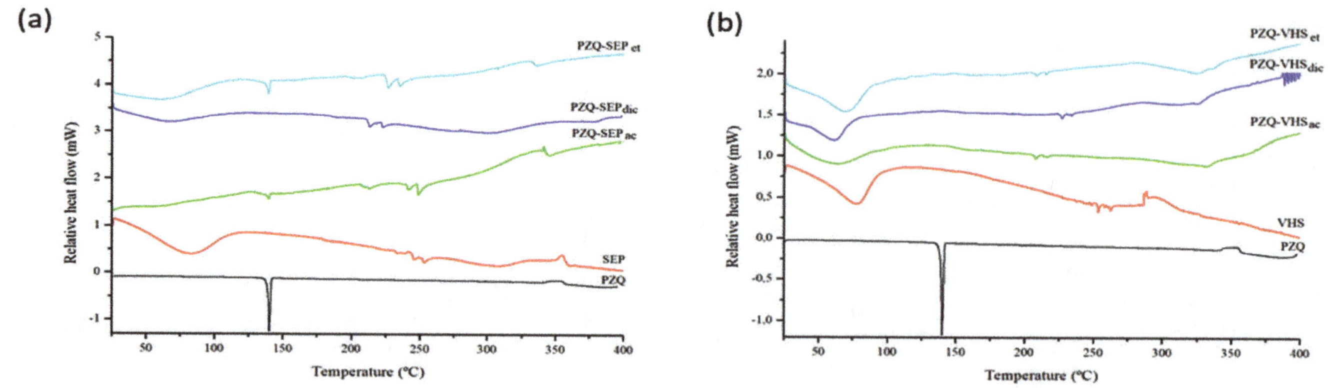

Figure 2. Differential Scanning Calorimetric (DSC) profiles of sepiolite and interaction products of sepiolite (**a**) and montmorillonite and interactions products of montmorillonite (**b**).

In Figure 2a, the PZQ–SEPet and PZQ–SEPac interaction product profiles presented a very low-intensity peak corresponding to the melting of the drug. This indicates that a small amount of PZQ crystallized outside of the channels in the interstitial spaces of solid. Specifically, the enthalpy of the endothermic peak (ΔH) at 144 °C was 3.9 and 1.3 J g^{-1} respectively, which can be compared with the enthalpy of 90.4 J g^{-1} of the melting peak of the pristine drug. Therefore, the ΔH melting (PZQ–SEP)/ΔH melting (pure PZQ), was 4.3% in PZQ–SEPet and 1.4% in PZQ–SEPac. On the contrary, in the PZQ–SEPdic profile, the complete disappearance of the melting peak of the drug was observed.

The DSC curves of PZQ–VHS interaction products showed the water evaporation of the raw materials until 100 °C, and no melting peak of PZQ was observed in all interaction products (PZQ–VHSet, PZQ–VHSdic and PZQ–VHSac) (Figure 2b).

Therefore, the lack of the peak of PZQ in the interaction products was observed probably due to the amorphization and no recrystallization of the drug after the complete interaction with the clay. This justified the lack of drug reflections in the PZQ–clay powder XRD patterns. Previous studies found similar results [21,31,33].

In summary, the appearance of a small peak of the drug in some of the samples is practically insignificant and its appearance or non-appearance depends on the variability of production, compared with previous results [33]. Therefore, in drug–clay interaction products, a practically complete amorphization of the drug occurs.

According to the first weight loss of the TGA profile, absorbed water of VHS and SEP accounted for 8% and 10% *w*/*w*, respectively (Figure 3). Zeolitic water loss of SEP occurred at 250–350 °C [45].

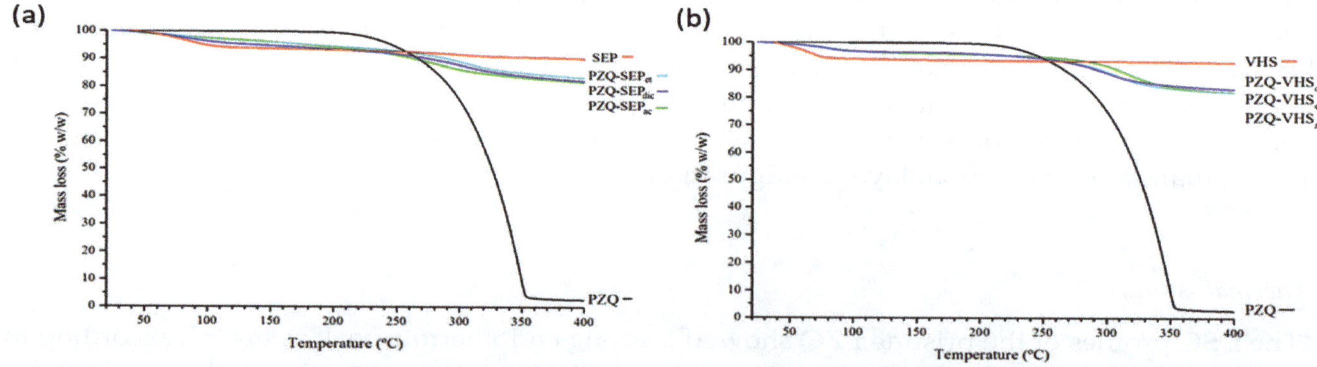

Figure 3. Thermogravimetric Analysis (TGA) profiles of the studied samples with sepiolite (**a**) and with montmorillonite (**b**).

In the interaction products both with sepiolite and montmorillonite, thermal decomposition of the drug resulted in weight losses in the range between 200 and 400 °C, corroborating the adsorption of the PZQ in these mineral solids (Figure 3).

3.3. Fourier Transform Infrared Spectroscopy

FTIR spectra of PZQ, SEP and VHS were previously described in detail [33,43,46,47]. In Figure 4, the two most intense bands of the PZQ appear at 1665–1621 cm^{-1}, which correspond to the ν(C=O) stretching vibration mode. The spectra of sepiolite and montmorillonite showed intense bands at 1200–800 cm^{-1}, corresponding to the ν(Si–O) and δ(MOHM′) (M, M′ = Al, Mg) vibrations [47].

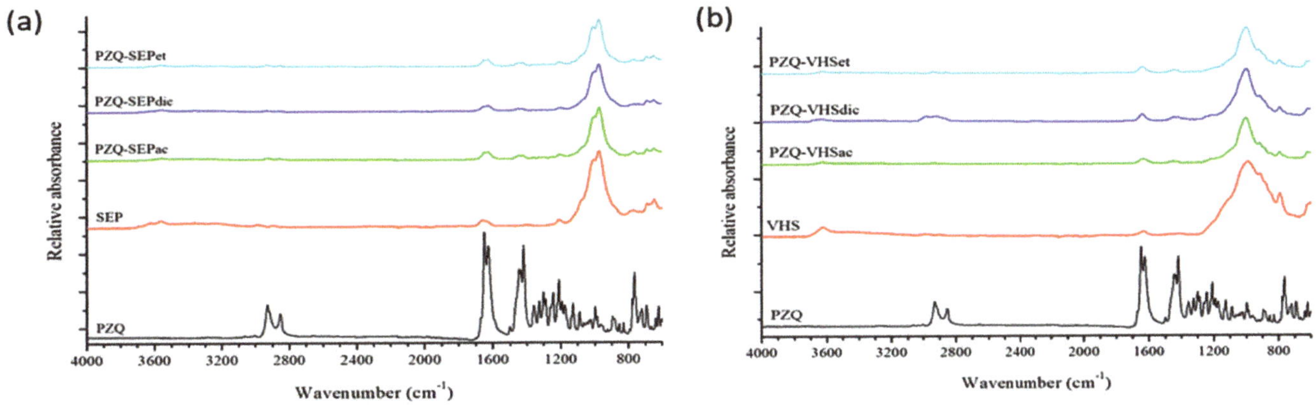

Figure 4. Fourier Transform Infrared (FTIR) spectra of sepiolite products (**a**) and of montmorillonite products (**b**).

In the interaction products prepared with sepiolite (Figure 4a) and montmorillonite (Figure 4b), the bands of the pristine PZQ were found, such as the bands that appeared at 1500–1400 cm^{-1}, which are characteristic of the δ(CH) bands of bending vibrations. This corroborated that the drug is present in the drug–clay interaction products regardless of the solvent used in the elaboration process, but the bands of the PZQ are masked by the clay in all cases, since the clay is in a much higher proportion.

3.4. In Vitro Release Studies

Drug release profiles of the interaction products with sepiolite (PZQ–SEPet, PZQ–SEPac and PZQ–SEPdic) and montmorillonite (PZQ–VHSet, PZQ–VHSac and PZQ–VHSdic) compared with the pristine PZQ were studied in sink conditions in acid aqueous medium with HCl 0.001 M (pH = 3) and in simulated intestinal fluid (pH = 6.8) (Figure 5).

The PZQ–SEP interaction products in acid medium revealed that all the products increased the dissolution rate of the PZQ drug. This enhance in the drug release profile is higher in the following order PZQ–SEPdic > PZQ–SEPet > PZQ–SEPac (Figure 5a). The same results were obtained in the SIF medium (Figure 5b). Therefore, the interaction products with sepiolite increase the dissolution rate of the PZQ greatly using any of the three solvents in the preparation method, with PZQ–SEPdic being the one that showed the best results in both media. This higher dissolution rate is due to the loss of crystallinity of PZQ that occurred during the intercalation in sepiolite. The amorphization overcomes the high cohesion energy in the packing of the PZQ crystal lattice [43] needed for its dissolution. In particular, this amorphization is higher in PZQ–SEPdic (Figure 2a) and, hence, its dissolution rate is the highest one.

The PZQ–VHS interaction products showed differences between them in acid medium (Figure 5c). In this medium, a strong increase in the dissolution rate of the drug was observed in the PZQ–VHSac product, whereas PZQ–VHSet showed only a slightly higher dissolution rate than the pristine PZQ. On the contrary, a surprising result of PZQ–VHSdic was found in acidic medium. In this case, the drug is released at a constant rate. This, in principle, leads to better control of plasma concentration and offers several advantages. Therefore, the PZQ–VHSdic in acidic medium showed a release that is interesting for new PZQ controlled release systems (Figure 5c). In simulated intestinal fluid, all the PZQ–VHS interaction products showed an increase in the dissolution rate with respect to the pristine PZQ drug. The material prepared with acetonitrile (PZQ–VHSac) presented the fastest release profile, followed by PZQ–VHSet and PZQ–VHSdic, which also presented a similar profile. In general, the increase in the dissolution rate of the PZQ–VHS interaction products also owes to the amorphization of PZQ. The peculiar behavior of PZQ–VHSdic at low pH can be due to a possible effect of the pH on the opening of the pores and interlayers of VHS that does not occur at higher pH, where the swelling is faster. Among the solvents used in this work, the dichloromethane is the only solvent non-miscible with water. It is likely that this behavior changed the macroscopic structure of the solid.

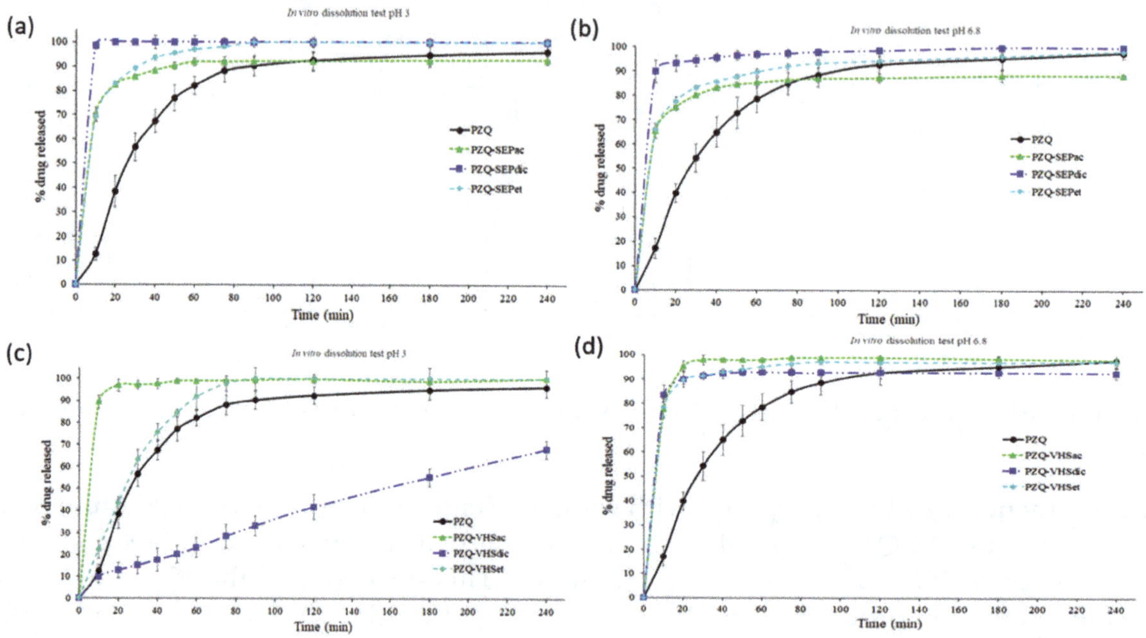

Figure 5. In vitro drug release profiles of sepiolite interaction products in HCl 0.001 M (**a**) and in simulated intestinal fluid (**b**), and of montmorillonite interaction products in HCl 0.001 M (**c**) and in simulated intestinal fluid (**d**); (mean values ± 6 SD; $n = 7$).

Moreover, in general, the PZQ–clay dissolution rate was higher in acidic medium (pH = 3) than in simulated intestinal fluid (pH = 6.8), in concordance with the results in no-sink conditions previously obtained in PZQ–clay interaction products prepared with ethanol [33]. Therefore, the interaction of the drug with the clay minerals induced an increase in dissolution rates with the independence of pH. This improvement was demonstrated in all interaction products with sepiolite in both media, and with montmorillonite in SIF medium. The interaction products with montmorillonite in acid medium showed a different behavior between them, with the PZQ–VHSac being the one with the highest dissolution rate.

Therefore, according to the results obtained in vitro, PZQ–VHS and PZQ–SEP interaction products might improve the oral bioavailability of the drug by increasing both dissolution rate and amount of drug dissolved in the medium that simulates the stomach, obtaining new accelerated oral release systems of the PZQ. Moreover, the PZQ–VHSdic in the acidic medium could be a new controlled release system of the drug.

Subsequently, the experimental dissolution data of PZQ, PZQ–SEP and PZQ–VHS interaction products were fitted to various kinetic models in order to analyze the drug release. The correlation coefficient (R^2) and Akaike Information Criterion (AIC) obtained from the dissolution model's fitting are summarized in Tables S1 and S2. In general, the results showed that zero-order and first-order models were not appropriate to study these dissolution kinetics. In the same way, Square Root (Higuchi) and Power Law (Peppas) are not appropriate for the adjustments of the experimental dissolution values since there are no sufficient values lower than 63.2% of the drug release to adjust a kinetic [37]. In Tables S1 and S2, correlation coefficient and AIC values of PZQ, PZQ–SEPac, PZQ–SEPdic, PZQ–SEPet, PZQ–VHSac, PZQ–VHSet in acid and SIF media suggested that the Weibull model could be considered as an adequate model to describe the release kinetic, because the R^2 obtained was the highest value and AIC value was the lowest once compared with the rest of the proposed models. The Weibull model presented an initial burst release [48,49], which is increased in the interaction products with clays. However, PZQ–VHSdic in an acid medium (pH = 3) showed a different dissolution profile, as can be seen in Table S2 and Figure 5c. In this case, the results suggested that the Cube Root (Hixson–Crowell) is the more accurate model to describe the release kinetics. Therefore, the PZQ–VHSdic IP in an acid medium (pH = 3) presented a release that is controlled by the dissolution rate of the drug particles and it is assumed that the particles of the interaction product are isometric and monodisperse. This geometric shape of the particles remains constant and there is a decrease in the surface area associated with the dissolution of the pharmaceutical form [50,51].

3.5. Solubility Studies

The PZQ–SEPet and PZQ–VHSet showed an increase in the solubility compared to the pristine drug in the studied media. The results in the acid aqueous medium with HCl 0.001 M (pH = 3) indicated that the solubility of the PZQ–SEPet and PZQ–VHSet interaction products were similar in both cases (0.71 and 0.74 mg/mL, respectively). Similar results are obtained in simulated intestinal fluid (pH = 6.8), where the solubility of PZQ–SEPet and PZQ–VHSet was 0.61 and 0.65 mg/mL, respectively. Therefore, the interaction products enhanced the solubility of the drug, and this increase was in the range of 36–48% with respect to pristine PZQ (Table 1).

Table 1. Solubility values (in mg/mL) of praziquantel (PZQ), PZQ–SEPet and PZQ–VHSet and increase solubility (in %) with respect to that of PZQ in acid and SIF media (solubility mean values ± 0.07 SD; $n = 3$).

	HCl 0.001 M Medium, pH = 3		SIF Medium, pH = 6.8	
	Solubility (mg/mL)	Increase (%)	Solubility (mg/mL)	Increase (%)
PZQ	0.50		0.45	
PZQ–SEPet	0.71	42	0.61	36
PZQ–VHSet	0.74	48	0.65	44

3.6. Cytotoxicity Studies

In vitro cytotoxicity tests in the HCT116 cell line were performed in PZQ, SEP, VHS, PZQ–SEPet and PZQ–VHSet products. The interaction products with ethanol were selected as a reference from the rest because they present an increase in the in vitro dissolution profile in sink conditions and in non-sink conditions, as demonstrated by previous work [33].

The raw material (PZQ, SEP and VHS) in concentrations between 6.4 nM and 100 µM were tested, demonstrating that they can be considered biocompatible toward HCT116 cell lines due to the fact that the percentage of the cell viability was slightly lower than the untreated cells in all cases (control) (Figure 6).

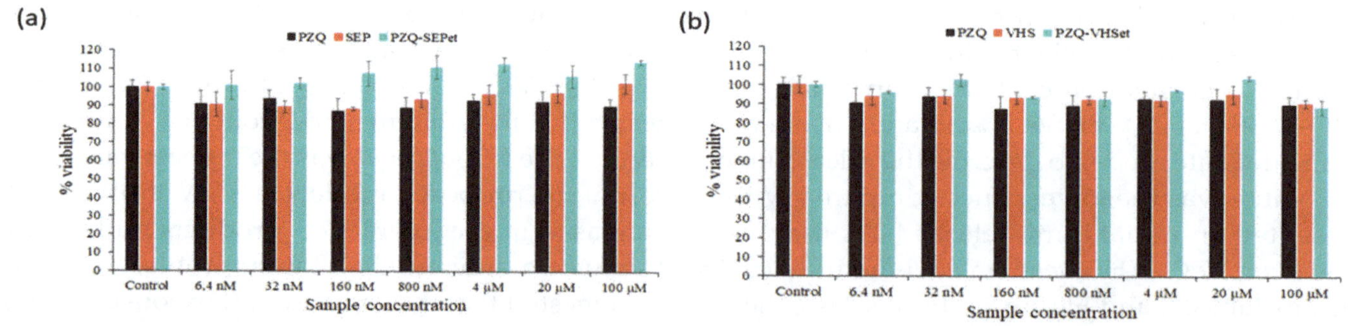

Figure 6. Cell viability of SEP and PZQ–SEPet (**a**), and VHS and PZQ–VHSet (**b**) compared to PZQ after 48 h of treatment. (Control: untreated cells in complete medium; mean values ± 8 SE; *n* = 3).

In the PZQ–SEPet interaction products, the loss of cell viability was not observed in any of the concentrations tested, even a positive effect in cell growth was observed with respect to the control, and pure SEP and PZQ. Therefore, the PZQ–SEPet revealed its biocompatibility with cell and had a positive effect on the cell viability compared to raw PZQ and SEP solids in these ranges of concentrations (Figure 6a). PZQ–SEPdic and PZQ–SEPac products are expected to behave similarly.

PZQ–VHSet showed a slight loss of cell viability like pure products, up to a maximum of 11% in the highest concentration tested. In this case, a positive effect on cell growth was not observed, but the viability of the PZQ–VHSet interaction product was similar to that of the pristine drug and VHS, therefore it can be considered biocompatible according to the in vitro results (Figure 6b). Likewise, PZQ–VHSdic and PZQ–VHSac products are expected to have similar behavior.

3.7. Cell Cycle Studies

The cell cycle tests by means of propidium iodide were performed to investigate the cell cycle corresponding to the Sub-G1 phase of the cells in contact with the interaction products prepared (PZQ–SEPet and PZQ–VHSet) and their raw materials (PZQ, SEP and VHS) (Figure 7). These studies allowed us to deduce if there is any alteration of any phase of the cell cycle despite the cell proliferation not being affected, after observing above that there is no significant loss in cell viability of the cells treated with the samples studied.

The control tests are shown in the upper part of the figure (Figure 7). Control tests demonstrated that, in comparison with cellular cycles of healthy, untreated cells ("not treated" cells in Figure 7), DMSO does not affect the cells, unlike etoposide (antineoplasic drug). As can be seen by the cell cycle analysis, the etoposide control group is severely affected and induces death to 64.3% of the cell population.

In Figure 7a, the results showed that the cell cycle was not affected when the cells were treated with PZQ, SEP and PZQ–SEPet, and only at high concentrations, the cell death was increased slightly, although not in a notable way. Furthermore, in none of the concentrations tested was it observed that the PZQ–SEPet interaction product produced a significantly higher percentage of cell death than that with the pure PZQ.

The results of PZQ, VHS and PZQ–VHSet samples are shown in Figure 7b. The PZQ–VHSet interaction product showed that the cellular cycle of the cells was not affected, and cell death was not observed at low sample concentration (0.8–4 µM). At high concentrations (20–100 µM), affectation of the cell cycle of the cells was observed as well as greater cell death. This damage in the cell cycle is very high at the 100 µM concentration. This is the same in pure VHS clay, therefore, this occurs in the interaction product due to the presence of the clay mineral.

In summary, the PZQ–SEPet interaction product showed that it does not affect, in any concentration, the cellular cycle of the cells, and its behavior is similar to the pure drug. However, the PZQ–VHSet interaction product showed that it affects, at high concentrations, the cellular cycle, so only the lower concentrations (<0.8–4 µM) do not affect the Sub-G1 phase of the cells (Figure 7).

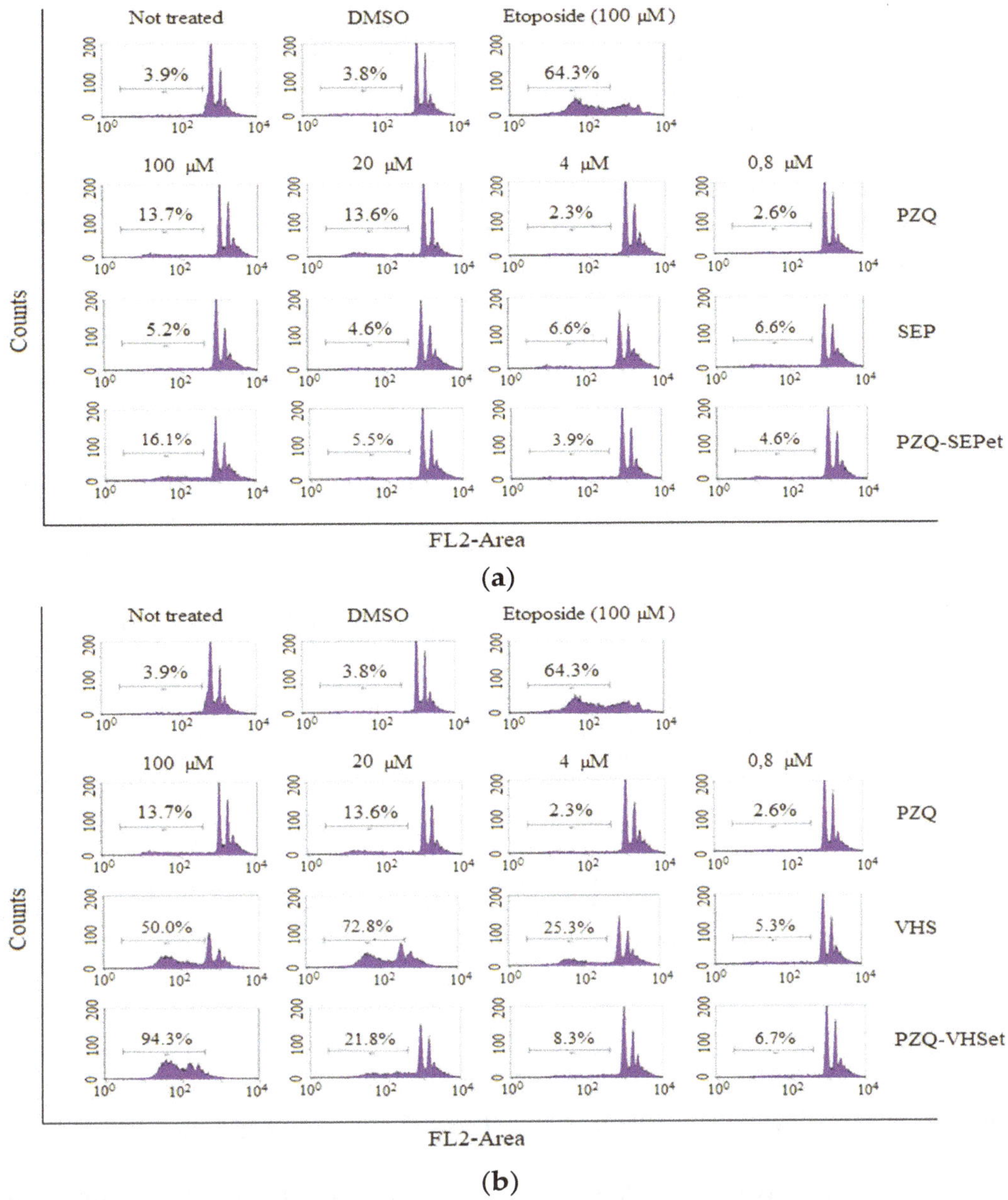

Figure 7. Cell cycle of the HCT116 line treated with the PZQ, SEP and PZQ–SEPet (**a**), and with the PZQ, VHS and PZQ–VHSet (**b**). The percentages indicate the number of cells in Sub-G1 (apoptotic or necrotic). Negative controls (Not treated and DMSO) and positive control (Etoposide) are also included.

4. Conclusions

The interaction products PZQ–SEP and PZQ–VHS prepared with ethanol, dichloromethane and acetonitrile allowed us to carry out an effective interaction of the low water-soluble drug with the clays. Therefore, this described methodology that uses organic solvents and clays can be used to prepare drug–clay complexes, with drugs that have low aqueous solubility. The characterization using different techniques of these interaction products showed that the drug is amorphized, reducing its crystallinity.

In vitro drug release profiles of the interaction products with sepiolite compared with the pristine PZQ in sink conditions in acid aqueous medium (pH = 3) and in simulated intestinal fluid (pH = 6.8) showed that in all products the dissolution rate of the drug improved, and specifically the PZQ–SEPdic was the one that most increased the rate dissolution. In the interaction products with montmorillonite, in acid medium (pH = 3), the PZQ–VHSac improved the dissolution rate of the drug, and the PZQ–VHSdic showed a controlled release of PZQ, which can be very interesting for another type of modified drug delivery system. In SIF medium (pH = 6.8), all the PZQ–VHS interaction products increased the dissolution rate of the drug.

Cytotoxicity and cell cycle studies were performed in the interaction products prepared with ethanol, and the interaction products with dichloromethane and acetonitrile are expected to have similar behavior. The PZQ–SEPet interaction product was biocompatible with the HTC116 line cells, and it did not produce a decrease in cell viability or alterations in the cell cycle. However, the PZQ–VHSet showed a slight loss of cell viability like pure products, but in the cell cycle study, the affectation of the cell cycle and damage of the cells were observed at the highest concentration tested, so low concentrations should be used.

Therefore, the methodology used with organic solvents is an interesting technological strategy for effective interaction between praziquantel and clays. In general, according to the results obtained, the PZQ–SEP interaction products increased more the dissolution rates of drug, without producing cytotoxicity or alterations in the cell cycle of HTC116 cells. These systems should be considered as promising pharmaceutical systems to improve the bioavailability of water low-soluble of praziquantel.

Author Contributions: Conceptualization, A.B.-S., C.V. and C.I.S.-D.; methodology, A.B.-S., C.V. and C.I.S.-D.; formal analysis, A.B.-S. and R.S.-E.; investigation, A.B.-S.; data curation, A.B.-S.; writing—original draft preparation, A.B.-S.; writing—review and editing, A.B.-S., R.S.-E., F.G.-V., C.V. and C.I.S.-D.; supervision, A.B.-S., C.V. and C.I.S.-D.; funding acquisition, C.V. and C.I.S.-D. All authors have read and agreed to the published version of the manuscript.

Acknowledgments: This project was supported by the Spanish research groups CTS-946 and RNM363. Technical support was provided by the Centro de Instrumentación Científica (University of Granada), the Instituto Andaluz de Ciencias de la Tierra (Consejo Superior de Investigaciones Científicas-University of Granada) and the Xtrem Biotech SL (Spin-off University of Granada).

References

1. World Health Organization (WTO). Available online: https://www.who.int/neglected_diseases/en/ (accessed on 1 June 2020).
2. World Health Organization (WTO). Available online: https://www.who.int/news-room/fact-sheets/detail/schistosomiasis (accessed on 1 June 2020).
3. Chitsulo, L.; Engels, D.; Montresor, A.; Savioli, L. The global status of schistosomiasis and its control. *Acta Trop.* **2000**, *77*, 41–51. [CrossRef]
4. Steinmann, P.; Keiser, J.; Bos, R.; Tanner, M.; Utzinger, J. Schistosomiasis and water resources development: Systematic review, meta-analysis, and estimates of people at risk. *Lancet Infect. Dis.* **2006**, *6*, 411–425. [CrossRef]
5. Wang, W.; Wang, L.; Liang, Y.-S. Susceptibility or resistance of praziquantel in human schistosomiasis: A review. *Parasitol. Res.* **2012**, *111*, 1871–1877. [CrossRef]
6. Andrews, P. Praziquantel: Mechanisms of anti-schistosomal activity. *Pharmacol. Ther.* **1985**, *29*, 129–156. [CrossRef]
7. Liu, Y.; Wang, X.; Wang, J.K.; Ching, C.B. Structural characterization and enantioseparation of the chiral compound praziquantel. *J. Pharm. Sci.* **2004**, *93*, 3039–3046. [CrossRef] [PubMed]
8. Borrego-Sánchez, A.; Viseras, C.; Aguzzi, C.; Sainz-Díaz, C.I. Molecular and crystal structure of praziquantel. Spectroscopic properties and crystal polymorphism. *Eur. J. Pharm. Sci.* **2016**, *92*, 266–275. [CrossRef]
9. U.S. Food and Drug Administration (FDA). Available online: https://www.fda.gov/AboutFDA/CentersOffices/OfficeofMedicalProductsandTobacco/CDER/ucm128219.htm (accessed on 1 June 2020).

10. Amidon, G.L.; Lennernäs, H.; Shah, V.P.; Crison, J.R. A theoretical basis for a biopharmaceutic drug classification: The correlation of in vitro drug product dissolution and in vivo bioavailability. *Pharm. Res.* **1995**, *12*, 413–420. [CrossRef]
11. González-Esquivel, D.; Rivera, J.; Castro, N.; Yepez-Mulia, L.; Helgi, J.C. In vitro characterization of some biopharmaceutical properties of praziquantel. *Int. J. Pharm.* **2005**, *295*, 93–99. [CrossRef]
12. Bergaya, F.; Lagaly, G. General introduction: Clays, clay minerals, and clay science. In *Developments in Clay Science*; Handbook of Clay Science, Elsevier: Amsterdam, The Netherlands, 2006; Volume 1, pp. 1–18. [CrossRef]
13. Guggenheim, S.; Adams, J.M.; Bain, D.C.; Bergaya, F.; Brigatti, M.F.; Drits, V.A.; Formoso, M.L.L.; Galán, E.; Kogure, T.; Stanjek, H. Summary of recommendations of nomenclature committees relevant to clay mineralogy: Report of the Association Internationale Pour l'Etude des Argiles (AIPEA) nomenclature committee for 2006. *Clays Clay Miner.* **2006**, *54*, 761–772. [CrossRef]
14. López-Galindo, A.; Viseras, C. Pharmaceutical and Cosmetic Applications of Clays. *Interface Sci. Technol.* **2004**, *1*, 267–289. [CrossRef]
15. Aguzzi, C.; Viseras, C.; Cerezo, P.; Rossi, S.; Ferrari, F.; López-Galindo, A.; Caramella, C. Influence of dispersion conditions of two pharmaceutical grade clays on their interaction with some tetracyclines. *Appl. Clay Sci.* **2005**, *30*, 79–86. [CrossRef]
16. Aguzzi, C.; Cerezo, P.; Viseras, C.; Caramella, C. Use of clays as drug delivery systems: Possibilities and limitations. *Appl. Clay Sci.* **2007**, *36*, 1–3. [CrossRef]
17. Viseras, C.; Cerezo, P.; Sánchez, R.; Salcedo, I.; Aguzzi, C. Current challenges in clay minerals for drug delivery. *Appl. Clay Sci.* **2010**, *48*, 291–295. [CrossRef]
18. Borrego-Sánchez, A.; Carazo, E.; Albertini, B.; Passerini, N.; Perissutti, B.; Cerezo, P.; Viseras, C.; Hernández-Laguna, A.; Aguzzi, C.; Sainz-Díaz, C.I. Conformational polymorphic changes in the crystal structure of the chiral antiparasitic drug praziquantel and interactions with calcium carbonate. *Eur. J. Pharm. Biopharm.* **2018**, *132*, 180–191. [PubMed]
19. Borrego-Sánchez, A.; Sánchez-Espejo, R.; Albertini, B.; Passerini, N.; Cerezo, P.; Viseras, C.; Sainz-Díaz, C.I. Ground calcium carbonate as a low cost and biosafety excipient for solubility and dissolution improvement of praziquantel. *Pharmaceutics* **2019**, *11*, 533.
20. Trofimov, A.D.; Ivanova, A.A.; Zyuzin, M.V.; Timin, A.S. Porous inorganic carriers based on silica, calcium carbonate and calcium phosphate for controlled/modulated drug delivery: Fresh outlook and future perspectives. *Pharmaceutics* **2018**, *10*, 167.
21. Rodrigues, S.G.; Chaves, I.S.; Melo, N.F.S.; de Jesus, M.B.; Fraceto, L.F.; Fernandes, S.A.; de Paula, E.; de Freitas, M.P.; Pinto, L.M.A. Computational analysis and physico-chemical characterization of an inclusion compound between praziquantel and methyl-β-cyclodextrin for use as an alternative in the treatment of schistosomiasis. *J. Incl. Phenom. Macrocycl. Chem.* **2010**, *70*, 19–28. [CrossRef]
22. Maragos, S.; Archontaki, H.; Macheras, P.; Valsami, G. Effect of cyclodextrin complexation on the aqueous solubility and solubility/dose ratio of praziquantel. *AAPS Pharm. Sci. Tech.* **2009**, *10*, 1444.
23. Becket, G.; Schep, L.J.; Tan, M.Y. Improvement of the in vitro dissolution of praziquantel by complexation with α-, β-, and γ-cyclodextrins. *Int. J. Pharm.* **1999**, *179*, 65–71.
24. De la Torre, P.; Torrado, S.; Torrado, S. Preparation, dissolution and characterization of Praziquantel solid dispersions. *Chem. Pharm. Bull.* **1999**, *47*, 1629–1633. [CrossRef]
25. Costa, E.D.; Priotti, J.; Orlandi, S.; Leonardi, D.; Lamas, M.C.; Nunes, T.G.; Diogo, H.P.; Salomon, C.J.; Ferreira, M.J. Unexpected solvent impact in the crystallinity of praziquantel/poly(vinylpyrrolidone) formulations. A solubility, DSC and solid-state NMR study. *Int. J. Pharm.* **2016**, *511*, 983–993. [CrossRef] [PubMed]
26. Passerini, N.; Albertini, B.; Perissutti, B.; Rodriguez, L. Evaluation of melt granulation and ultrasonic spray congealing as techniques to enhance the dissolution of praziquantel. *Int. J. Pharm.* **2006**, *318*, 92–102. [CrossRef] [PubMed]
27. Liu, Y.; Wang, T.; Ding, W.; Dong, C.; Wang, X.; Chen, J.; Li, Y. Dissolution and oral bioavailability enhancement of praziquantel by solid dispersions. *Drug Deliv. Transl. Res.* **2018**, *8*, 580–590. [CrossRef] [PubMed]
28. Cheng, L.; Lei, L.; Guo, S. In vitro and in vivo evaluation of praziquantel loaded implants based on PEG/PCL blends. *Int. J. Pharm.* **2010**, *387*, 129–138. [CrossRef]

29. Chaud, M.V.; Lima, A.C.; Vila, M.M.D.C.; Paganelli, M.O.; Paula, F.C.; Pedreiro, L.N.; Gremião, M.P.D. Development and evaluation of praziquantel solid dispersions in sodium starch glycolate. *Trop. J. Pharm. Res.* **2013**, *12*, 163–168. [CrossRef]
30. Mourao, S.C.; Costa, P.I.; Salgado, H.R.N.; Gremiao, M.P.D. Improvement of antischistosomal activity of praziquantel by incorporation into phosphatidylcholine-containing liposomes. *Int. J. Pharm.* **2005**, *295*, 157–162. [CrossRef]
31. Timóteo, T.R.R.; Melo, C.G.; Danda, L.J.A.; Silva, L.C.P.B.B.; Fontes, D.A.F.; Silva, P.C.D.; Aguilera, C.S.B.; Siqueira, L.P.; Rolim, L.A.; Neto, P.J.R. Layered double hydroxides of CaAl: A promising drug delivery system for increased dissolution rate and thermal stability of praziquantel. *Appl. Clay Sci.* **2019**, *180*, 105197. [CrossRef]
32. El-Feky, G.S.; Mohamed, W.S.; Nasr, H.E.; El-Lakkany, N.M.; Seif el-Din, S.H.; Botros, S.S. Praziquantel in a clay nanoformulation shows more bioavailability and higher efficacy against murine schistosoma mansoni infection. antimicrob. *Agents Chemother.* **2015**, *59*, 3501–3508.
33. Borrego-Sánchez, A.; Carazo, E.; Aguzzi, C.; Viseras, C.; Sainz-Díaz, C.I. Biopharmaceutical improvement of praziquantel by interaction with montmorillonite and sepiolite. *Appl. Clay Sci.* **2018**, *160*, 173–179. [CrossRef]
34. Sainz-Díaz, C.I.; Borrego-Sánchez, A.; Viseras, C.; Aguzzi, C. Method for Preparing a Nano-Structured Material of Praziquantel and a Silicate, Material Obtained and Use as an Antiparasitic. Patent WO/2020/012044, 15 January 2019.
35. Lauroba, J.; Doménech, J. La liberación como factor limitativo de la absorción gastrointestinal. In *Biofarmacia y Farmacocinética*; Lauroba, J., Doménech, J., Plá, J.M., Eds.; Síntesis: Madrid, Spain, 1998; Volume 2, pp. 241–274.
36. Costa, P.; Souza Lobo, J.M. Modeling and comparison of dissolution profiles. *Eur. J. Pharm. Sci.* **2001**, *13*, 123–133. [CrossRef]
37. Siepman, J.; Göpferich, A. Mathematical modeling of bioerodible, polymeric drug delivery systems. *Adv. Drug Deliv. Rev.* **2001**, *48*, 229–247. [CrossRef]
38. Cheikh, D.; García-Villén, F.; Majdoub, H.; Viseras, C.; Zayania, M.B. Chitosan/beidellite nanocomposite as diclofenac carrier. *Int. J. Biol. Macromol.* **2019**, *126*, 44–53. [CrossRef] [PubMed]
39. Akaike, H. A new look at the statistical model identification. *IEEE Trans. Automat. Contr.* **1974**, *19*, 716–723.
40. Gong, J.P.; Traganos, F.; Darzynkiewicz, Z. A selective procedure for DNA extraction from apoptotic cells applicable for gel electrophoresis and flow cytometry. *Anal. Biochem.* **1994**, *218*, 314–319. [CrossRef] [PubMed]
41. El-Subbagh, H.I.; Al-Badr, A.A. Praziquantel. In *Analytical Profiles of Drug Substances and Excipients*; Florey, K., Ed.; Academic Press Inc.: New York, NY, USA, 1998; Volume 25, pp. 463–500.
42. Meteleva, E.S.; Chistyachenko, Y.S.; Suntsova, L.P.; Khvostov, M.V.; Polyakov, N.E.; Selyutina, O.Y.; Tolstikova, T.G.; Frolova, T.S.; Mordvinov, V.A.; Dushkin, A.V.; et al. Disodium salt of glycyrrhizic acid–A novel supramolecular delivery system for anthelmintic drug praziquantel. *J. Drug Deliv. Sci. Technol.* **2019**, *50*, 66–77. [CrossRef]
43. Borrego-Sánchez, A.; Hernández-Laguna, A.; Sainz-Díaz, C.I. Molecular modeling and infrared and Raman spectroscopy of the crystal structure of the chiral antiparasitic drug Praziquantel. *J. Mol. Model.* **2017**, *23*, 106. [CrossRef]
44. Borrego-Sánchez, A.; Viseras, C.; Sainz-Díaz, C.I. Molecular interactions of praziquantel drug with nanosurfaces of sepiolite and montmorillonite. *Appl. Clay Sci.* **2020**, *197*, 105774.
45. Viseras, C.; López-Galindo, A. Pharmaceutical applications of some Spanish clays (sepiolite, palygorskite, bentonite): Some preformulation studies. *Appl. Clay Sci.* **1999**, *14*, 69–82. [CrossRef]
46. Frost, R.L.; Locos, O.B.; Ruan, H.; Kloprogge, J.T. Near-infrared and mid-infrared spectroscopic study of sepiolites and palygorskites. *Vib. Spectrosc.* **2001**, *27*, 1–13. [CrossRef]
47. Ortega-Castro, J.; Hernández-Haro, N.; Muñoz-Santiburcio, D.; Hernández-Laguna, A.; Sainz-Díaz, C.I. Crystal structure and hydroxyl group vibrational frequencies of phyllosilicates by DFT methods. *Theochem. J. Mol. Struct.* **2009**, *912*, 82–87. [CrossRef]
48. Langenbucher, F. Letters to the editor: Linearization of dissolution rate curves by the Weibull distribution. *J. Pharm. Pharmacol.* **1972**, *24*, 979–981. [CrossRef] [PubMed]
49. Weibul, W. Wide applicability. *J. Appl. Mech.* **1951**, *103*, 293–297.

50. Hixson, A.W.; Crowell, J.H. Dependence of reaction velocity surface and agitation. *Ind. Eng. Chem.* **1931**, *23*, 923–931. [CrossRef]
51. Neibergall, P.J.; Milosovich, G.; Goyan, J.E. Dissolution rate studies. II. Dissolution of particles under conditions of rapid agitation. *J. Pharm. Sci.* **1963**, *52*, 236–241.

7

Wound Healing Activity of Nanoclay/Spring Water Hydrogels

Fátima García-Villén [1,*], Angela Faccendini [2], Dalila Miele [2], Marco Ruggeri [2], Rita Sánchez-Espejo [3], Ana Borrego-Sánchez [3], Pilar Cerezo [1], Silvia Rossi [2], César Viseras [1,3] and Giuseppina Sandri [2]

1 Department of Pharmacy and Pharmaceutical Technology, Faculty of Pharmacy, University of Granada, Campus of Cartuja, 18071 s/n Granada, Spain; mcerezo@ugr.es (P.C.); cviseras@ugr.es (C.V.)
2 Department of Drug Sciences, Faculty of Pharmacy, University of Pavia, Taramelli Street 12, 27100 Pavia, Italy; angela.faccendini@gmail.com (A.F.); dalila.miele01@universitadipavia.it (D.M.); marco.ruggeri02@universitadipavia.it (M.R.); silvia.rossi@unipv.it (S.R.); g.sandri@unipv.it (G.S.)
3 Andalusian Institute of Earth Sciences, CSIC-UGR, Avenida de las Palmeras 4, Armilla, 18100 Granada, Spain; ritaespejo@hotmail.com (R.S.-E.); anaborrego@iact.ugr-csic.es (A.B.-S.)
* Correspondence: fgarvillen@ugr.es

Abstract: Background: hydrogels prepared with natural inorganic excipients and spring waters are commonly used in medical hydrology. Design of these clay-based formulations continues to be a field scarcely addressed. Safety and wound healing properties of different fibrous nanoclay/spring water hydrogels were addressed. Methods: in vitro biocompatibility, by means of MTT assay, and wound healing properties were studied. Confocal Laser Scanning Microscopy was used to study the morphology of fibroblasts during the wound healing process. Results: all the ingredients demonstrated to be biocompatible towards fibroblasts. Particularly, the formulation of nanoclays as hydrogels improved biocompatibility with respect to powder samples at the same concentration. Spring waters and hydrogels were even able to promote in vitro fibroblasts motility and, therefore, accelerate wound healing with respect to the control. Conclusion: fibrous nanoclay/spring water hydrogels proved to be skin-biocompatible and to possess a high potential as wound healing formulations. Moreover, these results open new prospects for these ingredients to be used in new therapeutic or cosmetic formulations.

Keywords: sepiolite; palygorskite; spring water; hydrogel; fibroblast; biocompatibility; wound healing

---

1. Introduction

Chronic wounds are a current health problem with devastating consequences for patients and contribute to major costs to healthcare systems and societies. This type of wound results from an impaired wound healing process and is usually characterized by prolonged or excessive inflammation, persistent infections and inability of the dermal and/or epidermal cells to respond to repair stimuli [1–3]. The USA total Medicare spending for all wound types has been estimated to range from $28.1 to $96.8 billion. Diabetic foot ulcers (one of the main chronic wounds) accounted for $6.1 to $18.7 billion [2], the main cost burden attributed to amputations [1]. The development and implementation of new wound healing management strategies and healthcare products is, therefore, imperative. In recent years, different technological strategies have been proposed, including clays, metals, polymers and lipid-based systems among others, as reviewed by Bernal-Chávez et al. and García-Villén et al. [4,5]. Particularly, clay-based dressings have been proven to be useful in wound healing [5–7]. Among the different clay-based formulations, those composed of a clay suspended in mineral medicinal water, known as therapeutic muds, are widely used in clinical medical hydrology [8–10]. The solid phase of these systems is frequently incorporated into spring water to obtain a semisolid formulation known as "artificial thermal mud" [11–14]. Thermal muds have demonstrated their clinical effectiveness against dermatological affections such as psoriasis [15–18], atopic dermatitis, vitiligo [19,20], seborrheic dermatitis, fungal infections, eczema [18,21–23] and acne [24]. These clinical effects have been traditionally associated with the liquid phase. Avène and La Roche-Posay spring waters increase the fluidity of plasma membranes on cultured human skin fibroblasts [25–28] and have been useful in the management of chronic inflammatory skin diseases. La Roche-Posay spring water protected cultured human skin fibroblasts against lipid peroxidation induced by ultraviolet A and B radiation [29]. Boron and manganese-rich thermal waters are used for the treatment of ulcers and chronic wounds [30–34].

The influence of the thermal mud's solid phase in the resulting clinical efficacy has not been studied in depth. The inorganic solid phase of thermal muds is mainly composed of clay minerals [8,10,35–37]. The clay mineral presence in wound healing formulations is supported by their already demonstrated biocompatibility with different types of skin cells [38–40]. The combination of clay minerals with other ingredients, such as polymers, allows the formation of scaffolding materials. In these occasions, clay minerals not only improved the mechanical strength and functionality of the polymers, but they also acted as synergistic ingredients for wound healing [41–44]. Biocompatibility of clay minerals such as halloysite, montmorillonite, palygorskite, sepiolite and imogolite have been widely studied [45–55]. Sasaki et al. reported that Mg^{2+} and Si^{4+} ions released by a synthetic Mg-rich smectite clay mineral can promote collagen formation and angiogenesis on skin wounds [56].

Moreover, palygorskite ("attapulgite") has been used as scaffolding material when included in poly(lactic-co-glycolic acid) nanofibers, being crucial for mesenchymal cell adhesion and proliferation [57]. Sepiolite and palygorksite inhibit lipid peroxidation and possess anti-inflammatory properties by reducing neutrophil migration and edema [58,59]. Pharmaceutical grade palygorskite (Pharmasorb® colloidal) did not only demonstrate to be biocompatible but also to protect fibroblasts from carvacrol cytotoxicity [6].

As discussed, both spring waters and clay minerals have been separately studied as potential wound healing ingredients. Synergistic effects would be expectable when both ingredients are formulated as spring-water/clay hydrogels. The role of these systems in wound healing studies has been scarcely addressed. The existing studies include a clinical study of diabetic gangrenous wounds treated with volcanic deposits muds [60], black-mud Dead Sea effects in wounded mice [61] and wound healing activity of emulsions prepared with a Brazilian clay [62].

With these premises, spring water hydrogels have been recently formulated and characterized, including mineralogical and chemical composition as well as textural and thermal properties, as a first step in the design of pharmaceutical-grade systems [63]. The second step would involve the study and evaluation of their biocompatibility. In this regard, the simplest starting point would include in vitro biocompatibility studies over skin cells like fibroblasts and in vitro wound healing studies.

Particularly, the in vitro biocompatibility and cell gap motility (wound healing) properties of two selected Spanish medicinal waters (obtained from Graena and Alicún de las Torres thermal stations), two clay minerals (palygorskite and sepiolite) and their corresponding hydrogels were studied. Additionally, particle size distribution and zeta potential measures as well as cation exchange capacities of the solid phases were carried out. In vitro wound healing tests were also evaluated by analyzing fibroblast F-actin microfilament organization by means of phalloidin staining. To the best of the authors' knowledge, this is the first time that nanoclay/spring water mineral medicinal hydrogels have been evaluated in terms of in vitro cytotoxicity and wound healing.

2. Materials and Methods

2.1. Materials

Two pharmaceutical grade clays granted by TOLSA company (Madrid, Spain)—magnesium aluminum silicate (PS9) and attapulgite (G30)—with mineralogical identification previously evaluated (Table 1) were used [63].

Table 1. Fibrous clay (PS9 and G30) mineralogical composition (modified from [63]).

	PS9		G30	
Mineralogical Composition	Sepiolite	92%	Palygorskite	58%
	Muscovite	8%	Quartz	26%
			Fluorapatite	7%
			Smectites and sepiolite	6%
			Calcite/dolomite	3%

Two medicinal waters from Graena (GR) and Alicún De Las Torres (ALI) thermal stations were used. Both spring sources are located in Granada (Andalusia, Spain) and are classified as hypothermal (ALI) and hyperthermal (GR), both of them having a strong mineralization [64,65]. Their pH, conductivity and elemental compositions have been determined in a previous study, and results are summarized in Table 2.

Table 2. Medicinal water characteristics and elemental composition determined by means of ICP-OES and ICP-MS (modified from [63]).

		ALI	GR
	pH ± s.d.	**7.90 ± 0.0472**	**8.02 ± 0.0823**
	Conductivity (μS/cm) ± s.d.	**2251.5 ± 6.74537**	**2465.5 ± 8.89482**
Elemental Composition	Ca (mg/L)	348.00	460.00
	Mg (mg/L)	109.0	88.00
	Na (mg/L)	57.00	27.40
	K (mg/L)	4.60	6.80
	B (μg/L)	25.00	12.00
	Ba (μg/L)	18.80	13.00
	Cr (μg/L)	4.3	1
	Zn (μg/L)	464.99	301.08
	Mn (μg/L)	<1	108.66
	Li (μg/L)	244.2	65.00
	Ni (μg/L)	9.4	5.20
	Fe (μg/L)	6.00	21.00
	Se (μg/L)	2.3	1.00

According to previous studies and characterizations [63], hydrogels were prepared mixing 10% *w/w* of each clay mineral with the corresponding spring water, by means of a turbine high-speed agitator (Silverson LT, Chesham, UK) at 8000 rpm for 10 min. The obtained hydrogels are summarized in Table 3.

Table 3. Thermal muds tested, identification codes and composition.

Identification Code	Composition
PS9ALI	10% *w/w* PS9, 90% *w/w* ALI
PS9GR	10% *w/w* PS9, 90% *w/w* GR
G30ALI	10% *w/w* G30, 90% *w/w* ALI
G30GR	10% *w/w* G30, 90% *w/w* GR

2.2. *Characterization of Inorganic Ingredients*

2.2.1. Particle Size

Particle size distribution was determined by a Malvern Mastersizer 2000 LF granulometer (Malvern InstrumentsTM). Measurements were performed in purified water after dispersing the solids by midst sonication for 30 s. The amount of sample added in each experiment was determined by the real-time laser obscuration degree indicated by "Mastersizer 2000" software. The optimal laser obscuration was delimited between 10–20%. Three replicates were performed for each sample, and statistical particle diameters (d_{10}, d_{50}, d_{90}) were calculated together with the SPAN factor as an index of the amplitude of particle size distribution calculated according to Equation (1).

$$\mathrm{SPAN} = \frac{d_{90} - d_{10}}{d_{50}} \tag{1}$$

2.2.2. Cation Exchange Capacity

Cation exchange capacity (CEC) of PS9 and G30 was determined by dispersing 1 g of dry powder in 25 mL of tetramethyl ammonium bromide (TMAB) aqueous solution (1 M). The resultant dispersions were shaken in a Roller Mixer for 24 h and subsequently centrifuged (8000 rpm, 30 min) and filtered (0.45 µm pore size, HAWP-Millipore filter). Three replicates were performed for each sample together with two blanks of pure TMAB (1 M). The CEC determination is based on the exchange between bromine (in the TMAB solution) and cations present in the clay. The main exchangeable cations released from the clay mineral, once the Br exchanged, are K^+, Na^+, Mg^{2+} and Ca^{2+}. Cations released, present in the resultant solution, were determined by ICP-OES (Optima 8300 ICP-OES Spectrometer, Perkin Elmer, Waltham, MA, USA), and CEC was calculated as the sum of exchangeable cations, expressed in mEq/100 g of clay mineral.

2.2.3. Zeta Potential

Zeta-potential (ζ-potential) measurements determine the electrical potential difference between the stationary layer of fluid surrounding the solid particles and the bulk (electric double layer). Zeta potentials of different concentrations of PS9 and G30, suspended in Dulbecco's modified Eagle medium, supplemented with 10% fetal bovine serum, 200 IU/mL penicillin and 0.2 mg/mL streptomycin, were also measured. Afterwards, ζ-potentials of the aforementioned suspensions were determined by using an electrophoretic light scattering (ELS) Zetasizer Naso-ZTM (Malvern Instruments, Worcestershire, UK). Samples were placed inside a folded capillary zeta potential cell (DTS1061, Malvern Instruments). Three replicates were obtained for each sample, and analyses were done at 25 ± 0.5 °C. During the analyses, 20 points were collected for each replicate and results expressed in mV.

2.3. *In Vitro Tests of Inorganic Ingredients, Spring Waters and Hydrogels*

2.3.1. Biocompatibility Tests

Normal human dermal fibroblasts (NHDFs) from juvenile foreskin (PromoCell GmbH, Heidelberg, Germany) were used. All cells were between the 10th and 13th passages. NHDFs were grown in Dulbecco's modified Eagle medium (DMEM, Sigma Aldrich®-Merck, Milan, Italy), supplemented with 10% fetal bovine serum (FBS, Euroclone, Milan, Italy), 200 IU/mL penicillin and 0.2 mg/mL streptomycin (PBI International, I), kept at 37 °C in a 5% CO_2 atmosphere with 95% relative humidity (RH). Fibroblasts were seeded in 96-well plates (area 0.34 cm^2/well) at a density of 10^5 cells/cm^2. Cells were grown 24 h to obtain sub-confluence. Then, cell substrates were washed with saline solution, and the cell substrates were put in contact with the samples. Biocompatibility of all samples was assessed after 24 h contact between samples and NHDF cultures. Powdered PS9 and G30 clay minerals were used in concentrations of 1000, 500, 50 and 5 μg/mL. ALI and GR medicinal waters were used in concentrations 0.25, 2.5, 25 and 50% *v/v*. Regarding PS9ALI, PS9GR, G30ALI and G30GR, cell contact concentrations were prepared in order to have equal amounts of clay mineral with respect to powdery samples, bearing in mind that hydrogels were prepared with 10% *w/w* of the corresponding clay. Since the final amount of clay fibroblasts was put in contact with the same as in the experiments with pristine clays, the same concentration codes (1000, 500, 50 and 5 μg/mL) were used. Briefly, clay and hydrogel samples were dispersed in sterile Hanks' Balanced Salt Solution (Sigma-Aldrich) and mixed with Ultra-Turrax® (S 25N, -18G, IKA, Staufen, Germany) for 5 min, 150,000 rpm. These initial suspensions were subsequently diluted in order to obtain samples having a concentration in the range previously mentioned. Eight replicates were assessed for all samples and for the control (NHDF cultures in pure DMEM phenol red).

After the 24 h contact, growth medium and samples were withdrawn from each well, and MTT (3-(4,5-dimethylthiazol-2-yl)-2,5-diphenyltetrazolium bromide) test was performed. This test is based on the activity of mitochondrial dehydrogenases of vital cells that convert MTT in formazan crystals. DMEM phenol red-free and 50 μL of MTT dissolution were added in each well, the final MTT concentration being 2.5 mg/mL. MTT-NHDF contact was maintained for 3 h before the whole supernatant was withdrawn and substituted by 100 μL of dimethyl sulfoxide solution (DMSO, Sigma-Aldrich®-Merck, Milan, Italy) to dissolve formazan purple salts. The absorbance was assayed at 570 nm by means of an ELISA plate reader (Imark Absorbance Reader, Bio-rad, Hercules, CA, USA), with a reference wavelength set at 655 nm. Cell viability was calculated as % ratio of the absorbance of each sample and the absorbance of the cells kept in contact with the growth medium (control).

2.3.2. Cell Motility Assay for Wound Healing

The gap closure cell motility assay is based on the employment of a Petri μ-Dish$^{35\ \mathrm{mm,\ low}}$ (Ibidi, Giardini, Italy) in which a silicone insert is enclosed. The insert comprises two chambers with a growth area of 0.22 cm^2 divided by a septum with a width of cell-free gap of 500 ± 50 μm. NHDFs were seeded in each chamber at 10^5 cells/cm^2 concentration and were grown until confluence in the same conditions described in Section 2.3.1. After 24 h, fibroblasts reached confluence, and the silicone inserts were subsequently removed with sterile tweezers, displaying two areas of cell substrates divided by the 500 μm (± 50) gap.

Cell substrates were washed with sterile phosphate buffer solution (PBS; 10% *v/v*) to eliminate debris. Then, they were put in contact with a final volume of 700 μL of phenol red DMEM in which samples were included at determined concentrations. These concentrations were selected according to MTT results. Particularly, PS9, G30, PS9ALI, PS9GR, G30ALI and G30GR were used in concentration B (50 μg/mL of clay mineral), and spring waters were used in 2.5% *v/v* concentrations. Cells kept in contact with pure growth medium were used as control.

Microphotographs were taken at prefixed time intervals (0, 24, 48 h) to evaluate cell growth inside the gap. Anoptical microscope (Leica, DMI3000-B model) equipped with LAS EZ software was used (Leica microsystems, Wetzlar, Germany). In order to analyze results in a more objective way, the full area of the wound healing space was photographed in all samples. Then, wound closure was monitored by measuring the remaining gap with ImageJ software. The percentage of wound closure was calculated according to Equation (2), where WS0 stands for "wound space at time 0" and WS24 is "wound space after 24 h", both of them measured as an area (μm^2).

$$\%\ \text{Wound closed after 24 h} = 100 - \frac{WS_{24}\left(\mu m^2\right)\cdot 100}{WS_0\left(\mu m^2\right)} \quad (2)$$

2.4. *Confocal Laser Scanning Microscopy*

An additional sequence of wound healing experiments was stopped at 24 h of growth in order to study the morphology of fibroblasts during the wound closure procedure. NDHFs were washed three times with PBS (10% *v/v*) and fixed with glutaraldehyde solution in PBS (3% *v/v*, 800 μL; Sigma-Aldrich®-Merck, Milan, Italy). Contact with glutaraldehyde was maintained for 2 h (4–8 °C), and all samples were protected from light. Three PBS washes were once again performed prior to fibroblast permeabilization. Permeabilization was performed by adding Triton X-10 (0.1% *w/v*) for 10 min at room temperature. Triple PBS wash was again performed. Fluorescein isothiocyanate (FITC, λ_{ex} = 495 nm; λ_{em} = 513 nm)-labeled phalloidin (Phalloidin-FITC, Sigma-Aldrich) was used to mark polymerized F-actin in the cytoplasm of NHDF (50 μg/mL, darkness, 40 min at room temperature). The procedure was defined according to fabricant indications. After several PBS washings aiming to eliminate unbound phalloidin-FITC, fibroblast nuclei staining was done. Blue fluorescence nucleic acid stain 4′,6-diamidino-2-phenylindole (DAPI, Sigma-Aldrich) was used. This molecule binds to double-stranded DNA, thus labelling nuclei (λ_{ex} = 485 nm; λ_{em} = 552 nm). Contact between DAPI and cells was maintained for 10 min at room temperature in darkness. Finally, samples were washed and preserved in PBS (10% *v/v*) to avoid dryness. Confocal Laser Scanning Microscopy (CLSM) microphotographs were obtained by a Leica TCS SP2 (Leica Microsystems, Milan, Italy). Images were processed with ImageJ software.

2.5. Statistical Analysis

The statistical differences were determined by means of non-parametric Mann–Whitney (Wilcoxon) W test. In all cases, SPSS Statistic software was used, and differences were considered significant at *p*-values ≤ 0.05. Only significant differences are reported.

3. Results and Discussion

3.1. Caracterization of Inorganic Ingredients

3.1.1. Particle Size

The granulometric distribution of PS9 and G30 is plotted in Figure 1. Both samples were unimodal and, therefore, homogeneous. PS9 showed to be finer than G30 (Table 4), the latter one slightly asymmetric. Calculated SPAN factors showed that the amplitude of particle size distribution for both samples had no significant difference (Table 4).

Table 4. Statistical particle diameters, SPAN factor (average ± s.d.; n = 3) and main modes of PS9 and G30 clay minerals.

	PS9	G30
d_{10} (μm)	4.0 ± 0.07	4.8 ± 0.03
d_{50} (μm)	9.9 ± 0.15	20.2 ± 0.03
d_{90} (μm)	23.9 ± 0.2	49.3 ± 0.10
SPAN Factor	2.0 ± 0.02	2.2 ± 0.01
Main Mode (μm)	8.9	28.3

In terms of hydrogels, the finer the particles of the solid phase, the higher the stability of the resultant semisolid system (no phase separation) and the better the textural properties (smoothness). Mineralogical composition of G30 (Table 1) included 26% *w/w* of quartz. The presence of this mineral could influence rheology and textural properties of hydrogels. Particularly, it infers an abrasive texture to the preparation if quartz particle sizes are big. Particle sizes higher than 150 μm could be abrasive, particularly when they have remarkable hardness, such in the case of quartz [66]. Despite the presence of 26% of quartz mineral in G30, its particles were smaller than 100 μm (Figure 1), which means that resultant hydrogels possessed smooth textures, which are crucial for the acceptance of the patients [67].

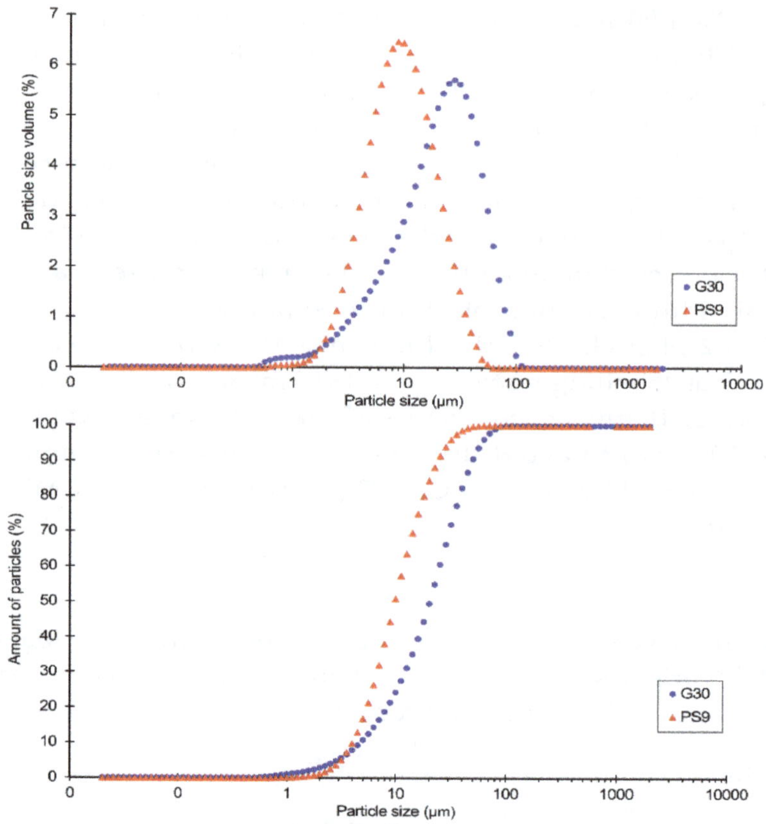

Figure 1. Particle size analysis of PS9 and G30. Differential analysis (up) and cumulative percentage of particles (down).

3.1.2. Cation Exchange Capacity

The individual exchangeable elements and total CEC of PS9 and G30 are summarized in Table 5. Total CEC values were inside the expected CEC limits for sepiolite (9.18 mEq/100 g) and palygorskite (16.29 mEq/100 g) [68,69]. Sepiolite and palygorskite CEC are usually <25 mEq/100 g [70] with higher values usually related to impurities [71–81]. The higher CEC showed by G30 with respect to PS9 could be explained by the presence of 6% *w/w* of smectites and/or sepiolite in G30, as previously described.

Table 5. CEC results of PS9 and G30 (average mEq/100 g ± s.d.; n = 3).

mEq/100g	PS9	G30
Na^+	0.70 ± 0.045	1.68 ± 0.071
K^+	0.33 ± 0.023	0.13 ± 0.032
Mg^{2+}	3.62 ± 0.341	7.61± 0.326
Ca^{2+}	4.53 ± 0.123	6.87± 0.186
Total	9.18	16.29

The main exchangeable cations for both clays were Mg^{2+} and Ca^{2+}, which was in agreement with the chemical composition of PS9 and G30 showed by X-ray fluorescence analysis [63], though Na^+ and K^+ were also detected in small amounts. Na^+, K^+, Mg^{2+} and Ca^{2+} are essential elements since they are widely found inside and outside human cells [82–84]. The presence of suitable levels of ions such as calcium, magnesium, sodium and potassium in the wound bed are important to enhance the healing process. They allow the activity of the enzymes involved in the healing process, leading to the cascade of the repairing and regenerative processes. Specifically, calcium and magnesium levels should raise during the first 5 d of wound healing in order to promote granulation tissue formation and epidermal cell proliferation [85]. Moreover, during the restoration of the trans-epithelial potential of cells in the damaged tissue, Na^+, K^+ and/or Ca^{2+} play a crucial role [86]. The bioavailability of these cations in the wound site should promote the healing process and contribute to fasten the damaged area reparation.

Mg^{2+} cations, abundant in both ALI and GR, have demonstrated remarkable properties for tissue regeneration and repair, particularly in the promotion of collagen formation and angiogenesis on skin wounds [56,87]. For this reason, it is conceivable that ALI and GR should perform wound healing effects, as previously remarked. The maximum exchangeable amount of Mg^{2+} from PS9 and G30 corresponded to 17.67 and 37.14 mg/L, respectively (Table 5). Magnesium concentration due to the spring water was 5–12 mg/L, and this proved to be effective during wound healing by Sasaki et al. [56]. Consequently, both PS9 and G30 were considered as potentially effective minerals due to their exchangeable Mg^{2+} content.

Normal homeostasis of mammalian skin is also maintained by elements such as calcium, modulating keratinocyte and fibroblast proliferation and differentiation [88]. Certain skin disorders, such as psoriasis, have been related to Ca^{2+} disorders in keratinocytes [89,90]. Extracellular calcium is a determinant factor in the differentiation and maturation of fibroblasts, and its effectiveness is dose-dependent [89] Another recent study on wound healing demonstrated that calcium cations released from a calcium alginate wound dressing promoted endothelial cell growth and proliferation [91].

Zinc is also important during wound healing steps [85,88], though it was not detected as an exchangeable cation of PS9 nor G30 through the ICP-OES measurements performed. However, both ALI and GR waters contained Zn (Table 2).

Potassium has also demonstrated to favor wound healing (fibroblast differentiation, re-epithelialization, migration and proliferation of dermal cells), so its presence both in spring waters and hydrogels is considered as a positive feature [92,93].

3.1.3. Zeta Potential

Zeta-potential results of PS9 and G30 at different concentrations are presented in Figure 2. Regarding ζ potential of minerals in pH 7 buffer, PS9 and G30 results were in agreement with other sepiolite and palygorskite samples previously studied [94–96]. In particular, the zeta potential of PS9 in aqueous pH 7 solution was more negative (higher) than that of G30.

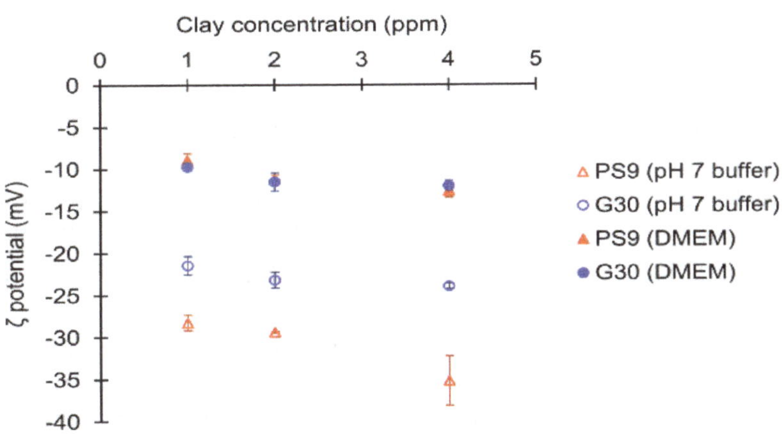

Figure 2. Zeta potential variations of PS9 and G30 (mean values ± s.d.; n = 3) in pH 7 buffer and complete DMEM culture medium at different concentrations.

It has been demonstrated that surface charge of nanoparticles has the potential to influence cell viability [97]. The importance of clay particle zeta potentials during biocompatibility and wound healing tests lies in the fact that cells possess a negative surface zeta potential. Negative zeta potential is one of the most decisive factors of biocompatible materials, showing higher cell viability [98,99]. It is known that particles with positive zeta potentials interact and/or penetrate cells easily due to their opposite charge, thus being one of the main strategies to improve transfection efficiency [100,101].

Negatively charged particles have also proved to interact with cells up to a certain extent and even be able to enter by endocytosis-mediated mechanisms [102,103], although this happens with higher difficulty for negative particles than for positive ones. The uncontrolled entrance of certain substances into the cells could jeopardize their viability, thus inferring that positively charged materials are more likely to put the cell viability at risk.

Another factor by which nanoparticle surface charge demonstrated to influence cell viability is due to their agglomeration state [99]. Berg and co-workers revealed that hepatocytes showed less viability when exposed to metal nanoparticles with zeta potentials close to their isoelectric point [97]. This change in zeta potential was also strongly related to the agglomeration state of the very same particles. That is, the more neutral the nanoparticles are, the more easily they aggregate and, subsequently, the faster their precipitation over the cell tapestry and/or their interaction with the negatively charged cell membranes.

Cell media, such as DMEM, have demonstrated to significantly modify zeta potential of different suspended particles [104–106]. These changes are ascribed to the presence of a wide variety of charged molecules such as amino acids and vitamins, among others. The interaction of clay particles with these molecules changes the zeta potential of the former ones. In fact, PS9 and G30 suffered a significant change of zeta potential when added to full DMEM culture medium (Figure 2). In this occasion, no significant differences were found between PS9 and G30 values, thus confirming that the resultant surface charges of the particles is governed by the culture medium. Therefore, during biocompatibility and wound healing tests, clay particles should maintain a −10 mV zeta potential. The reduction of zeta potential strength would reduce the stability of the clay suspensions, making them less flocculated and, consequently, more prone to precipitation phenomena. Precipitation of clay particles could hinder cell viability by cell suffocation. Nonetheless, the fact that they still showed a negative surface charge would hinder the entrance of clay particles inside cells. These results will be confirmed by MTT analysis.

3.2. *In Vitro Tests of Inorganic Ingredients, Spring Waters and Hydrogels*

3.2.1. Biocompatibility Tests

Biocompatibility results on NHDF treated with medicinal ALI and GR waters for 24 h are plotted in Figure 3. No significant differences were found, even when multiple comparisons were performed. In fact, ALI and GR viability results were around 100% for all water dilutions. Therefore, mineral medicinal waters studied in this work did not hinder dermal fibroblasts viability, thus determining their biocompatibility. Internal comparisons between ALI and GR concentrations were also performed. Mann–Whitney marked differences in ALI viability were between 50% vs. 0.25% and 25% vs. 0.25% (Figure 3). Su et al. detected an optimal dilution of a concentrated underground mineral spring water that made skin cells to grow better in comparison with other dilutions [107]. By the same token, ALI concentrations higher than 25% (*v*/*v*) could allow slightly better NHDF growth performances with respect to more diluted samples.

PS9 clay mineral and corresponding peloids PS9ALI and PS9GR are plotted in Figure 4 (left) as well as G30 and its corresponding peloids G30ALI and G30GR Figure 4 (right). In a general view, the lower the sample concentration (either clay or thermal mud), the higher the cell viability. None of the samples nor their concentrations presented a cellular viability below 80%. This fact indicated the absence of drastic cellular cytotoxicity within 24 h. With respect to PS9 and G30 clays, it was possible to observe a slight reduction of the cellular viability (with respect to GM) as the clay concentration increased. In fact, when the clay mineral concentration corresponded to 1 mg/mL, cellular viability was close to 80% (for both pristine clays and thermal muds). Nonetheless, statistical analyses indicated no significant differences between PS9 and G30 1000 μg/mL concentrations vs. GM, which confirmed that PS9 and G30 were highly biocompatible against NHDF cells. G30 5 μg/mL concentration showed significant differences vs. GM. Notably, the lower the concentration of the clay, the better the cellular proliferation. It has been suggested by some studies that the precipitation of clay minerals could hinder cell viability by some sort of physical effect [50,103]. The biocompatibility of Veegum HS © (Bentonite clay) was evaluated by Salcedo et al., finding that at 167 μg/mL of Veegum HS © concentration the viability of Caco-2 cells reduced approximately to 50% [50]. This effect was ascribed to the precipitation of clay particles, which blocked cell membrane channels. According to the authors, montmorillonite had a particle size ranging from 45–75 μm [50], which is a particle size range very similar to that of PS9 and G30. In these conditions, it was argued that if the precipitation of clay particles occurred, cell viability could be compromised at concentrations ≥160 μg/mL. On the contrary, neither PS9 nor G30 showed fibroblasts viabilities lower than 50% even at the highest concentration tested, thus demonstrating to possess a remarkable biocompatibility.

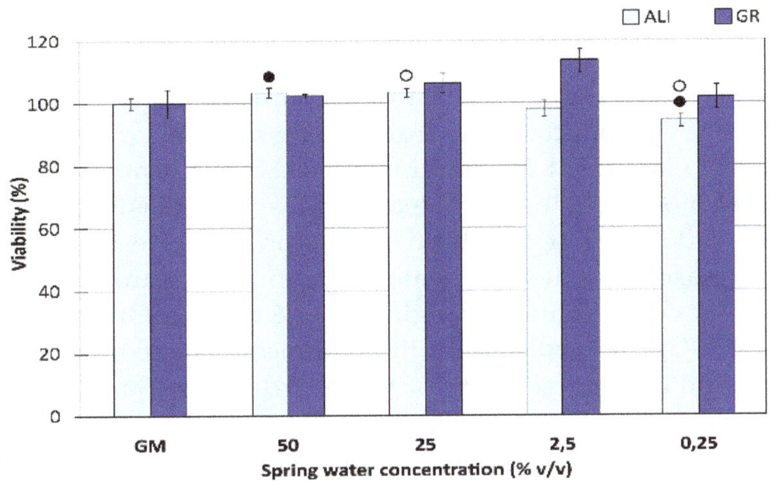

Figure 3. Biocompatibility tests (contact time 24 h) of ALI and GR medicinal waters. Viability (%) vs. medicinal water concentration (% *v/v*) toward NHDF. GM stands for "growth medium" and refers to control test. Mean values ± s.d.; n = 8. Significant differences are marked as (•) ALI 50% (*v/v*) vs. ALI 0.25% (*v/v*); (○) ALI 25% (*v/v*) vs. ALI 0.25% (*v/v*). Mann–Whitney (Wilcoxon) W tests, *p* values ≤ 0.05.

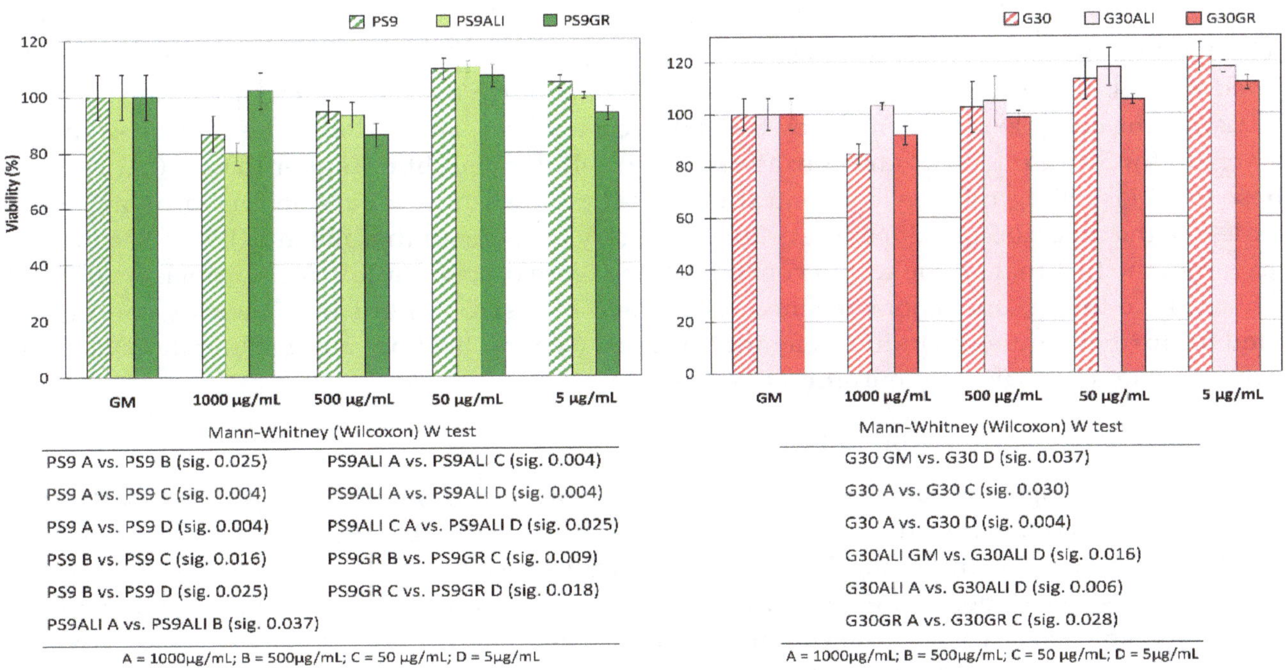

Figure 4. Biocompatibility tests (contact time 24 h) of PS9, PS9ALI and PS9GR (left) and G30, G30ALI and G30GR (right). Viability (%) vs. clay concentrations toward NHDF. GM stands for "growth medium" and refers to control test. Mean values ± s.d.; n = 8. Significant differences were reported within the figure (down) as "sig" which refers to "*p*-values".

Internal statistical studies for PS9 and G30 results detected significant differences in G30 1000 μg/mL vs. 50 μg/mL and 5 μg/mL. For PS9, concentrations of PS9 1000 and 500 μg/mL differed both between them as well as with 50 and 5 μg/mL (see Figure 4). These findings mean that, for both clays, smaller clay amounts in contact with fibroblasts were characterized by a higher degree of fibroblast biocompatibility. The biocompatibility results obtained for both clays were in agreement with the existing literature. Sepiolite clay mineral (Pangel S9) has been previously tested by Fukushima et al. towards fibroblasts and osteoblasts [108]. In this case, authors combined 10% of sepiolite with poly(butylene adipate-co-terephthalate) reporting no cytotoxicity. A Tolsa's Group sepiolite clay was also employed by Fernandes et al. [109]. In this case, they reported a reduction of HeLa cell viability of 50% when sepiolite was present in 1000 μg/mL concentration. No such a reduction was found in this work when PS9 was used at the same concentration. Nonetheless, these differences could be ascribed to differences in the type of cell culture [110]. Apart from anti-inflammatory, antibacterial and anti-oxidant properties of a natural Spanish palygorskite, its cytotoxicity against murine macrophages has been reported to start from 300 μg/mL onwards [58,59]. Particularly, authors reported a reduction of 20% viability at the aforementioned concentration. Once again, in the present study, G30 showed higher biocompatibility (at least against fibroblasts) because, even at 500 μg/mL concentration, fibroblasts did not show a viability reduction. In more recent studies, pharmaceutical grade palygorskite (Pharmasorb® colloidal) was able to protect human dermal fibroblasts against carvacrol cytotoxicity at clay concentrations ranging from 8 to 12 μg/mL [6].

Neither PS9ALI nor PS9GR showed significant differences between GM and tested concentrations, thus demonstrating the total biocompatibility of these hydrogels. Statistically, PS9ALI and PS9GR thermal mud showed similar significant differences between concentrations, following the same trend previously described for PS9. In fact, 50 and 5 μg/mL clay concentrations apparently favored cellular viability (Figure 4, left). The agreement among PS9ALI, PS9GR and PS9 biocompatibility results allowed the confirmation of their reproducibility. Both PS9ALI and PS9GR, as well as PS9, shared significant differences of concentration 50 μg/mL due to the higher viability results obtained at this concentration (Figure 4, left).

Regarding G30ALI and G30GR peloids, Mann–Whitney statistical analysis pointed out significant discrepancy in activity between G30ALI GM and 1000 μg/mL concentration vs. 5 μg/mL and between G30GR 1000 μg/mL vs. 50 μg/mL (as specified in Figure 4, right). Since the same trend has been reported for G30 samples, once again it was possible to confirm the reproducibility of the results.

Despite the complexity generated by the statistical analysis, all solid samples (Figure 4) showed a better result for 50 μg/mL concentration, always with cellular viabilities higher than 100%. According to these findings, 50 μg/mL clay concentration was the safest/most ideal one for fibroblast cultures, regardless of the type (PS9 or G30) or the origin of the clay (powder or thermal mud). It is also important not to forget the fact that all the tested concentrations were biocompatible for fibroblasts within 24 h of contact. Due to the conclusions reached with the MTT test, 50 μg/mL was the clay concentration selected for further studies including cell motility assay (wound healing) and proliferation CLSM tests. For spring waters, 50% *v*/*v* concentration was used.

3.2.2. Cell Motility Assay for Wound Healing

Microscopy images of gap closure results are reported in Figures 5–7. ALI and GR samples were tested at 50% (*v*/*v*) concentration, while PS9, G30, PS9ALI, PS9GR, G30ALI and G30GR were tested at 50 μg/mL of clay mineral. The microphotographs taken at zero time (0 h) showed for all the samples the presence of defined gaps mimicking wounds. Normal fibroblasts grown at confluence were clearly visible in each side of the wound. The time 0 gaps were reported to measure approximately 500 μm, which was in agreement with the variability of the silicone inserts of the Petri μ-Dishes used (500 ± 50 μm). Insoluble clay particles were visible in the cultures treated with PS9, G30 and hydrogels PS9ALI, PS9GR, G30ALI and G30GR, unlike GM, ALI and GR. In all cases, after 24 h, fibroblasts started to invade the gap and even established contact with the cells of the opposite side in certain points of some samples. NHDF cells also maintained their typical fusiform morphology during the whole experiment. These facts confirmed that the presence of spring waters, clay or hydrogels did not impair cell growth. This was in line with the biocompatibility results previously discussed. In all cases, fibroblasts crossed the empty zone after 48 h, thus forming anastomosis. In spring water ALI and GR samples, fibroblasts of both sides of the wound established contact within 24 h (Figure 5). In comparison with the control (GM), it was clear that the addition of ALI and GR favored wound closure, since the contact points between fibroblasts were more numerous. According to the measurements of the wounded area performed by image analysis, ALI and GR samples covered, respectively, 62.9% and 59.1% of the initial wounded area, whereas GM covered about 31.8% of the wound (Figure 8). After 48 h all the cell substrates reached confluence, and this further supports the biocompatibility of the hydrogels and their components in vitro. Previous works have claimed that the presence of elements such as B^{3+} and Mn^{+2} in keratinocyte culture mediums induced the migration of these cells [30]. They tested boron and manganese at different concentrations (500–1000 µg/L and 100–1500 µg/L, respectively). In fact, keratinocytes in contact with these elements were able to cover the artificial gap (scratch-assay method) with 20% more efficiency with respect to the control group (without B^{3+} and Mn^{+2}) in 24 h. ALI and GR chemical compositions have been previously reported by Aguzzi et al. [111] and García-Villén et al. [63] (Table 3). The absence of significant differences between GR, ALI and GM groups further confirmed the biocompatibility of both mineral medicinal waters since they did not hinder wound closure. The presence of B^{3+} and Mn^{+2} in both GR and ALI could explain why they did not interfere with cell motility during wound healing in a significant manner. Other elements such as As^{3+} and Fe^{2+} (both presents in ALI and GR waters) have also demonstrated to improve wound healing, particularly of the nasal mucosa [112]. General skin regenerative properties of spring waters have been reported in the literature [32–34,113]. The study of Liang et al. demonstrated that skin regenerative properties of Nagano spring water were related to the spring water chemical composition, with no influence of microorganisms [31]. Another beneficial effect that could be ascribed to ALI and GR according to their chemical composition is the protective effect against oxidative stress due to the presence of sulfur [114].

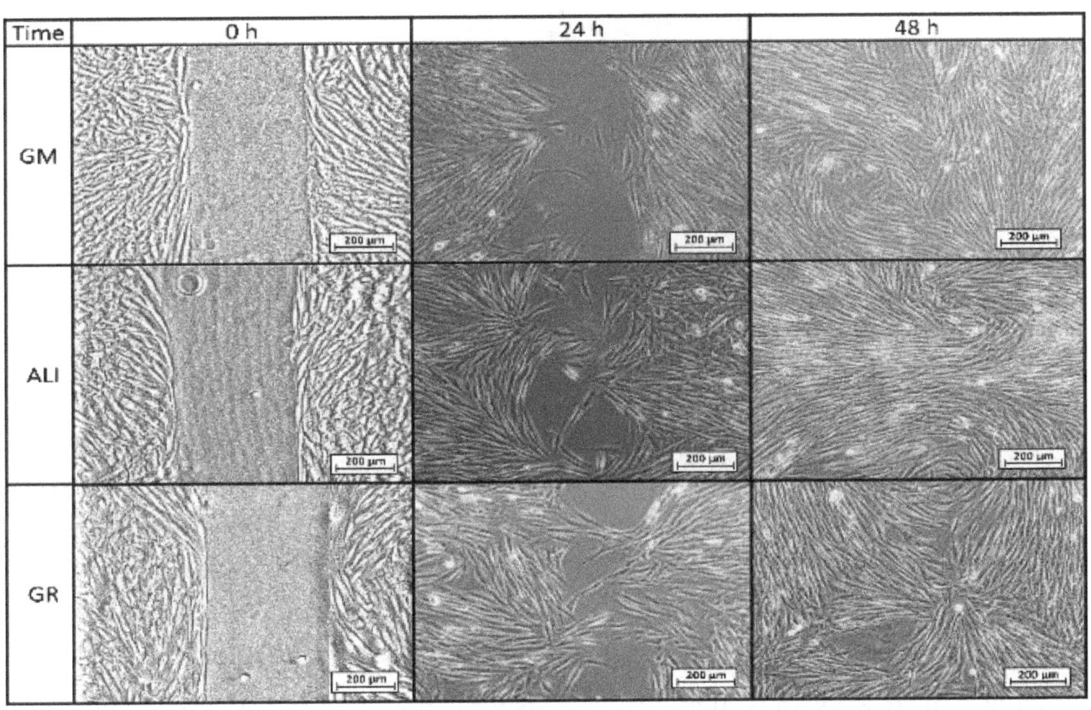

Figure 5. Optical microscopy of wound healing tests for control group (GM) and spring waters (ALI and GR) at 50% (*v*/*v*) culture concentration.

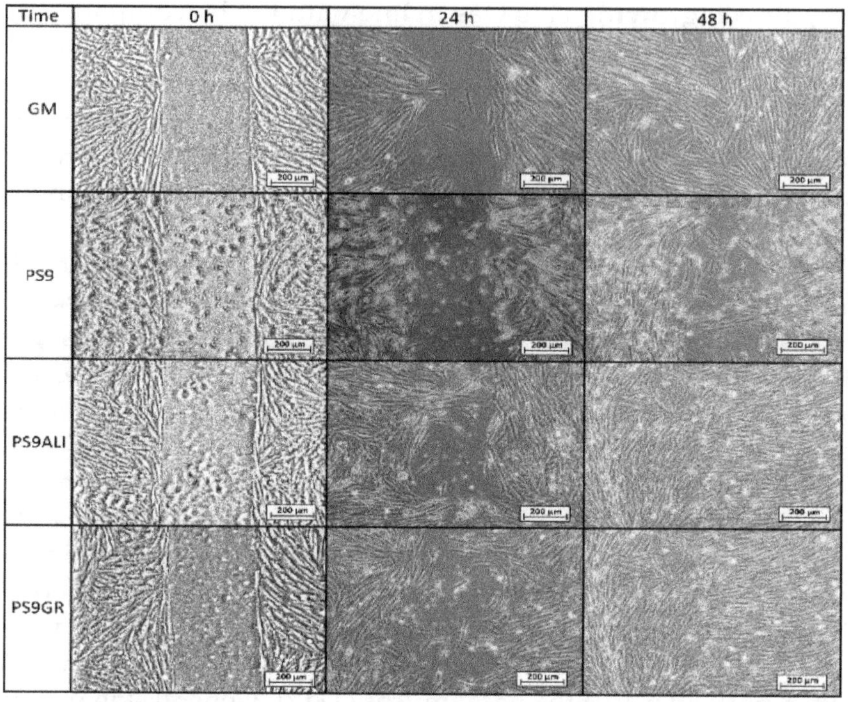

Figure 6. Optical microscopy of wound healing tests for control group (GM), PS9 clay mineral and corresponding peloids PS9ALI and PS9GR, all of them with a clay concentration of 50 µg/mL.

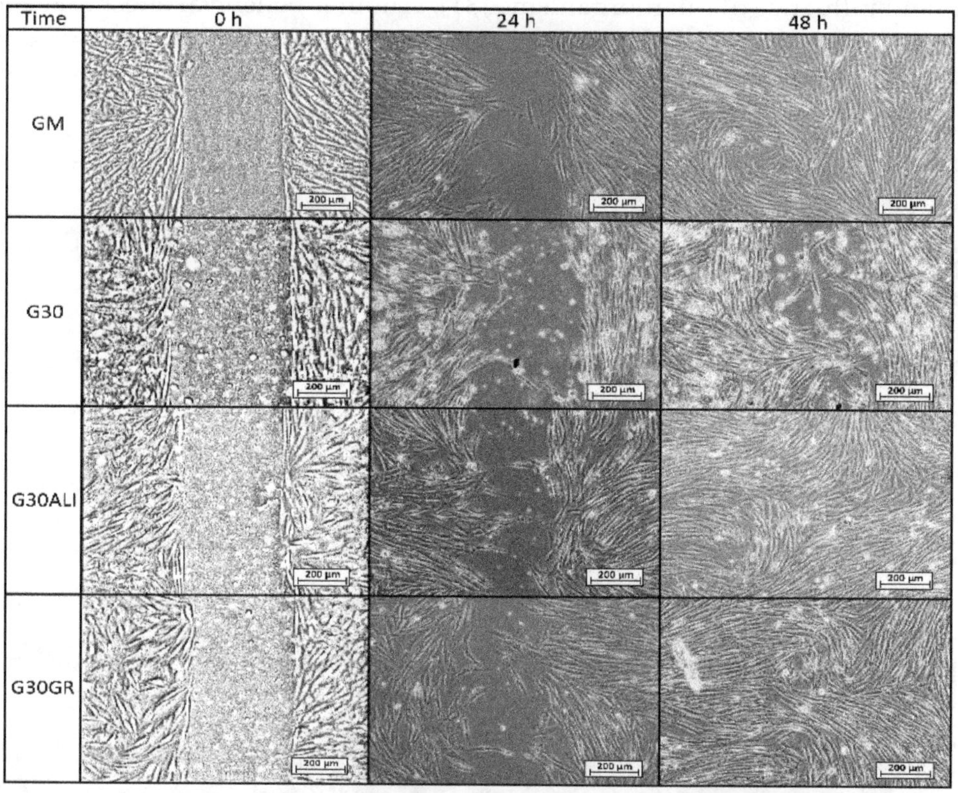

Figure 7. Optical microscopy of wound healing tests for control group (GM), G30 clay mineral and corresponding peloids G30ALI and G30GR, all of them with a clay concentration of 50 µg/mL.

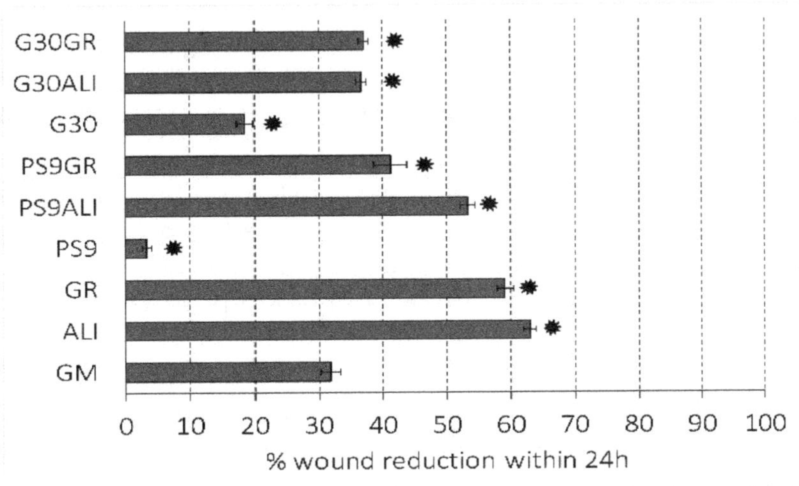

Figure 8. Histogram of % wound reduction after 24 h, calculated according to Equation (2). Mean values ± s.d. (n = 6). Significant differences between samples and GM are marked with *.

Regarding PS9 and G30 clay samples (Figures 6 and 7), it was not possible to find zones with full fibroblast confluence after 48 h, though both sides of the wound were able to establish contact at this time. Fibroblast contacts of PS9 and G30 samples in the culture medium were slower with respect to GM. According to MTT results (Section 3.2.1), which were also performed for 24 h, pristine clays did not hinder cell viability. However, their presence seemed to impede fibroblast mobility during the wound healing assay, slowing down the total gap closure with respect to GM and studied peloids. In fact, the uncovered gap width after 24 h was significantly higher for PS9 and G30 with respect to the rest of the samples (Figure 8), thus indicating a slower coverage of the wounded area. For these similar samples, the majority of insoluble particles visible within the cell substrate were concentrated adjacent to or over/inside fibroblasts. It is well known that cell membranes are negatively charged and can be penetrated by positive substances. Negatively charged particles can also interact and even penetrate cells by endocytosis-mediated mechanisms [102,103,115]. According to the zeta potential results previously reported (Figure 2), PS9 and G30 had a negative net charge in the major part of the pH range tested. These clay particles could interact between them (thus forming bigger aggregates) and with cells by establishing interactions such as Van der Waals forces. This hypothesis was the starting point of Abduljauwad and Ahmed, who proposed that the interaction between clay minerals and cells would hinder cell migration [116]. They evaluated the roles of montmorillonite, hectorite and palygorskite particles in cancer cell migration and demonstrated these materials could prevent cellular metastasis. Results of scratch-induced wound healing assays reported by these authors demonstrated that clay mineral particles significantly delayed the gap closure in comparison with control experiments. For instance, while the control showed full gap closure within 24 h, palygorskite showed a mean gap closure of 59 ± 3% after 24 h. Polymeric composite films containing montmorillonite were evaluated by Salcedo et al. [50] and Mishra et al. [117]. The scratch assay showed, in both cases, that the presence of montmorillonite particles alone was able to alter cell behavior (Caco-2 and fibroblasts, respectively for each study), slowing down the gap closure. Similar results were reported by Vaiana et al. on montmorillonite and keratinocytes [118]. These results were in agreement with PS9 and G30 performances during wound healing: though clays were not cytotoxic, more time would be necessary to obtain complete cell confluence within the artificial wound (gap) in their presence. The biocompatibility and safety of natural clay minerals such as palygorskite during wound healing was also supported by in vivo studies. A natural Brazilian palygorskite was tested for in vivo wound healing of rats [119]. In comparison with functionalized clay minerals, the natural one provided more advanced and safer wound healing, since histological cuts demonstrated the presence of dermal papilla and hair follicles after 14 d of treatment [119].

The presence of hydrogels promoted in vitro fibroblast mobility during wound healing processes. In fact, coverage of the artificial gap was faster for PS9ALI, PS9GR, G30ALI and G30GR with respect to GM and pristine clays (Figure 8). It is worth to note that all therapeutic muds were used in concentrations equal to the powdered clay samples. That is, the amount of peloid within the culture medium was higher in order to compensate for them only possessing a 10% *w/w* of clay mineral. Whatsoever the nature of the interaction between clay particles and fibroblasts, responsible for the gap closure deceleration (observed in PS9 and G30 tests), it was reduced to a minimum when it came to thermal mud formulations. In fact, significant differences were found between gap closures of peloids vs. GM, demonstrating that the evaluated hydrogels induced a positive effect during wound healing.

These results are supported by previous studies in which clay minerals have reported to exert neutral or positive wound healing effects when combined with other substances [44,120]. For instance, no significant changes have been found during in vitro wound healing studies of montmorillonite–chitosan–silver sulfadiazine nanocomposites with respect to the control. That is, the presence of the clay mineral did not hinder the gap closure procedure and did not affect fibroblast phenotypes [54]. On the other hand, better skin re-epithelialization and reorganization have been found when halloysite and chitosan were combined to form a nanocomposite with respect to the use of both materials independently [47]. In vivo infected wound treatment with silver nanoparticles was improved by the use of montmorillonite as a carrier, which reduced the drug cytotoxicity [121]. Montmorillonite also demonstrated to exert a wound healing effect when combined with chitosan and polyvinylpyrrolidone polymers [48]. The nanocomposite films containing bentonite increased the in vivo wound healing processes in mice when compared with the formulations without the clay. For instance, wound closure after 16 d was 92–93% for samples without clay and 95–97% for those with montomorillonite, and all of them were higher than the negative control at the same time (84%) [48].

Despite the scarce literature regarding the use of therapeutic muds in skin regenerative properties, the existing studies were also in agreement with the present observations. Thermal mud treatments with volcanic deposits of Azerbaijan facilitated the healing of chronic gangrenous wounds of diabetic patients [60]. The major part of the patients subjected to pelotherapy reached total wound recovery by the end of the treatment. Two natural Dead Sea black mud samples were evaluated by Abu-al-Basal for their in vivo wound healing properties [61]. One of them was used in its pristine state, while the other was formulated in form of a facial mask by adding plant extracts and vitamin E. Both samples accelerated the wound healing process by enhancing granulation, wound contraction, epithelialization, angiogenesis and collagen deposition. Another in vivo wound healing study was performed by Dário et al. [62]. They evaluated a natural peloid extracted from Ocara Lake (northeast of Brazil), which was sieved, solid-state characterized and sterilized. The solid fraction was mainly composed of quartz, illite and kaolinite, and it was formulated as an emulsion. The emulsion was put in contact with injured Wistar rats. The formulation including the Ocara Lake solid fraction induced histological changes in the deep dermis that allowed an effective healing with respect to control groups. On the other hand, there is evidence in literature about the anti-inflammatory properties of peloids [122]. Moreover, a recent study focusing on fibrous clays suggests that sepiolite and palygorskite, the main components of PS9 and G30, respectively, did not influence the in vitro NO (inflammation signal) production of murine macrophages (RAW 264.7). Furthermore, both clays decreased the leucocyte infiltration shortly after exposure in vivo on mouse ear edema (12-O-tetradecanoylphorbol-13-acetate (TPA) as inflammatory agent). In particular, sepiolite and palygorskite caused decreases on the number of infiltrated cells per field [59]. Analogously, other clay minerals, as halloysite and montmorillonite, proved macrophage cytocompatibility and negligible secretion of TNFa, as proinflammatory cytokines [123]. The anti-inflammatory properties of clays could control the inflammatory phase in the healing process, shortening healing time and avoiding wound chronicity.

3.3. Confocal Laser Scanning Microscopy

CLSM microphotograph results (Figure 9) showed fluorescence of fibroblast nuclei and cytoplasm. Green fluorescence is due to the binding of phalloidin specifically with F-actin, and the blue one is due to 4′,6-diamidino-2-phenylindole (DAPI) bounded to DNA. Morphology of fibroblasts during wound healing is very important, since it gives information about migration and adhesion of cells. F-actin filaments facilitate cell–cell interaction and tissue regeneration [124]. In all samples, regardless of the type of sample with which fibroblasts were put in contact with, NHDF showed typical fusiform morphology. Moreover, fibroblasts located in the wounded area possessed typical morphology of migrating cells. Therefore, it was possible to identify retraction/protrusion parts of fibroblasts due to the position of F-actin. Typical actin filament structures were detectable in all samples: lamellipodia, filopodia and stress fibers (dorsal stress fibers and transverse arcs). Moreover, fibroblasts in mitosis were also visible in some points.

Regarding the speed of wound closure, the CLSM results were in agreement with those obtained by optical microscopy. GM control after 24 h demonstrated that NHDFs were able to make contact and started to close the gap, though yet some empty zones were clearly visible. The number of cells inside the wound gap in ALI and GR samples was higher than that in GM. PS9 and G30 showed the worst result in terms of "gap closure", which confirmed the previous results. Once again, it was possible to observe that the "slowing down" effect of PS9 and G30 did not happen when both clays were formulated in form of nanoclay/spring water hydrogels. Particularly, hydrogels G30ALI, G30GR, PS9ALI and PS9GR induced a faster wound healing with respect to the rest of the samples.

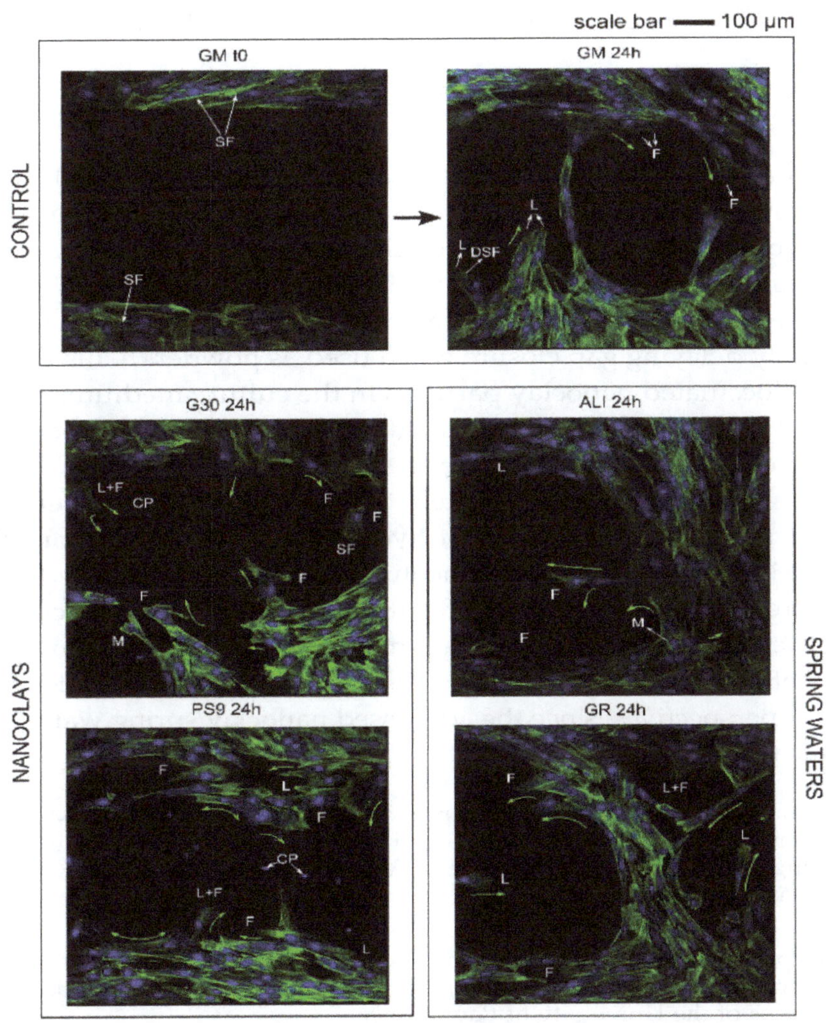

Figure 9. *Cont.*

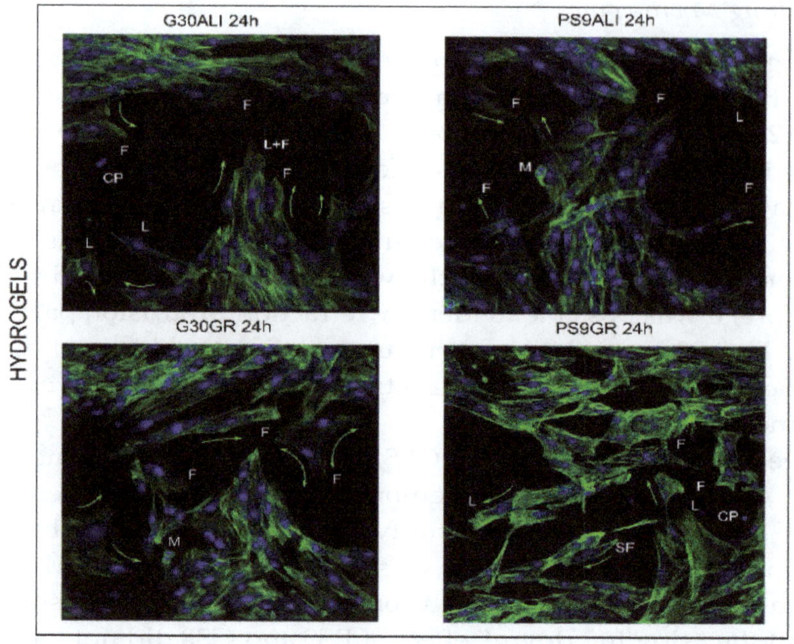

Figure 9. CLSM microphotographs during wound healing. NHDMs were stained with phalloidin-FITC (green, F-actin filaments) and DAPI (blue, nucleus). Green arrows indicate the migration direction; different F-actin structures have been identified by L (lamellipodia), F (filopodia), SF (stress fibers) and DSF (dorsal stress fibers). Additionally, M stands for (mitosis) and CP stands for (clay particles).

4. Conclusions

Fibroblast biocompatibility and wound healing efficacy of inorganic hydrogels formulated with two nanoclays in two natural spring waters have been studied. Both spring waters were fully biocompatible and favored wound healing, inducing faster gap closure with respect to control. The studied nanoclays did not interfere with cell viability to a great extent (≥80% of cell viability), thus not being cytotoxic at the studied concentrations. Nonetheless, they interfered with the in vitro wound healing processes, slightly delaying gap closure when used as powders. This effect could be ascribed to the presence of non-flocculated nanoclay particles in the culture medium. Hydrogels formulated with the aforementioned ingredients did not hindered gap closure and reported a higher percentage of wound closure after 24 h with respect to the control.

In conclusion, this study has demonstrated the usefulness and potential of PS9 and G30 clay minerals as excipients in the preparation of hydrogels intended for wound healing and other therapeutic uses. Maximum in vitro wound healing effects were achieved by using PS9 in the formulation of the hydrogels. These promising results encourage the use of clay minerals as wound healing ingredients. Thermal center treatments are mostly focused on the physical effects of thermal muds, which are very effective against musculoskeletal disorders. Nonetheless, the findings of this study have opened new perspectives, since the addressed nanoclay/spring water hydrogels could also be used to treat chronic wounds.

Author Contributions: Data curation, F.G.-V.; Funding acquisition, C.V. and G.S.; Methodology, F.G.-V., A.F., D.M. and M.R.; Project administration, C.V. and G.S.; Supervision, A.F. and D.M.; Writing—original draft, F.G.-V.; Writing—review & editing, R.S.-E., A.B.-S., P.C., S.R., C.V. and G.S. All authors have read and agreed to the published version of the manuscript.

Acknowledgments: This project was supported by an FPU grant (MECD), the Spanish research group CTS-946 and the program for international mobility of PhD students (University of Granada). Special thanks to the Department of Drug Sciences of the University of Pavia (Italy).

References

1. Olsson, M.; Järbrink, K.; Ni, G.; Sönnergren, H.; Schmidtchen, A.; Pang, C.; Bajpai, R.; Car, J. The humanistic and economic burden of chronic wounds: A protocol for a systematic review. *Syst. Rev.* **2017**, *6*, 15.
2. Nussbaum, S.R.; Carter, M.J.; Fife, C.E.; DaVanzo, J.; Haught, R.; Nusgart, M.; Cartwright, D. An Economic Evaluation of the Impact, Cost, and Medicare Policy Implications of Chronic Nonhealing Wounds. *Value Health* **2018**, *21*, 27–32. [CrossRef] [PubMed]
3. Fonder, M.A.; Lazarus, G.S.; Cowan, D.A.; Aronson-Cook, B.; Kohli, A.R.; Mamelak, A.J. Treating the chronic wound: A practical approach to the care of nonhealing wounds and wound care dressings. *J. Am. Acad. Dermatol.* **2008**, *58*, 185–206. [CrossRef] [PubMed]
4. Bernal-Chávez, S.; Nava-Arzaluz, M.G.; Quiroz-Segoviano, R.I.Y.; Ganem-Rondero, A. Nanocarrier-based systems for wound healing. *Drug Dev. Ind. Pharm.* **2019**, *45*, 1389–1402. [CrossRef]
5. García-Villén, F.; Souza, I.M.S.; de Melo Barbosa, R.; Borrego-Sánchez, A.; Sánchez-Espejo, R.; Ojeda-Riascos, S.; Viseras, C. Natural inorganic ingredients in wound healing. *Curr. Pharm. Des.* **2020**, *26*, 621–641. [CrossRef]
6. Tenci, M.; Rossi, S.; Aguzzi, C.; Carazo, E.; Sandri, G.; Bonferoni, M.C.; Grisoli, P.; Viseras, C.; Caramella, C.M.; Ferrari, F. Carvacrol/clay hybrids loaded into in situ gelling films. *Int. J. Pharm.* **2017**, *531*, 676–688. [CrossRef]
7. García-Villén, F.; Faccendini, A.; Aguzzi, C.; Cerezo, P.; Bonferoni, M.C.; Rossi, S.; Grisoli, P.; Ruggeri, M.; Ferrari, F.; Sandri, G.; et al. Montmorillonite-norfloxacin nanocomposite intended for healing of infected wounds. *Int. J. Nanomed.* **2019**, *14*, 5051–5060. [CrossRef]
8. Mefteh, S.; Khiari, I.; Sánchez-Espejo, R.; Aguzzi, C.; López-Galindo, A.; Jamoussi, F.; Viseras, C. Characterisation of Tunisian layered clay materials to be used in semisolid health care products. *Mater. Technol.* **2014**, *29*, B88–B95. [CrossRef]
9. García-Villén, F.; Sánchez-Espejo, R.; Carazo, E.; Borrego-Sánchez, A.; Aguzzi, C.; Cerezo, P.; Viseras, C. Characterisation of Andalusian peats for skin health care formulations. *Appl. Clay Sci.* **2018**, *160*, 201–205. [CrossRef]
10. Khiari, I.; Sánchez-Espejo, R.; García-Villén, F.; Cerezo, P.; Aguzzi, C.; López-Galindo, A.; Jamoussi, F.; Viseras, C. Rheology and cation release of tunisian medina mud-packs intended for topical applications. *Appl. Clay Sci.* **2019**, *171*, 110–117. [CrossRef]
11. Rebelo, M.; Viseras, C.; López-Galindo, A.; Rocha, F.; da Silva, E.F. Rheological and thermal characterization of peloids made of selected Portuguese geological materials. *Appl. Clay Sci.* **2011**, *52*, 219–227. [CrossRef]
12. Rebelo, M.; Viseras, C.; López-Galindo, A.; Rocha, F.; da Silva, E.F. Characterization of Portuguese geological materials to be used in medical hydrology. *Appl. Clay Sci.* **2011**, *51*, 258–266. [CrossRef]
13. Sánchez-Espejo, R.; Aguzzi, C.; Cerezo, P.; Salcedo, I.; López-Galindo, A.; Viseras, C. Folk pharmaceutical formulations in western Mediterranean: Identification and safety of clays used in pelotherapy. *J. Ethnopharmacol.* **2014**, *155*, 810–814. [CrossRef]
14. Viseras, C.; Cerezo, P. Aplicación de peloides y fangos termales. In *Técnicas y Tecnologías en Hidrología Médica e Hidroterapia*; Hernández-Torres, A., Alcázar-Alcázar, R., Eds.; Agencia de Evaluación de Tecnologías Sanitarias - Instituto de Salud Carlos III - Ministerio de Sanidad y Consumo: Madrid, Spain, 2006; pp. 141–146, ISBN 84-95463-33-4.
15. Elkayam, O.; Ophir, J.; Brener, S.; Paran, D.; Wigler, I.; Efron, D.; Even-Paz, Z.; Politi, Y.; Yaron, M. Immediate and delayed effects of treatment at the Dead Sea in patients with psoriatic arthritis. *Rheumatol. Int.* **2000**, *19*, 77–82. [CrossRef] [PubMed]
16. Delfino, M.; Russo, N.; Migliaccio, G.; Carraturo, N. Experimental study on efficacy of thermal muds of Ischia Island combined with balneotherapy in the treatment of psoriasis vulgaris with plaques. *Clin. Ter.* **2003**, *154*, 167–171. [PubMed]
17. Cozzi, F.; Raffeiner, B.; Beltrame, V.; Ciprian, L.; Coran, A.; Botsios, C.; Perissinotto, E.; Grisan, E.; Ramonda, R.; Oliviero, F.; et al. Effects of mud-bath therapy in psoriatic arthritis patients treated with TNF inhibitors. Clinical evaluation and assessment of synovial inflammation by contrast-enhanced ultrasound (CEUS). *Jt. Bone Spine* **2015**, *82*, 104–108. [CrossRef] [PubMed]
18. Harari, M. Beauty is not only skin deep: The Dead Sea features and cosmetics. *An. Hidrol. Médica* **2012**, *5*, 75–88.

19. Huang, A.; Seité, S.; Adar, T. The use of balneotherapy in dermatology. *Clin. Dermatol.* **2018**, *36*, 363–368. [CrossRef]
20. Riyaz, N.; Arakkal, F. Spa therapy in dermatology. *Indian J. Dermatol. Venereol. Leprol.* **2011**, *77*, 128. [CrossRef]
21. Comacchi, C.; Hercogova, J. A single mud treatment induces normalization of stratum corneum hydration, transepidermal water loss, skin surface pH and sebum content in patients with seborrhoeic dermatitis. *J. Eur. Acad. Dermatol. Venereol.* **2004**, *18*, 372–374. [CrossRef]
22. Williams, L.B.; Haydel, S.E.; Giese, R.F., Jr.; Eberl, D.D. Chemical and Mineralogical Characteristics of French Green Clays Used for Healing. *Clays Clay Miner.* **2008**, *56*, 437–452. [CrossRef] [PubMed]
23. López-Galindo, A.; Viseras, C.; Aguzzi, C.; Cerezo, P. Pharmaceutical and cosmetic uses of fibrous clays. In *Developments in Clay Science*; Galán, E., Singer, A., Eds.; Elsevier: Amsterdam, The Netherlands, 2011; Volume 3, pp. 299–324, ISBN 9780444536075.
24. Argenziano, G.; Delfino, M.; Russo, N. Mud and baththerapy in the acne cure. *Clin. Ter.* **2004**, *155*, 125.
25. Cézanne, L.; Gaboriau, F.; Charveron, M.; Morlière, P.; Tocanne, J.F.; Dubertret, L. Effects of the Avène spring water on the dynamics of lipids in the membranes of cultured fibroblasts. *Skin Pharmacol.* **1993**, *6*, 231–240. [CrossRef] [PubMed]
26. Mahe, Y.F.; Perez, M.J.; Tacheau, C.; Fanchon, C.; Martin, R.; Rousset, F.; Seite, S. A new Vitreoscilla filiformis extract grown on spa water-enriched medium activates endogenous cutaneous antioxidant and antimicrobial defenses through a potential Toll-like receptor 2/protein kinase C, zeta transduction pathway. *Clin. Cosmet. Investig. Dermatol.* **2013**, *6*, 191–196.
27. Mahé, Y.F.; Martin, R.; Aubert, L.; Billoni, N.; Collin, C.; Pruche, F.; Bastien, P.; Drost, S.S.; Lane, A.T.; Meybeck, A. Induction of the skin endogenous protective mitochondrial MnSOD by Vitreoscilla filiformis extract. *Int. J. Cosmet. Sci.* **2006**, *28*, 277–287. [CrossRef]
28. Castex-Rizzi, N.; Charveron, M.; Merial-Kieny, C. Inhibition of TNF-alpha induced-adhesion molecules by Avène Thermal Spring Water in human endothelial cells. *J. Eur. Acad. Dermatol. Venereol.* **2011**, *25*, 6–11. [CrossRef]
29. Moysan, A.; Morlière, P.; Marquis, I.; Richard, A.; Dubertret, L. Effects of selenium on UVA-Induced lipid peroxidation in cultured human skin fibroblasts. *Skin Pharmacol. Physiol.* **1995**, *8*, 139–148. [CrossRef]
30. Chebassier, N.; Ouijja, E.H.; Viegas, I.; Dreno, B. Stimulatory effect of boron and manganese salts on keratinocyte migration. *Acta Derm. Venereol.* **2004**, *84*, 191–194. [CrossRef]
31. Liang, J.; Kang, D.; Wang, Y.; Yu, Y.; Fan, J.; Takashi, E. Carbonate ion-enriched hot spring water promotes skin wound healing in nude rats. *PLoS ONE* **2015**, *10*, e0117106. [CrossRef]
32. Chiarini, A.; Dal Pra, I.; Pacchiana, R.; Zumiani, G.; Zanoni, M.; Armato, U. Comano's (Trentino) thermal water interferes with interleukin-6 production and secretion and with cytokeratin-16 expression by cultured human psoriatic keratinocytes: Further potential mechanisms of its anti-psoriatic action. *Int. J. Mol. Med.* **2006**, *18*, 1073–1079. [CrossRef]
33. Faga, A.; Nicoletti, G.; Gregotti, C.; Finotti, V.; Nitto, A.; Gioglio, L. Effects of thermal water on skin regeneration. *Int. J. Mol. Med.* **2012**, *29*, 732–740. [CrossRef] [PubMed]
34. Nicoletti, G.; Saler, M.; Pellegatta, T.; Tresoldi, M.M.; Bonfanti, V.; Malovini, A.; Faga, A.; Riva, F. Ex vivo regenerative effects of a spring water. *Biomed. Rep.* **2017**, *7*, 508–514. [PubMed]
35. Sánchez-Espejo, R.; Aguzzi, C.; Salcedo, I.; Cerezo, P.; Viseras, C. Clays in complementary and alternative medicine. *Mater. Technol.* **2014**, *29*, B78–B81. [CrossRef]
36. Sánchez-Espejo, R.; Cerezo, P.; Aguzzi, C.; López-Galindo, A.; Machado, J.; Viseras, C. Physicochemical and in vitro cation release relevance of therapeutic muds "maturation". *Appl. Clay Sci.* **2015**, *116–117*, 1–7. [CrossRef]
37. Khiari, I.; Mefteh, S.; Sánchez-Espejo, R.; Cerezo, P.; Aguzzi, C.; López-Galindo, A.; Jamoussi, F.; Viseras Iborra, C. Study of traditional Tunisian medina clays used in therapeutic and cosmetic mud-packs. *Appl. Clay Sci.* **2014**, *101*, 141–148. [CrossRef]
38. Lizarbe, M.A.; Olmo, N.; Gavilanes, J.G. Outgrowth of fibroblasts on sepiolite-collagen complex. *Biomaterials* **1987**, *8*, 35–37. [CrossRef]
39. Olmo, N.; Lizarbe, M.A.; Gavilanes, J.G. Biocompatibility and degradability of sepiolite-collagen complex. *Biomaterials* **1987**, *8*, 67–69. [CrossRef]

40. Kommireddy, D.S.; Ichinose, I.; Lvov, Y.M.; Mills, D.K. Nanoparticle Multilayers: Surface Modification for Cell Attachment and Growth. *J. Biomed. Nanotechnol.* **2006**, *1*, 286–290. [CrossRef]
41. Kokabi, M.; Sirousazar, M.; Hassan, Z.M. PVA-clay nanocomposite hydrogels for wound dressing. *Eur. Polym. J.* **2007**, *43*, 773–781. [CrossRef]
42. Dawson, J.I.; Oreffo, R.O.C. Clay: New opportunities for tissue regeneration and biomaterial design. *Adv. Mater.* **2013**, *25*, 4069–4086. [CrossRef]
43. Aguzzi, C.; Sandri, G.; Cerezo, P.; Carazo, E.; Viseras, C. Health and medical applications of tubular clay minerals. In *Developments in Clay Science*; Elsevier: Amsterdam, The Netherlands, 2016; Volume 7, pp. 708–725, ISBN 9780081002933.
44. Sandri, G.; Bonferoni, M.C.; Rossi, S.; Ferrari, F.; Aguzzi, C.; Viseras, C.; Caramella, C. Clay minerals for tissue regeneration, repair, and engineering. In *Wound Healing Biomaterials*; Ågren, M.S., Ed.; Elsevier: Amsterdam, The Netherlands, 2016; pp. 385–402, ISBN 9781782424567.
45. Ishikawa, K.; Akasaka, T.; Abe, S.; Yawaka, Y.; Suzuki, M.; Watari, F. Application of Imogolite, Almino-Silicate Nanotube, as Scaffold for the Mineralization of Osteoblasts. *Bioceram. Dev. Appl.* **2010**, *1*, 1–3. [CrossRef]
46. Ishikawa, K.; Akasaka, T.; Yawaka, Y.; Watari, F. High functional expression of osteoblasts on imogolite, aluminosilicate nanotubes. *J. Biomed. Nanotechnol.* **2010**, *6*, 59–65. [CrossRef] [PubMed]
47. Sandri, G.; Aguzzi, C.; Rossi, S.; Bonferoni, M.C.; Bruni, G.; Boselli, C.; Cornaglia, A.I.; Riva, F.; Viseras, C.; Caramella, C.; et al. Halloysite and chitosan oligosaccharide nanocomposite for wound healing. *Acta Biomater.* **2017**, *57*, 216–224. [CrossRef]
48. Shanmugapriya, K.; Kim, H.; Saravana, P.S.; Chun, B.S.; Kang, H.W. Fabrication of multifunctional chitosan-based nanocomposite film with rapid healing and antibacterial effect for wound management. *Int. J. Biol. Macromol.* **2018**, *118*, 1713–1725. [CrossRef] [PubMed]
49. Vergaro, V.; Abdullayev, E.; Lvov, Y.M.; Zeitoun, A.; Cingolani, R.; Rinaldi, R.; Leporatti, S. Cytocompatibility and uptake of halloysite clay nanotubes. *Biomacromolecules* **2010**, *11*, 820–826. [CrossRef] [PubMed]
50. Salcedo, I.; Aguzzi, C.; Sandri, G.; Bonferoni, M.C.; Mori, M.; Cerezo, P.; Sánchez, R.; Viseras, C.; Caramella, C. In vitro biocompatibility and mucoadhesion of montmorillonite chitosan nanocomposite: A new drug delivery. *Appl. Clay Sci.* **2012**, *55*, 131–137. [CrossRef]
51. Li, P.-R.; Wei, J.-C.; Chiu, Y.-F.; Su, H.-L.; Peng, F.-C.; Lin, J.-J. Evaluation on cytotoxicity and genotoxicity of the exfoliated silicate nanoclay. *ACS Appl. Mater. Interfaces* **2010**, *2*, 1608–1613. [CrossRef]
52. Rotoli, B.M.; Guidi, P.; Bonelli, B.; Bernardeschi, M.; Bianchi, M.G.; Esposito, S.; Frenzilli, G.; Lucchesi, P.; Nigro, M.; Scarcelli, V.; et al. Imogolite: An aluminosilicate nanotube endowed with low cytotoxicity and genotoxicity. *Chem. Res. Toxicol.* **2014**, *27*, 1142–1154. [CrossRef]
53. Lai, X.; Agarwal, M.; Lvov, Y.M.; Pachpande, C.; Varahramyan, K.; Witzmann, F.A. Proteomic profiling of halloysite clay nanotube exposure in intestinal cell co-culture. *J. Appl. Toxicol.* **2013**, *33*, 1316–1329. [CrossRef]
54. Sandri, G.; Bonferoni, M.C.; Ferrari, F.; Rossi, S.; Aguzzi, C.; Mori, M.; Grisoli, P.; Cerezo, P.; Tenci, M.; Viseras, C.; et al. Montmorillonite-chitosan-silver sulfadiazine nanocomposites for topical treatment of chronic skin lesions: In vitro biocompatibility, antibacterial efficacy and gap closure cell motility properties. *Carbohydr. Polym.* **2014**, *102*, 970–977. [CrossRef]
55. Maisanaba, S.; Pichardo, S.; Puerto, M.; Gutiérrez-Praena, D.; Cameán, A.M.; Jos, A. Toxicological evaluation of clay minerals and derived nanocomposites: A review. *Environ. Res.* **2015**, *138*, 233–254. [CrossRef] [PubMed]
56. Sasaki, Y.; Sathi, G.A.; Yamamoto, O. Wound healing effect of bioactive ion released from Mg-smectite. *Mater. Sci. Eng. C. Mater. Biol. Appl.* **2017**, *77*, 52–57. [CrossRef] [PubMed]
57. Wang, Z.; Zhao, Y.; Luo, Y.; Wang, S.; Shen, M.; Tomás, H.; Zhu, M.; Shi, X. Attapulgite-doped electrospun poly(lactic-co-glycolic acid) nanofibers enable enhanced osteogenic differentiation of human mesenchymal stem cells. *RSC Adv.* **2015**, *5*, 2383–2391. [CrossRef]
58. Cervini-Silva, J.; Nieto-Camacho, A.; Gómez-Vidales, V. Oxidative stress inhibition and oxidant activity by fibrous clays. *Colloids Surf. B Biointerfaces* **2015**, *133*, 32–35. [CrossRef]
59. Cervini-Silva, J.; Nieto-Camacho, A.; Ramírez-Apan, M.T.; Gómez-Vidales, V.; Palacios, E.; Montoya, A.; Ronquillo de Jesús, E. Anti-inflammatory, anti-bacterial, and cytotoxic activity of fibrous clays. *Colloids Surf. B Biointerfaces* **2015**, *129*, 1–6. [CrossRef]

60. Nasirov, M.I.; Efendieva, F.M.; Ismaĭlova, D.A. The influence of peloids from volcanic deposits in Azerbaijan on the dynamics of sugar content in blood and urine and the wound healing in patients at the early stages of diabetic gangrene of the lower extremities. *Vopr. Kurortol. Fizioter. Lech. Fiz. Kult.* **2009**, 42–43.
61. Abu-al-Basal, M.A. Histological evaluation of the healing properties of Dead Sea black mud on full-thickness excision cutaneous wounds in BALB/c mice. *Pakistan J. Biol. Sci.* **2012**, *15*, 306–315. [CrossRef]
62. Dário, G.M.I.; Da Silva, G.G.; Gonçalves, D.L.; Silveira, P.; Junior, A.T.; Angioletto, E.; Bernardin, A.M. Evaluation of the healing activity of therapeutic clay in rat skin wounds. *Mater. Sci. Eng. C* **2014**, *43*, 109–116. [CrossRef]
63. García-Villén, F.; Sánchez-Espejo, R.; López-Galindo, A.; Cerezo, P.; Viseras, C. Design and characterization of spring water hydrogels with natural inorganic excipients. *Appl. Clay Sci.* **2020**. Manuscript under review.
64. Diputación Provincial de Granada; Instituto Tecnológico Geominero de España. Atlas Hidrogeológico de la Provincia de Granada. 1990. Available online: http://aguas.igme.es/igme/publica/libro75/lib_75.htm (accessed on 24 April 2020).
65. Maraver Eyzaguirre, F.; Armijo de Castro, F. *Vademécum II de Aguas Mineromedicinales Españolas*; Maraver Eyzaguirre, F., Armijo Castro, F., Eds.; Editorial Complutense: Madrid, Spain, 2010; ISBN 9788474919981.
66. Klinkenberg, M.; Rickertsen, N.; Kaufhold, S.; Dohrmann, R.; Siegesmund, S. Abrasivity by bentonite dispersions. *Appl. Clay Sci.* **2009**, *46*, 37–42. [CrossRef]
67. Quintela, A.; Costa, C.; Terroso, D.; Rocha, F. Abrasiveness index of dispersions of Portuguese clays using the Einlehner method: Influence of clay parameters. *Clay Miner.* **2014**, *49*, 27–34. [CrossRef]
68. Ganfoud, R.; Puchot, L.; Fouquet, T.; Verge, P. H-bonding supramolecular interactions driving the dispersion of kaolin into benzoxazine: A tool for the reinforcement of polybenzoxazines thermal and thermo-mechanical properties. *Compos. Sci. Technol.* **2015**, *110*, 1–7. [CrossRef]
69. Santos, S.C.R.; Boaventura, R.A.R. Adsorption of cationic and anionic azo dyes on sepiolite clay: Equilibrium and kinetic studies in batch mode. *J. Environ. Chem. Eng.* **2016**, *4*, 1473–1483. [CrossRef]
70. Álvarez, A.; Santarén, J.; Esteban-Cubillo, A.; Aparicio, P. Current Industrial Applications of Palygorskite and Sepiolite. In *Developments in Palygorskite-Sepiolite Research. A New Outlook of These Nanomaterials*; Galán, E., Singer, A., Eds.; Elsevier B.V: Oxford, UK, 2011; pp. 281–298, ISBN 978-0-444-53607-5.
71. McLean, S.A.; Allen, B.L.; Craig, J.R. The Occurrence of Sepiolite and Attapulgite on the Southern High Plains. *Clays Clay Miner.* **1972**, *20*, 143–149. [CrossRef]
72. Galan, E. Properties and applications of palygorskite-sepiolite clays. *Clay Miner.* **1996**, *31*, 443–453. [CrossRef]
73. Zeng, H.F.; Lin, L.J.; Xi, Y.M.; Han, Z.Y. Effects of raw and heated palygorskite on rumen fermentation in vitro. *Appl. Clay Sci.* **2017**, *138*, 125–130. [CrossRef]
74. Lobato-Aguilar, H.; Uribe-Calderón, J.A.; Herrera-Kao, W.; Duarte-Aranda, S.; Baas-López, J.M.; Escobar-Morales, B.; Cauich-Rodríguez, J.V.; Cervantes-Uc, J.M. Synthesis, characterization and chlorhexidine release from either montmorillonite or palygorskite modified organoclays for antibacterial applications. *J. Drug Deliv. Sci. Technol.* **2018**, *46*, 452–460. [CrossRef]
75. Shariatmadari, H. Sorption of Selected Cationic and Neutral Organic Molecules on Palygorskite and Sepiolite. *Clays Clay Miner.* **1999**, *47*, 44–53. [CrossRef]
76. Rytwo, G.; Nir, S.; Crespin, M.; Margulies, L. Adsorption and Interactions of Methyl Green with Montmorillonite and Sepiolite. *J. Colloid Interface Sci.* **2000**, *222*, 12–19. [CrossRef]
77. Lemić, J.; Tomašević-Čanović, M.; Djuričić, M.; Stanić, T. Surface modification of sepiolite with quaternary amines. *J. Colloid Interface Sci.* **2005**, *292*, 11–19. [CrossRef]
78. Shirvani, M.; Shariatmadari, H.; Kalbasi, M.; Nourbakhsh, F.; Najafi, B. Sorption of cadmium on palygorskite, sepiolite and calcite: Equilibria and organic ligand affected kinetics. *Colloids Surf. A Physicochem. Eng. Asp.* **2006**, *287*, 182–190. [CrossRef]
79. Al-Futaisi, A.; Jamrah, A.; Al-Rawas, A.; Al-Hanai, S. Adsorption capacity and mineralogical and physico-chemical characteristics of Shuwaymiyah palygorskite (Oman). *Environ. Geol.* **2007**, *51*, 1317–1327. [CrossRef]
80. Chang, P.-H.; Li, Z.; Yu, T.-L.; Munkhbayer, S.; Kuo, T.-H.; Hung, Y.-C.; Jean, J.-S.; Lin, K.-H. Sorptive removal of tetracycline from water by palygorskite. *J. Hazard. Mater.* **2009**, *165*, 148–155. [CrossRef] [PubMed]
81. Rhouta, B.; Zatile, E.; Bouna, L.; Lakbita, O.; Maury, F.; Daoudi, L.; Lafont, M.C.; Amjoud, M.; Senocq, F.; Jada, A.; et al. Comprehensive physicochemical study of dioctahedral palygorskite-rich clay from Marrakech High Atlas (Morocco). *Phys. Chem. Miner.* **2013**, *40*, 411–424. [CrossRef]

82. Paolisso, G.; Barbagallo, M. Hypertension, diabetes mellitus, and insulin resistance. The role of intracellular magnesium. *Am. J. Hypertens.* **1997**, *10*, 346–355. [CrossRef]
83. Tateo, F.; Ravaglioli, A.; Andreoli, C.; Bonina, F.; Coiro, V.; Degetto, S.; Giaretta, A.; Menconi Orsini, A.; Puglia, C.; Summa, V. The in-vitro percutaneous migration of chemical elements from a thermal mud for healing use. *Appl. Clay Sci.* **2009**, *44*, 83–94. [CrossRef]
84. De Gomes, C.S.F.; Silva, J.B.P. Minerals and clay minerals in medical geology. *Appl. Clay Sci.* **2007**, *36*, 4–21. [CrossRef]
85. Lansdown, A.B.G.; Sampson, B.; Rowe, A. Sequential changes in trace metal, metallothionein and calmodulin concentrations in healing skin wounds. *J. Anat.* **1999**, *195*, 375–386. [CrossRef]
86. Dubé, J.; Rochette-Drouin, O.; Lévesque, P.; Gauvin, R.; Roberge, C.J.; Auger, F.A.; Goulet, D.; Bourdages, M.; Plante, M.; Germain, L.; et al. Restoration of the transepithelial potential within tissue-engineered human skin in vitro and during the wound healing process in vivo. *Tissue Eng. Part A* **2010**, *16*, 3055–3063. [CrossRef]
87. Ma, J.; Zhao, N.; Zhu, D. Biphasic responses of human vascular smooth muscle cells to magnesium ion. *J. Biomed. Mater. Res. Part A* **2016**, *104*, 347–356. [CrossRef]
88. Lansdown, A.B.G. Calcium: A potential central regulator in wound healing in the skin. *Wound Repair Regen.* **2002**, *10*, 271–285. [CrossRef] [PubMed]
89. Fairley, J.A.; Marcelo, C.L.; Hogan, V.A.; Voorhees, J.J. Increased calmodulin levels in psoriasis and low Ca++ regulated mouse epidermal keratinocyte cultures. *J. Investig. Dermatol.* **1985**, *84*, 195–198. [CrossRef] [PubMed]
90. Karvonen, S.L.; Korkiamäki, T.; Ylä-Outinen, H.; Nissinen, M.; Teerikangas, H.; Pummi, K.; Karvonen, J.; Peltonen, J. Psoriasis and altered calcium metabolism: Downregulated capacitative calcium influx and defective calcium-mediated cell signaling in cultured psoriatic keratinocytes. *J. Investig. Dermatol.* **2000**, *114*, 693–700. [CrossRef]
91. Gao, Y.; Jin, X. Needle-punched three-dimensional nonwoven wound dressings with density gradient from biocompatible calcium alginate fiber. *Text. Res. J.* **2019**, *89*, 2776–2788. [CrossRef]
92. Hotta, E.; Hara, H.; Kamiya, T.; Adachi, T. Non-thermal atmospheric pressure plasma-induced IL-8 expression is regulated via intracellular K + loss and subsequent ERK activation in human keratinocyte HaCaT cells. *Arch. Biochem. Biophys.* **2018**, *644*, 64–71. [CrossRef] [PubMed]
93. Shim, J.H.; Lim, J.W.; Kim, B.K.; Park, S.J.; Kim, S.W.; Choi, T.H. KCl mediates K+ channel-activated mitogen activated protein kinases signaling in wound healing. *Arch. Plast. Surg.* **2015**, *42*, 11–19. [CrossRef]
94. Li, Y.; Wang, M.; Sun, D.; Li, Y.; Wu, T. Effective removal of emulsified oil from oily wastewater using surfactant-modified sepiolite. *Appl. Clay Sci.* **2018**, *157*, 227–236. [CrossRef]
95. Di Credico, B.; Tagliaro, I.; Cobani, E.; Conzatti, L.; D'Arienzo, M.; Giannini, L.; Mascotto, S.; Scotti, R.; Stagnaro, P.; Tadiello, L. A Green Approach for Preparing High-Loaded Sepiolite/Polymer Biocomposites. *Nanomaterials* **2019**, *9*, 46. [CrossRef]
96. Middea, A.; Spinelli, L.S.; Souza, F.G.; Neumann, R.; da Gomes, O.F.M.; Fernandes, T.L.A.P.; de Lima, L.C.; Barthem, V.M.T.S.; de Carvalho, F.V. Synthesis and characterization of magnetic palygorskite nanoparticles and their application on methylene blue remotion from water. *Appl. Surf. Sci.* **2015**, *346*, 232–239. [CrossRef]
97. Berg, J.M.; Romoser, A.; Banerjee, N.; Zebda, R.; Sayes, C.M. The relationship between pH and zeta potential of ~30 nm metal oxide nanoparticle suspensions relevant to in vitro toxicological evaluations. *Nanotoxicology* **2009**, *3*, 276–283. [CrossRef]
98. Spriano, S.; Sarath Chandra, V.; Cochis, A.; Uberti, F.; Rimondini, L.; Bertone, E.; Vitale, A.; Scolaro, C.; Ferrari, M.; Cirisano, F.; et al. How do wettability, zeta potential and hydroxylation degree affect the biological response of biomaterials? *Mater. Sci. Eng. C* **2017**, *74*, 542–555. [CrossRef] [PubMed]
99. Honary, S.; Zahir, F. Effect of zeta potential on the properties of nano-drug delivery systems—A review (Part 2). *Trop. J. Pharm. Res.* **2013**, *12*, 265–273.
100. Takeuchi, K.I.; Ishihara, M.; Kawaura, C.; Noji, M.; Furuno, T.; Nakanishi, M. Effect of zeta potential of cationic liposomes containing cationic cholesterol derivatives on gene transfection. *FEBS Lett.* **1996**, *397*, 207–209. [CrossRef]
101. Bengali, Z.; Pannier, A.K.; Segura, T.; Anderson, B.C.; Jang, J.-H.; Mustoe, T.A.; Shea, L.D. Gene delivery through cell culture substrate adsorbed DNA complexes. *Biotechnol. Bioeng.* **2005**, *90*, 290–302. [CrossRef] [PubMed]

102. Zhang, Y.; Yang, M.; Portney, N.G.; Cui, D.; Budak, G.; Ozbay, E.; Ozkan, M.; Ozkan, C.S. Zeta potential: A surface electrical characteristic to probe the interaction of nanoparticles with normal and cancer human breast epithelial cells. *Biomed. Microdevices* **2008**, *10*, 321–328. [CrossRef] [PubMed]
103. Wang, X.; Du, Y.; Luo, J. Biopolymer/montmorillonite nanocomposite: Preparation, drug-controlled release property and cytotoxicity. *Nanotechnology* **2008**, *19*, 065707. [CrossRef]
104. Sabuncu, A.C.; Grubbs, J.; Qian, S.; Abdel-Fattah, T.M.; Stacey, M.W.; Beskok, A. Probing nanoparticle interactions in cell culture media. *Colloids Surf. B Biointerfaces* **2012**, *95*, 96–102. [CrossRef]
105. da Silva, J.; Jesus, S.; Bernardi, N.; Colaço, M.; Borges, O. Poly(D, L-lactic Acid) nanoparticle size reduction increases its immunotoxicity. *Front. Bioeng. Biotechnol.* **2019**, *7*, 1–10. [CrossRef]
106. de Souza e Silva, J.M.; Hanchuk, T.D.M.; Santos, M.I.; Kobarg, J.; Bajgelman, M.C.; Cardoso, M.B. Viral inhibition mechanism mediated by surface-modified silica nanoparticles. *ACS Appl. Mater. Interfaces* **2016**, *8*, 16564–16572. [CrossRef]
107. Su, Y.; Liao, J.L.; Wang, F. Effect of Orient House-Chuen, a concentrate of deep underground mineral spring water, on proliferation and tyrosinase activity of melanocytes. *Chin. J. Biol.* **2010**, *23*, 964–966.
108. Fukushima, K.; Rasyida, A.; Yang, M.C. Characterization, degradation and biocompatibility of PBAT based nanocomposites. *Appl. Clay Sci.* **2013**, *80–81*, 291–298. [CrossRef]
109. Fernandes, A.C.; Antunes, F.; Pires, J. Sepiolite based materials for storage and slow release of nitric oxide. *New J. Chem.* **2013**, *37*, 4052–4060. [CrossRef]
110. Toledano-Magaña, Y.; Flores-Santos, L.; Montes de Oca, G.; González-Montiel, A.; Laclette, J.-P.; Carrero, J.-C. Effect of Clinoptilolite and Sepiolite Nanoclays on Human and Parasitic Highly Phagocytic Cells. *Biomed Res. Int.* **2015**, *2015*, 164980. [CrossRef] [PubMed]
111. Aguzzi, C.; Sánchez-Espejo, R.; Cerezo, P.; Machado, J.; Bonferoni, C.; Rossi, S.; Salcedo, I.; Viseras, C. Networking and rheology of concentrated clay suspensions "matured" in mineral medicinal water. *Int. J. Pharm.* **2013**, *453*, 473–479. [CrossRef]
112. Staffieri, A.; Marino, F.; Staffieri, C.; Giacomelli, L.; D'Alessandro, E.; Maria Ferraro, S.; Fedrazzoni, U.; Marioni, G. The effects of sulfurous-arsenical-ferruginous thermal water nasal irrigation in wound healing after functional endoscopic sinus surgery for chronic rhinosinusitis: A prospective randomized study. *Am. J. Otolaryngol.* **2008**, *29*, 223–229. [CrossRef]
113. Davinelli, S.; Bassetto, F.; Vitale, M.; Scapagnini, G. *Thermal Waters and the Hormetic Effects of Hydrogen Sulfide on Inflammatory Arthritis and Wound Healing*; Elsevier Inc.: Amsterdam, The Netherlands, 2019; ISBN 9780128142530.
114. Guzmán, R.; Campos, C.; Yuguero, R.; Masegù, C.; Gil, P.; Moragón, Á.C. Protective effect of sulfurous water in peripheral blood mononuclear cells of Alzheimer's disease patients. *Life Sci.* **2015**, *132*, 61–67. [CrossRef]
115. Lin, F.H.; Chen, C.H.; Cheng, W.T.K.; Kuo, T.F. Modified montmorillonite as vector for gene delivery. *Biomaterials* **2006**, *27*, 3333–3338. [CrossRef]
116. Abduljauwad, S.N.; Ahmed, H.-R. Enhancing cancer cell adhesion with clay nanoparticles for countering metastasis. *Sci. Rep.* **2019**, *9*, 5935. [CrossRef]
117. Mishra, R.K.; Ramasamy, K.; Lim, S.M.; Ismail, M.F.; Majeed, A.B.A. Antimicrobial and in vitro wound healing properties of novel clay based bionanocomposite films. *J. Mater. Sci. Mater. Med.* **2014**, *25*, 1925–1939. [CrossRef]
118. Vaiana, C.A.; Leonard, M.K.; Drummy, L.F.; Singh, K.M.; Bubulya, A.; Vaia, R.A.; Naik, R.R.; Kadakia, M.P. Epidermal growth factor: Layered silicate nanocomposites for tissue regeneration. *Biomacromolecules* **2011**, *12*, 3139–3146. [CrossRef]
119. de Gois da Silva, M.L.; Fortes, A.C.; Oliveira, M.E.R.; de Freitas, R.M.; da Silva Filho, E.C.; de La Roca Soares, M.F.; Soares-Sobrinho, J.L.; da Silva Leite, C.M. Palygorskite organophilic for dermopharmaceutical application. *J. Therm. Anal. Calorim.* **2014**, *115*, 2287–2294. [CrossRef]
120. Ninan, N.; Muthiah, M.; Park, I.K.; Wong, T.W.; Thomas, S.; Grohens, Y. Natural polymer/inorganic material based hybrid scaffolds for skin wound healing. *Polym. Rev.* **2015**, *55*, 453–490. [CrossRef]
121. Chu, C.-Y.; Peng, F.-C.; Chiu, Y.-F.; Lee, H.-C.; Chen, C.-W.; Wei, J.-C.; Lin, J.-J. Nanohybrids of Silver Particles Immobilized on Silicate Platelet for Infected Wound Healing. *PLoS ONE* **2012**, *7*, e38360. [CrossRef]

122. Carretero, M.I. Clays in pelotherapy. A review. Part II: Organic compounds, microbiology and medical applications. *Appl. Clay Sci.* **2020**, *189*, 105531. [CrossRef]
123. Sandri, G.; Faccendini, A.; Longo, M.; Ruggeri, M.; Rossi, S.; Bonferoni, M.C.; Miele, D.; Prina-Mello, A.; Aguzzi, C.; Viseras, C.; et al. Halloysite-and montmorillonite-loaded scaffolds as enhancers of chronic wound healing. *Pharmaceutics* **2020**, *12*, 179. [CrossRef] [PubMed]
124. Lehtimaki, J.; Hakala, M.; Lappalainen, P. Actin filament structures in migrating cells. *Handb. Exp. Pharmacol.* **2017**, *235*, 1–30.

8

Cellular Analysis and Chemotherapeutic Potential of a Bi-Functionalized Halloysite Nanotube

Yangyang Luo [1], Ahmed Humayun [1], Teresa A. Murray [1], Benjamin S. Kemp [1], Antwine McFarland [1], Xuan Liu [1] and David K. Mills [2,*]

1 Molecular Sciences & Nanotechnology, Louisiana Tech University, Ruston, LA 71272, USA; yangyang317luo@gmail.com (Y.L.); ah.humayun@gmail.com (A.H.); tmurray@latech.edu (T.A.M.); bscott.kemp@gmail.com (B.S.K.); awm011@latech.edu (A.M.); Xliu@latech.edu (X.L.)

2 School of Biological Sciences and the Center for Biomedical Engineering, Louisiana Tech University, Ruston, LA 71272, USA

* Correspondence: dkmills@latech.edu

Abstract: The surface of halloysite nanotubes (HNTs) was bifunctionalized with two ligands—folic acid and a fluorochrome. In tandem, this combination should selectively target cancer cells and provide a means for imaging the nanoparticle. Modified bi-functionalized HNTs (bi-HNTs) were then doped with the anti-cancer drug methotrexate. bi-HNTs were characterized and subjected to in vitro tests to assess cellular growth and changes in cellular behavior in three cell lines—colon cancer, osteosarcoma, and a pre-osteoblast cell line (MC3T3-E1). Cell viability, proliferation, and cell uptake efficiency were assessed. The bi-HNTs showed cytocompatibility at a wide range of concentrations. Compared with regular-sized HNTs, reduced HNTs (~6 microns) were taken up by cells in more significant amounts, but increased cytotoxicity lead to apoptosis. Multi-photon images confirmed the intracellular location of bi-HNTs, and the method of cell entry was mainly through caveolae-mediated endocytosis. The bi-HNTs showed a high drug loading efficiency with methotrexate and a prolonged period of release. Most importantly, bi-HNTs were designed as a drug carrier to target cancer cells specifically, and imaging data shows that non-cancerous cells were unaffected after exposure to MTX-doped bi-HNTs. All data provide support for our nanoparticle design as a mechanism to selectively target cancer cells and significantly reduce the side-effects caused by off-targeting of anti-cancer drugs.

Keywords: targeted drug delivery; halloysite nanotube; osteosarcoma; methotrexate; surface modification

---

1. Introduction

Cancer is the second leading cause of death in the United States [1]. While radiation and surgery treatments have advanced cancer treatment, chemotherapy is still one of the leading treatment modalities [2]. Unfortunately, current chemotherapeutic agents adversely affect healthy cells at the target site and elsewhere in the body [3]. Chemotherapy drugs work by impairing cell division and are effective treatments for early-stage tumors when cancer cells are rapidly multiplying. However, they also produce a range of unpleasant side effects. Systemic toxicity is an undesired consequence for most chemotherapeutic drugs [1,2]. The development of a multi-functional drug delivery system (DDS) with an ability to provide extended, controlled, and selective drug release is at the forefront of current cancer therapy research [2,3]. Targeting chemotherapeutic drugs directly at the tumor cells would increase drug effectiveness and reduce side effects.

Methotrexate (MTX) is a folic acid antagonist. It has an anti-cancer effect on lymphoblastic leukemia, lymphoma, osteosarcoma, and breast, lung, head, and neck cancers [4–6]. MTX restricts cancer cell growth by disrupting transmethylation reactions, which are essential in forming proteins, lipids, and myelin [7]. However, the high dose administration of MTX can damage cells in bone marrow, gastrointestinal mucosa, and hair follicles. Severe side effects, including renal failure, neurotoxicity, hematologic toxicity, mucocutaneous toxicity, and pulmonary toxicity, may result after high dose MTX treatments [8]. Accordingly, a targeted MTX drug delivery system designed to improve its target delivery and reduce destruction to healthy cells seems like a promising approach.

Halloysite nanotubes (HNTs) have attracted significant attention in drug delivery due to its biocompatibility, physicochemical stability, and unique structural properties. HNTs are naturally occurring nanoscale tubes composed of $Al_2O_3{\cdot}2SiO_2{\cdot}nH_2O$. In the process of aluminosilicate rolling, Al–OH groups are folded inside, and Si-O-Si groups are exposed to the outer surface. At neutral pH, the inner surface of HNTs is positively charged, and the outer surface is negatively charged [9]. Depending on the geological origin, the lumen and outer diameters of HNTs range between 10–15 nm and 50–80 nm, respectively [9]. While the length of HNTs averages between 0.5–2 μm. With specific surface modification, active agents can be conjugated on the surface or encapsulated in the empty HNT lumen. Curcumin [10], doxorubicin [11], irinotecan [12], and resveratrol [13] have been successfully doped into HNTs and shown to have an anti-cancer effect.

In a previous study, we demonstrated that the HNT surface could be functionalized with *N*-[3-(trimethoxysilyl)propyl) ethylenediamine (DAS) for grafting folic acid (FA) and fluorescein isothiocyanate (FITC) resulting in a bifunctionalized HNTs (bi-HNT). We used FA as a ligand for targeted drug delivery and FITC as a visual tracking agent. Surface modification using FA and FITC was further confirmed by FTIR, 13C CPMAS NMR spectrum, and UV-Vis. Folic acid directed HNTs adhered to folate receptors, which are overexpressed in numerous cancers but rarely expressed or nonexistent in most normal tissues [14–16].

In this study, we focused on identifying the cellular uptake mechanism and intracellular location of bi-HNTs after endocytosis. We further studied cellular interactions after exposure to bi-HNTs, including cell viability, proliferation, and cell uptake efficiency. When colon cancer cells (CT26WT) were co-cultured with bi-HNTs, cell viability decreased at higher doses. Further analysis showed that cell death was due to apoptosis. Also, size reduced bi-HNTs resulted in higher cell mortality. MTX loaded into bi-HNTs (MTX-bi-HNTs) was analyzed for its specific targeting ability in vitro after co-culturing with three different cell types. Our results show that bi-HNTs provided a high loading capacity for the cytotoxic cancer drug MTX and, bi-HNTs specifically targeted osteosarcoma cells and released MTX and inhibited cell proliferation. Interestingly, in the presence of MTX, non-osteosarcoma cells were unaffected.

2. Materials and Methods

2.1. Materials

All cell culture materials and reagents (including MTX, chlorpromazine and filipin) were purchased from Sigma Aldrich, St. Louis, MO, USA. Cell culture dishes, pipettes and other disposable plastics were purchased from Mid Sci, St. Louis, MO, USA. The *MTT* and XTT Cell Viability Assay Kit was obtained from Biotium, New York, NY, USA. The Annexin V-FITC Apoptosis Kit was purchased from Enzo Life Sciences, Inc. (New York, NY, USA) and DiOC18(7) from ThermoFisher Scientific (Waltham, MA, USA). All three-cell lines used colon cancer (CT26WT), and osteosarcoma (K7M2-WT) and a pre-osteoblast cell line (MC3T3-E1) were purchased from ATCC (Manassas, VA, USA).

2.2. Production of Shortened HNTs

Commercial-grade HNTs (10 g, Sigma Aldrich, St. Louis, MO, USA) were immersed in 50 mL PBS for 24 h and ultra-sonicated for 30 min using a sonicator (Qsonica, Newtown, CT, USA) at 70% power. The solution was allowed to set for 30 min, HNTs were then ultra-sonicated for another 30 min. Then, the mixture was transferred to 50 mL centrifuge tube and centrifuged at 100× *g* for 10 min. The pelleted deposits were collected and dried at 60 °C for 2 days. See Figure 1 for details regarding this procedure.

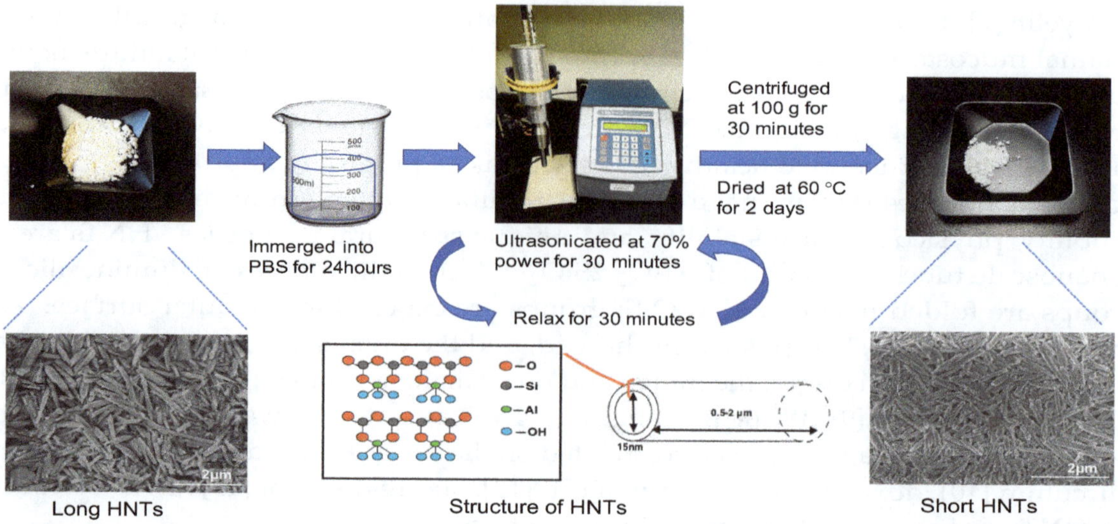

Figure 1. The process of reducing the length of halloysite nanotubes (HNTs). Between each step, the composites were washed and filtered using methanol, sodium chloride, a sodium bicarbonate solution, and distilled water (DI).

2.3. *bi-HNTs Synthesis*

bi-HNTs were synthesized using the same methods as described in a previous study (Figure 2) [16]. Briefly, HNTs (Sigma Aldrich, St. Louis, MO, USA) were reacted at reflux with *N*-[3-(trimethoxysilyl) propyl] ethylenediamine (DAS) (Sigma Aldrich, St. Louis, MO., USA) in toluene for 24 h. Then, the HNT-DAS composite was reacted with FA (Sigma Aldrich, St. Louis, MO, USA) in the presence of 1-ethyl-3-(3-dimethylaminopropyl) carbodiimide (EDC) (Sigma Aldrich, St. Louis, MO, USA) in DI water overnight. Finally, the HNT-DAS-FA composite was complexed with FITC (Sigma Aldrich, St. Louis, MO, USA) in acetone (Granger, Lake Forest, IL, USA) overnight.

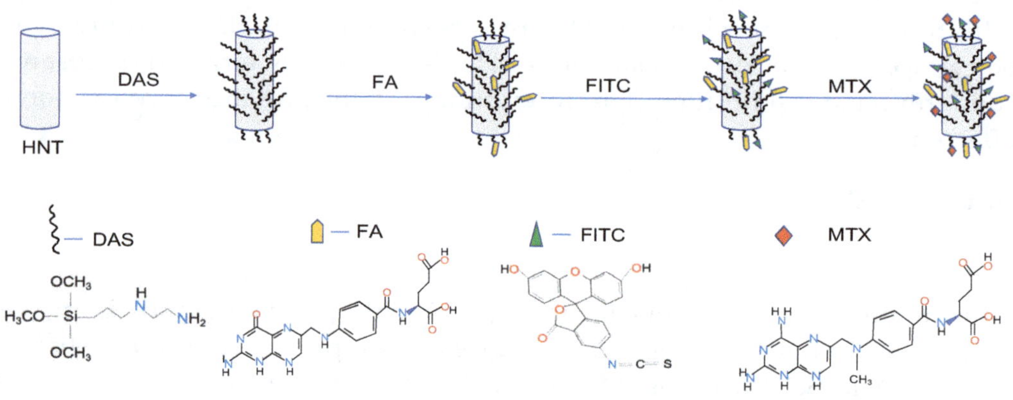

Figure 2. Schematic representation of the conjugation of both FA and FITC to DAS which is attached to the HNT surface. Methotrexate (MTX) was vacuum-doped into the HNT lumen. DAS = *N*-[3-(trimethoxysilyl)propyl) ethylenediamine, FA = folic acidity, FITC = fluorescein isothiocyanate.

2.4. *bi-HNTs Characterization*

2.4.1. Fourier-Transform Infrared Spectroscopy (FTIR)

The Infrared spectrum was recorded at a resolution of 4 s^{-1} with 16 scans using a Thermo Scientific NICOLET™ IR100 FT-IR Spectrometer (Thermo Fisher Scientific; Waltham, MA, USA). Thermo Scientific OMNIC™ software (Waltham, MA., USA) was used to study the stretched bands.

2.4.2. Scanning Electron Microscopy (SEM)

SEM images of original size of HNTs and shortened HNTs were analyzed by ImageJ (NIH, Rockville, MD, USA) and also used to measure particle size.

2.4.3. X-ray Diffraction (XRD)

XRD patterns of HNTs were obtained by Bruker D8 Discover diffractometer (San Jose, CA, USA) equipped with a copper anode X-ray source and a general area detector. The power applied for all tests was 40 kV with 40mA.

2.5. Cell Culture

Murine colorectal cancer CT26WT, osteosarcoma cells K7M2-WT, and pre-osteoblast cells MC3T3-E1 came cryopreserved from ATCC. Cryovials were thawed and allowed to equilibrate in a water bath, all the cells were cultured in 25 cm^2 tissue culture flask and incubated at 37 °C under humidified 5% CO_2 and 95% air. CT26WT cells were cultured in RPMI 1640 medium, osteosarcoma cells were cultured in DMEM (Thermo Fisher Scientific, Waltham, MA, USA) and pre-osteoblast cells were cultured in alpha-MEM (Thermo Fisher Scientific, Waltham, MA, USA), all the medium containing 10% FBS and 1% penicillin. Subconfluent cells were passaged with 0.25% trypsin, collected by centrifugation, suspended in cell culture medium and cultured at a 1:4 split into 25 cm^2 tissue culture flasks. All three types of cells through passaged four times before use.

2.6. MTS Assay

Cells were seeded into 48-well plate at a concentration of 1×10^5 cells/well and cultured for 24 h. Then cells were incubated in cell media that contained different concentrations of pure HNTs or functionalized HNTs (0, 50, 100, 150, 200, 250 μg/mL), respectfully. MTS stock solution (Thermo Fisher Scientific, Waltham, MA, USA) (40 μL) were added to each well and cultured for 2 h at 37 °C in darkness. 200 μL of supernatant of each sample were transferred to 96-well plates and read absorbance values at 490 nm by microplate reader (Thermo Fisher Scientific, Waltham, MA, USA).

2.7. XTT Assay

Cells were seeded into 48-well plate at a concentration of 1×10^5 cells/well and cultured for 24 h. 100 μL of cell suspension were added into 96-well tissue culture plates, then added with 25 μL activated XTT solution (XTT Cell Viability Assay Kit, Biotium, Fremont, CA, USA) and incubated for 2 h. Absorbance values were measured at 450 nm; background absorbance was measured at 630 nm. The final normalized absorbance values were obtained by subtracting background absorbance from signal absorbance.

2.8. Cell Uptake Efficiency

CT26WT cells were seeded into 48 wells at the concentration of 1.5×10^5 cells/well and incubated for 24 h. Then, bi-HNTs were added into cell culture medium at finial concentration of 25 μg/mL and incubated for another 24 h. After three times wash with fresh RPMI 1640, cell fluorescent intensities were measured by fluorescent microplate reader at 490/525 nm (Ex/Em). The cell numbers were measured.

2.9. Cell Uptake Mechanism

CT26WT cells were seeded into 24 wells at the concentration of 2×10^5 cells/well and cultured for 24 h. Two inhibitors, chlorpromazine and filipin, were selected to evaluate the bi-HNTs cell uptake mechanism. Chlorpromazine selectively inhibits clathrin-dependent endocytosis and filipin inhibits caveolae-dependent endocytosis. Cells were pre-cultured with CPZ (Sigma Aldrich, St. Louis, MO, USA) (7 μg/mL) or filipin (5 μg/mL) for 2 h. Cells treated without any inhibitor set as the control.

bi-HNTs (25 μg/mL) were added to each well and incubated for another 24 h. Fluorescent intensities expressed by cells were measured as above.

2.10. Multi-Photon Imaging

CT26WT cells were seeded on a glass slide at a concentration of 1×10^5 cells/mL and cultured for 24 h. bi-HNTs were added to the cell culture plate (25 μg/mL) and continually incubated for 12 h. DiOC18(7) (DiR) (ThermoFisher Scientific) working solution was prepared by following the company provided protocol. Cells were washed with DPBS for 3 times, then the DiR working solution was added into cell culture well (1 μL/mL) and incubated for 2 h. Cells were then fixed by 4% paraformaldehyde (Sigma Aldrich, St. Louis, MO, USA) for imaging by an in-house assembled multi-photon microscopy. Three-dimensional images were acquired using a Vivo-2 upright, multiphoton microscope system (Intelligent Imaging Innovations, Inc. (3i), Denver, Colorado, USA) with GaAsP photomultipliers (Hamamatsu, Tokyo, Japan), a Pockels cell (Conoptics, Inc., Danbury, CT, USA) to control laser power, and an ELWD 40×/0.6 NA objective lens (Nikon Instruments, Inc., Tokyo, Japan). Excitation of fluorescence was provided by a Chameleon Vision-2 multiphoton laser (80 MHz, Coherent. Inc., Santa Clara, CA, USA) tuned to 850 nm. Slidebook 6 software (3i) (Conoptics, Inc., Danbury, CT, USA) was used to control the microscope and multiphoton laser systems and to acquire images. Images were scanned in three dimensions with x- and y-dimensions of 248 μm (1024 × 1024-pixel resolution), with z-steps of 2 μm (z stack) to produce z stacks of 36 and 46 μm to ensure that all cells were captured within the volume. Pixel dwell time was set to 2 μL with pixel averaging of 5/scan to acquire z stack images [17,18].

2.11. Apoptosis and Necrosis

CT26WT cells were seeded into 24 wells at a concentration of 2×10^5 cells/well and cultured for 24 h. Then, a high dosage of bi-HNTs were added into the cell culture medium (150 μg/mL) and incubated for 24 h. Then 3×10^5 cells were collected and suspended in 500 μL of 1× binding Buffer, then mixed with 5 μL of Annexin V-FITC and 5 μL of propidium iodide (Sigma Aldrich, St. Louis, MO, USA). Cell suspension mixtures were incubated in the dark at room temperature for 5 min. Then samples were examined by flow cytometry (Thermo Fisher Scientific, Waltham, MA, USA) at 488/530 nm (Ex/Em). Beside the resuspended cells, we kept a portion of attached cells in 24 wells and stained by 5 μL of Annexin V-FITC and 5 μL of propidium iodide as well.

2.12. Drug Loading

Methotrexate (MTX) (Sigma Aldrich, St. Louis, MO, USA) was dissolved in PBS (1 mg/10 mL) and mixed with bi-HNTs (200 mg) and keep stirring for 12 h, then, the mixture was vacuumed for 24 h. After centrifugation, the supernatant liquid was collected and stored at −20 °C for drug loading efficiency determination, and the bottom deposited bi-HNTs were washed by PBS for 3 times and air-dried, the final product was collected for further study.

2.13. Drug Loading Efficiency

The supernatant was diluted with PBS at ratio of 1 (supernatant): 20 (PBS). Then the drug concentration in supernatant was determined by MTX Elisa kit (ENZ-KIT 142-0001, Enzo Life Science, Farmingdale, NY, USA). Experiment procedure followed the manufactory product manual. First, MTX standard (S1-S6) was prepared by diluting the company supplied lyophilized MTX to suggested concentrations (1000 ng/mL, 166.7 ng/mL, 27.8 ng/mL, 4.6 ng/mL, 0.77 ng/mL, 0.13 ng/mL). Then, 100 μL of standard solution and samples were added into 96 wells, 100 μL of assay buffer 13 was added to one well and set as S0 (0 ng/mL standard), and 150 μL of assay buffer 13 was added to another well set as NSB well. 50 μL of MTX antibody was added to all wells except for the NSB and blank, and this 96 well plat was sealed and incubated at room temperature on a plate shaker (Thermo Fisher Scientific, Waltham, MA, USA) for 30 min at ~500 rpm.

Then, all the wells were washed by wash buffer for 3 times. Followed with addition of 100 μL of MTX conjugated solution to all the wells except the blank, this plate was incubated at room temperature as before. After another 3 times wash, 100 μL of substrate solution was added to all wells and went through the final incubation as same as above. Finally, add 100 μL of stop solution to all wells and read the plate at 450 nm. According to the standard curve to calculate the MTX concentration of supernatant.

The drug loading efficiency was determined by following equation:

$$\text{Loading Efficiency} = (\text{Total amount of MTX} - \text{supernatant MTX})/\text{Total amount of MTX} \times 100\% \quad (1)$$

2.14. *Drug Release Profile*

MTX-loaded bi-HNTs (20 mg) were mixed with 2 mL PBS in a tube and incubated at room temperature on a rocking shaker. After incubated for different time periods (0.5, 1, 2, 4, 6, 8, 14, 24, 32, 48, 56, 64, 72, 80, 88, and 96 h) tube was centrifuged and 1 mL of supernatant was collected, and 1 mL fresh PBS refilled to tube. The collected samples were stored at −20 °C until all the time periods samples were collected and measured by MTX Elisa kit as above.

2.15. *MTX-bi-HNTs Targeting*

Methotrexate loaded bi-HNTs (50 μg/mL) were co-cultured with CT26WT, K7M2-WT, and MC3T3-E1 pre-osteoblasts separately in 48 wells tissue culture plates (1×10^5 cells/well). After 24 h incubation, cell viability of each cell type was assessed by MTS agent as above. Cells cultured without HNTs set as control.

2.16. *Statistical Analysis*

Data were obtained from three parallel experiments and are expressed as mean ± standard deviation (S.D.). Each experiment was repeated for three times to check the reproducibility if not otherwise stated. Statistical analysis was performed by two-tailed Student's *t*-tests between two groups. The significant level was set as $p < 0.05$.

3. Results

3.1. *Optimal Dosage Determination*

In our previous study [16], we assessed bi-HNTs cytotoxicity and observed that cytotoxicity increased with bi-HNT concentration. In order to confirm the optimal dosage range for bi-HNTs, we used an MTS assay and XTT assay to assess cell proliferation and viability with cells co-cultured with pure HNTs and bi-HNTs at different concentrations. Both tests presented similar results: cell viability changed with the concentration of HNTs nanoparticles. In the MTS assay (Figure 3A,B), cell proliferation was improved when the concentration of nanoparticles was below 100 mg/mL. However, when the concentration was increased to 150 mg/mL, the proliferation ability decreased by 20%. XTT assay showed similar results (Figure 3C,D), cell viability decreased with the increasing concentration of HNTs. However, the XTT assay showed that CT26WT cells have some tolerance to higher concentrations of HNTs, with significant cytotoxicity exhibited above 200 mg/mL. The cumulative results suggest that the highest dosage of bi-HNTs is 150 mg/mL.

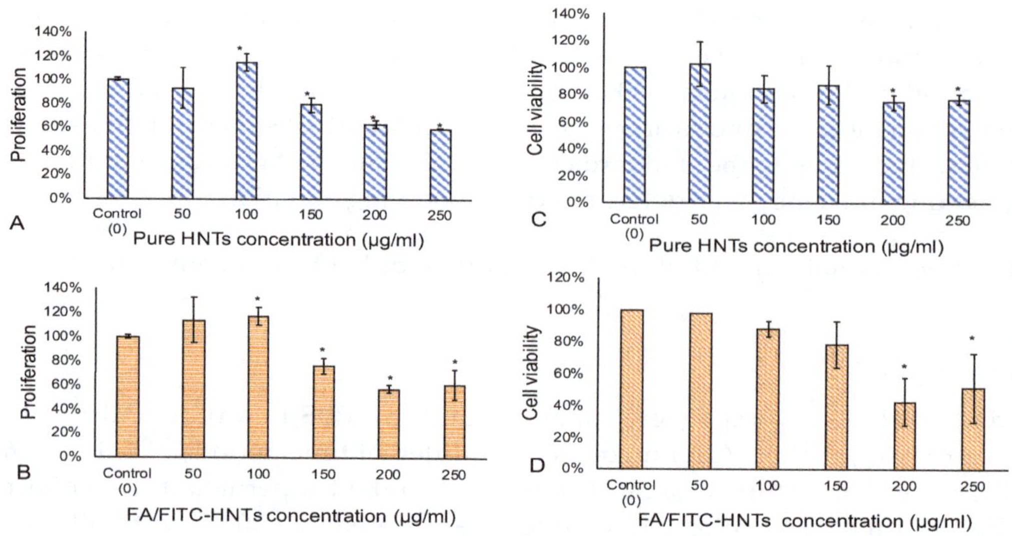

Figure 3. XTT Cell Proliferation Assay. CT26WT cells were cultured with pure HNTs (**A**) and bi-HNTs (**B**) at different concentrations. Cell proliferation at each different concentration was calculated with comparison to the control group. CT26WT cells cultured with pure HNTs (**C**) and bi-HNTs (**D**) at different concentrations. Cell viability at each different concentration point was calculated by comparison to the control group. (error bar with standard deviation, $n = 6$, * represents $p < 0.05$).

3.2. The Effect of Nanoparticle Size on the Interaction between bi-HNTs and Cells

3.2.1. Nanoparticle Size Determination

Halloysite nanotubes are naturally formed nanoparticles with an original length between 1–1.5 μm. Recently, several studies have used shortened HNTs [11,19,20]. Rong et al. introduced a detailed procedure to produce HNTs that are uniform in length [20]. We fabricated shortened HNTs by ultra-sonication (Figure 1). Dynamic light scattering (DLS) is the most commonly used.

Technique to determine nanoparticle size, however, DLS analysis requires spherical nanoparticles instead of virgate nanotubes. Thus, we used SEM micrographs of our HNT samples NIH Image J to measure their size and plotted the data into histogram graph (Figure 4). As it showed in Figure 4, the length of commercial purchased HNTs distributes in a very wide range with the average size of 0.914 ± 0.45 μm, $n = 102$ (Figure 4A), while the size of shorten HNTs was 0.715 ± 0.25 μm, $n = 80$ (Figure 4B). Comparing the two different sources of HNTs, we observed the size distribution of shortened HNTs to be more restricted in variation, which means they are more uniform in overall size. HNTs with a uniform size will provide a more accurate means for evaluating its effect on cellular behavior.

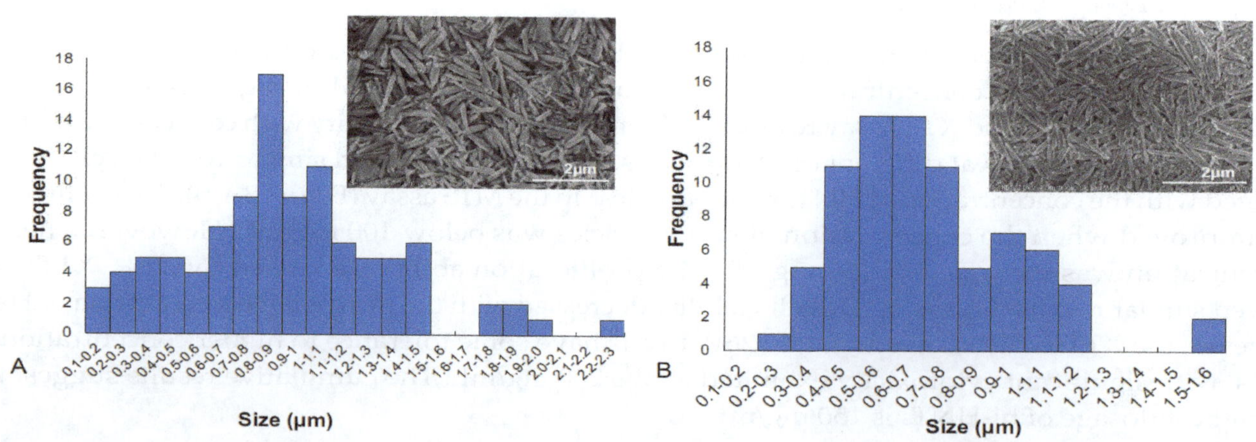

Figure 4. Histogram graph of size distribution of long HNTs (**A**) and shortened HNTs (**B**).

3.2.2. Cellular Interaction after Exposure to Long and Shortened HNTs

We hypothesized that different sized HNTs would affect cellular behavior, including our bi-functionalized HNTs. Cell up taking efficiency for two different sized HNTs was analyzed. We monitored the fluorescent intensity changes of cells (cell number = 4.46 × 105 ± 0.063 × 105) in 24 h (Figure 5A). Cellular uptake efficiency for both sizes of HNTs exhibited similar changes along with time. In the end, higher amounts of shortened HNTs are detected in cells, indicating that the smaller size of HNTs is more easily absorbed by cells.

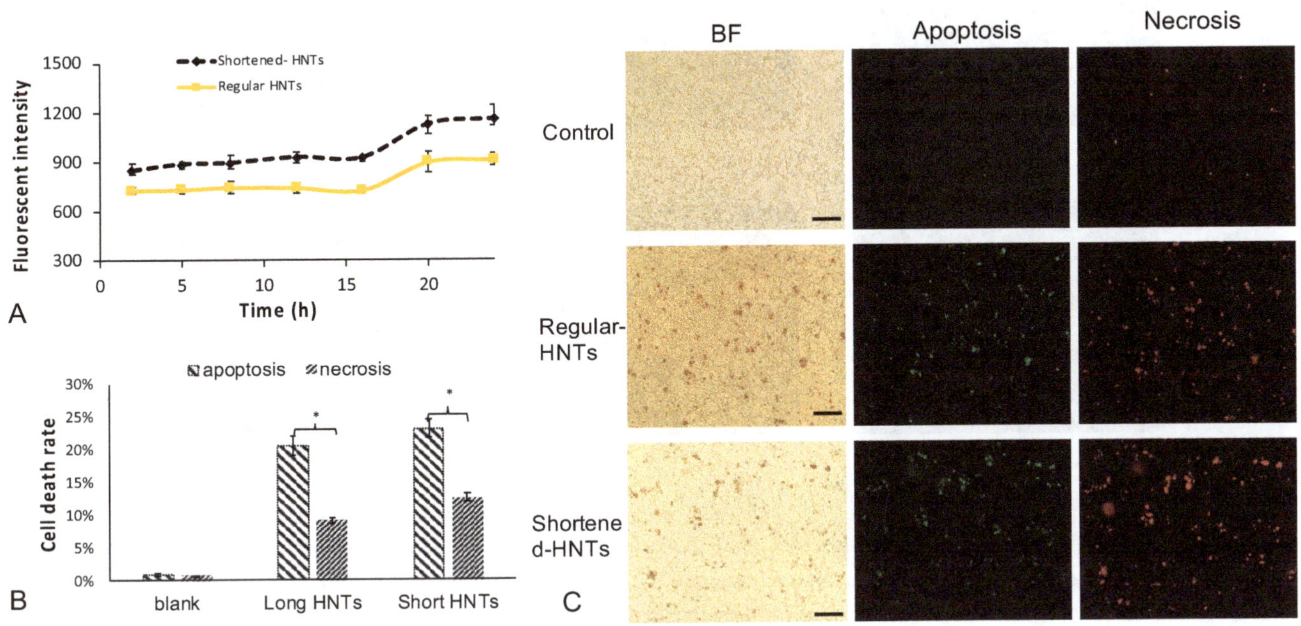

Figure 5. (**A**). Fluorescent intensity of FITC detected from CT26WT cells after 24 h incubation time (cell number for each test = $4.46 \times 10^5 \pm 0.063 \times 10^5$, each group had 9 tests, error bar with standard deviation). (**B**). The summary of flow cytometry results for apoptosis and necrosis analysis. The detailed flow cytometry results showed in Supplementary Information Figure S1. (cell number for each test = 3×10^5, each group had 6 tests, error bar with standard deviation, * represents $p < 0.05$) (**C**). Fluorescent pictures for apoptosis & necrosis analysis, the green color represents apoptosis and the red color represents necrosis. The first column represents brightfield images (scale bar with 100 μm).

3.2.3. Apoptosis and Necrosis

Previous cell cytotoxicity studies showed that cell viability decreased significantly when the concentration of HNTs reached 150 mg/mL [16]. To distinguish the mechanism of cell death, we examined cell death due to apoptosis or necrosis. CT26WT cells were incubated with long and short bi-HNTs; cell death was assessed using the Annexin V-FITC Apoptosis Kit. Apoptosis and necrosis were assessed by flow cytometry. The detail res as shown in Figure 5B, 20% ± 1.5% of cell death was caused by apoptosis and 10% ± 0.5% was due to necrosis when cells were cultured with long bi-HNTs. Cells cultured with shorted bi-HNTs showed apoptotic cell death at 23% ± 1.3% and 13% ± 0.6% due to necrosis. Thus, cell death was primarily due to apoptosis for long and shortened bi-HNTs. As seen in Figure 5, cells accumulated intracellularly shorter bi-HNTs as compared to long bi-HNTs and shortened bi-HNTs resulted in an overall higher cell death suggesting excessive cellular accumulation of bi-HNTs leads to apoptosis.

3.3. *Intracellular Location of bi-HNTs*

In order to confirm the intracellular location of bi-HNTs, we co-cultured bi-HNTs with CT26WT cells for 24 h and cells were then incubated with DiR for another 2 h. Multi-photon microscopy imaging showed cell were stained red with each reddish circular structure representing the plasma membrane;

the yellow particles represent bi-HNTs (Figure 6). Multi-photon images of labeled cells showed that many bi-HNTs were present within the plasma membrane and some had accumulated in the cytoplasm. The results further confirmed the targeting capacity of bi-HNTs in vitro.

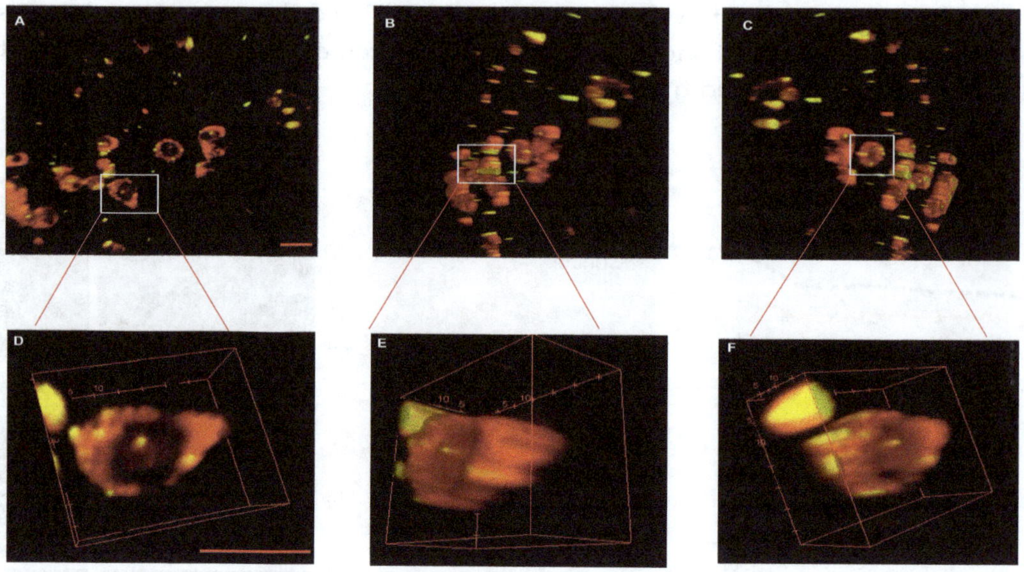

Figure 6. Multi-photon pictures of cells after exposure to bi-HNTs, pictures were analyzed with NIH Image J. Cell membranes were stained by DiR dye and exhibited a red color at wavelength of 850 nm. At this wavelength FITC exhibited a yellow color. The 3D pictures were captured at 36 microns in z with a 2 micron separation in each z step. (**A**) is the front view of the 3D picture for multiple cells, (**B**,**C**) are side views of the 3D picture. (**D**–**F**) are the zoom in pictures of the marked cell. (Scale bar with 50 μm).

3.4. *Targeted Drug Delivery*

The experiments described above support the observation that our bi-HNTs were successfully taken up by colon carcinoma cells (CT26WT). As the bi-HNTs were designed as a drug delivery system, we selected methotrexate (MTX) as model drug and loaded into bi-HNTs. Methotrexate is a commonly used anti-cancer drug to osteosarcoma. However, it is well-known for severe side effects. A cancer target drug delivery system is a promising strategy to reduce side effects and improve drug efficiency.

3.4.1. Folic Acid Coating and Drug Releasing

The chemical modification of bi-HNTs were detected by FTIR. Halloysite is an aluminosilicate clay mineral ($Al_2Si_2O_5(OH)_4$), the Si-O stretching vibrations and Al–OH vibrations were represented at 1000–1130 cm^{-1}. Folic acid, FITC and MTX containing –NH and –OH bonds, their characteristic absorption is in the range of 3300–3500 cm^{-1}, NH_2 scissoring at 1550 cm^{-1} and NH associated bending at 1652 cm^{-1}. The deformation in 3300–3500 cm^{-1} and 1652 cm^{-1} indicated the successful grafting of FA, FITC, and MTX (Figure 7A) [21]. The XRD patterns also present similar results. In Figure 7B, except for the HNTs profile there is a sharp peak appeared at $2\theta = 17.8°$ for other groups, which is the diffraction peaks of folic acid. The slight shift of this peak at HNTs + FA + FITC + MTX profile may due to the methotrexate loading. The loading efficiency of MTX in bi-HNTs was 34.74% ± 3.5%. Its drug release profile is presented in Figure 7D. Even through, there was a burst release during the first 20 h, this drug delivery system provided sustained drug release for more than 96 h.

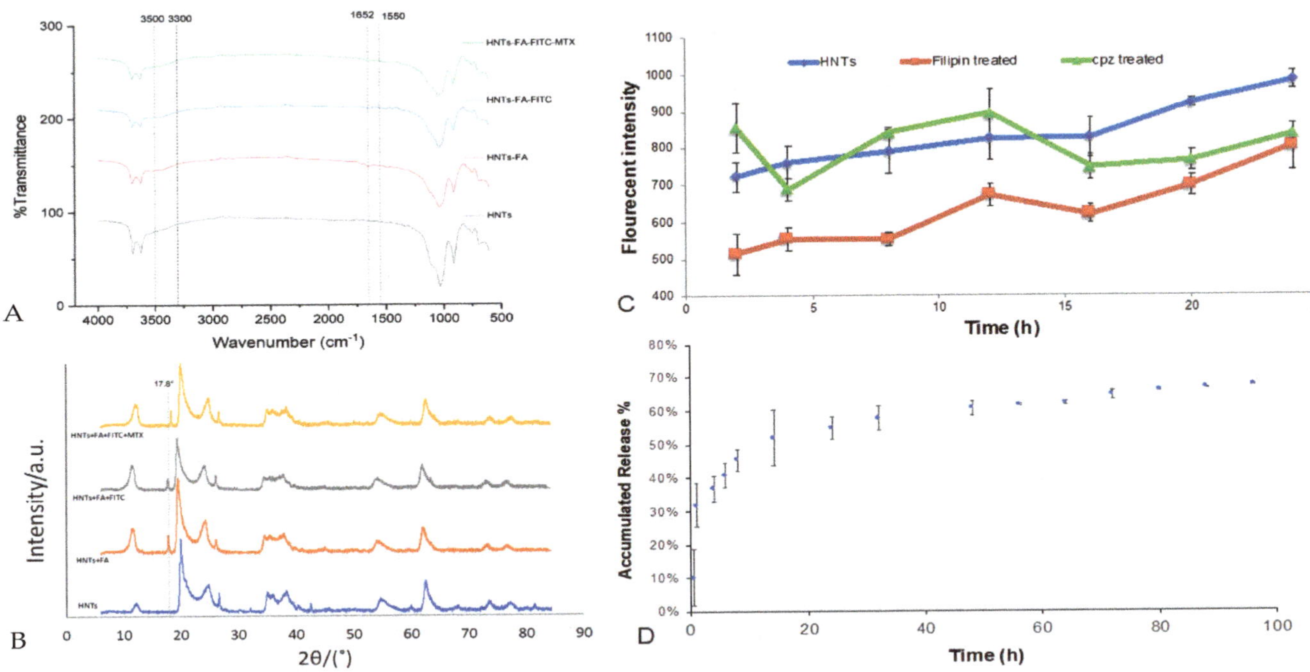

Figure 7. (**A**) FTIR detection of pure HNTs, HNTs-FA, FA/FITC-HNTs and FA/FTIC/MTX-HNTs. (**B**) XRD patterns of pure HNTs, HNTs-FA, FA/FITC-HNTs and FA/FTIC/MTX-HNTs. (**C**) Fluorescent intensity of FITC included in cells that pretreated by chlorpromazine (CPZ) or filipin and co-cultured with bi-HNTs for different time periods. (error bar with standard deviation, $n = 6$) (**D**) Accumulated drug release profile of methotrexate in 96 h. (Error bar with standard deviation, $n = 3$).

3.4.2. Cellular Uptake Mechanisms

Folic acid coated on bi-HNTs was designed to bind to folate receptors expressed by cancer cells. In the binding process, folic acid initiates cellular uptake mechanisms in two different ways: clathrin-mediated endocytosis or caveolae-mediated endocytosis. Chlorpromazine (CPZ) has the ability to disrupt clathrin-mediated endocytosis; while filipin inhibits caveolae formation. CT26WT cells were pretreated with these inhibitors and co-cultured in the presence of bi-HNTs. Their final fluorescent intensity was recorded, and the results are shown in Figure 7C. The addition of CPZ promoted HNT uptake in first 12 h, then the cell uptake decreased over time. On the other hand, filipin provided uptake inhibition during the entire testing time period. This indicates cellular absorption of bi-HNTs may mainly depend on caveolae-mediated endocytosis assist by clathrin-mediated endocytosis.

3.4.3. In Vitro Targeted Drug Release-Cellular Specificity

The bi-HNTs drug delivery system was designed to deliver drugs to specific cancer cells. Methotrexate is one of the most widely used drugs in treating osteosarcoma. Like many cancer drugs, it does have adverse side effects. In this experiment, the specific targeting of cancer cells versus normal cells was addressed. A pre-osteoblast cell line (MC3T3-E1), and two cancer cell lines, a colon cancer cell (CT26WT) and an osteosarcoma cell line (K7M2-WT), were selected to assess the targeting potential of bi-HNTs, and drug effectiveness in inhibiting cellular proliferation, the main effect of MTX (Figure 8A). The results suggest that MTX-loaded bi-HNTs (MTX-bi-HNTs) significantly inhibited osteosarcoma cell proliferation, and, at a low concentration (50 μg/mL). The other two cell types were not significantly affected by exposure to MTX (Figure 8B).

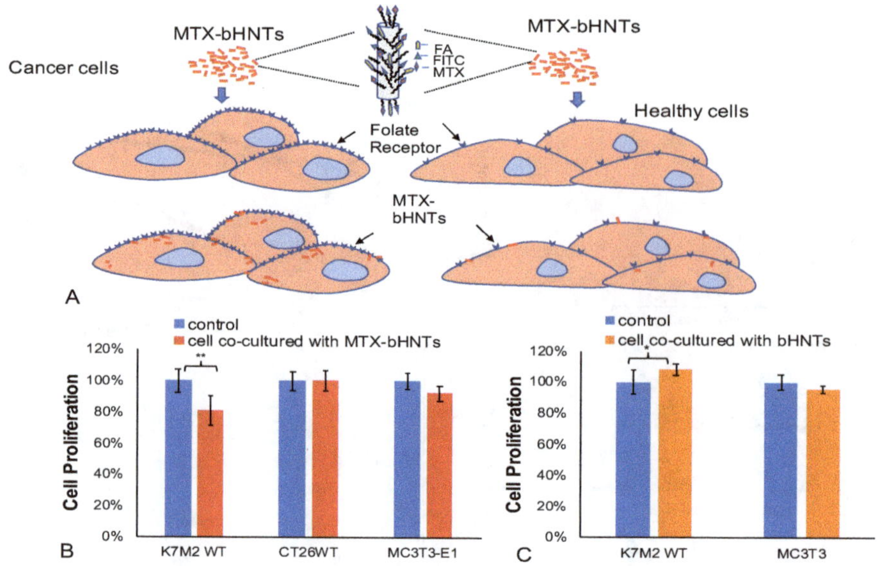

Figure 8. (**A**) Graphic depiction of osteosarcoma cells (K7M2WT), murine colon carcinoma cells (CT26WT) and preosteoblast cells (MC3T3) co-cultured with bi-HNTs. (**B**) Cell proliferation data after all three cell types were co-cultured with 50 μg/mL drug loaded bi-HNTs for 24 h. (**C**) Cell proliferation of above 3 types of cells after co-cultured with 50 μg/mL bi-HNTs for 24 h. (* represents $p < 0.05$, ** represents $p < 0.005$).

In order to clarify that inhibition of cell growth was caused by MTX instead of bi-HNTs, we analyzed cell viability by co-culturing cells with bi-HNTs but without MTX. The results showed that none of the osteosarcoma (K7M2-WT) or pre-osteoblast cells (MC3T3-E1) were affected by bi-HNTs (Figure 8C). This finding is consistent with our previous study using CT26WT; a low dose of bi-HNTs did not elicit any cytotoxicity (Figure 3). Collectively, these results demonstrate the effectiveness of MTX loaded bi-HNTs in selectively targeting osteosarcoma cells in delivery of MTX, inhibiting cell proliferation.

4. Discussion

Many studies have exploited halloysite as a nanocontainer loading chemotherapeutic agents into the HNT lumen [19–22] and adding doped HNTs to a range of polymers for anti-cancer drug delivery [23–26]. Other studies have focused on using surface modification of HNTs for use as a nanocarrier for anti-cancer drug delivery [20,27–29]. A commonly used strategy is to functionalize HNTs with an –NH2 group by using aminopropyltriethoxysilane (APTES). In a study by Guo et al. (2012), FA and magnetite nanoparticles (Fe_3O_4) were successfully grafted onto the HNT surface. The coated Fe_3O_4@HNTs exhibited a pH-sensitive drug release under the electrostatic interaction between the cationic and HNTs [20]. Coating nanotubes with a polymer shell is another mechanism, as shown by Li et al. (2018). They examined the potential of chitosan grafted onto HNTs as a nano-formulation for the anti-cancer drug curcumin [27].

Fewer studies have attempted to use modified HNTs as a mechanism for the intracellular delivery of anti-cancer agents [16,28–30] Dzamukova et al. (2015) used physically adsorbed dextrin end stoppers to secure the intracellular release of brilliant green [28]. Tagged halloysite nanotubes were also used as carriers for intercellular delivery to brain microvascular endothelium [29]. Kamalieva et al. (2018) studied the intracellular pathway of HNTs for potential application for antitumor drug delivery using human adenocarcinoma epithelial cells (A549) [30].

MTX is an FDA approved anti-cancer drug commonly used in the treatment of osteosarcoma. In a recent study, MTX-doped HNTs were coated with polyelectrolytes (PE), polyvinylpyrrolidone, and polyacrylic acid, and methotrexate [31] was infused within the coated layers. MTX release and cytotoxicity studies showed effectiveness in inhibiting osteosarcoma cell growth, and inhibition continued after PE/MTX-coated halloysite nanotubes were added to a polymer, Nylon-6.

Due to high chemical similarity in the structure between MTX and FA, several studies have shown that MTX modified nanoparticles have specificity for tumor cells [32–34]. Folic acid has a high binding affinity for the folate receptor, which is overexpressed in numerous cancers, including ovarian, endometrial, and renal carcinoma, lung, breast, and brain cancers [35]. MTX-loaded PEGylated chitosan nanoparticles had a higher cellular uptake efficiency compared to the FA-tagged group [36]. The high receptor affinity and overexpression enables folate-based nanoparticles to be highly specific, targeting tumor sites, and have great potential as a therapeutic application. FA-conjugated chitosan oligosaccharide-magnetic HNTs were studied as a delivery system for camptothecin, an anti-cancer drug [37]. Wu et al. (2018) also functionalized the HNT surface with APTES for conjugation of PEG and folic acid and subsequently loaded HNTs with doxorubicin [38]. The limitation of their study was the reported low drug loading efficiency, which was only 3%. In contrast, in this study, the loading efficiency of methotrexate was over 30%. In a recent report, HNTs had a loading efficiency of indocyanine green (ICG) as high as above 60% [39]. The variation in drug loading capability may be related to the different modification strategies used and the molecular size of drugs loaded.

The intracellular uptake pathway of HNTs was previously studied by Liu et al. [40]. HNTs were modified with APTES and labeled with FITC. Cells were treated with four different inhibitors, respectively, and then co-cultured with the FITC functionalized HNTs. They found both clathrin- and caveolae- dependent endocytosis were involved in the internalization of HNTs [40]. Liu's group also found that microtubules and actin microfilaments transported HNTs with the involvement of the Golgi apparatus and lysosome. Our results are consistent with their study. However, we observed that caveolae-mediated endocytosis was the primary mechanism of cellular import, and clathrin-mediated endocytosis was a secondary mechanism. Different surface modification strategies and cell types may be the possible explanation for the different results obtained in these studies and those reported here.

Even after pretreatment with chlorpromazine (CPZ), cytoplasmic accumulation of bi-HNTs was much more significant than the control group after the initial 12 h incubation time. One possible explanation is that disruption of clathrin-mediated endocytosis caused by CPZ induced caveolae to expand or more endocytic vesicles formed to internalize bi-HNTs. However, the overloading capability of caveolae reached capacity after several hours. Cells were unable to process the bi-HNTs loaded vesicles, so some were released from the cells. There is no report on the interaction between clathrin-and caveolae-mediated endocytosis during HNT uptake. Therefore, the detailed mechanism behind this phenomenon remains to be determined.

Our data further confirmed that bi-HNTs served well as a drug carrier and provided sustained MTX release time and showed selective binding to osteosarcoma cells. In contrast, non- osteosarcoma cells exposed to MTX were unaffected. We further showed that HNT size was also played a critical role in cellular uptake. Cellular uptake of smaller sized bi-HNTs was observed in greater amounts than unmodified HNTs. Increased intracellular accumulation may contribute to cell death through disruption of normal cellular metabolism resulting in cell death. Therefore, the application dosage of bi-HNTs should decrease with the size diminution; in other words, the smaller size of bi-HNTs has a higher working efficiency.

Even though the drug-loaded bi-HNTs has targeted FA receptors and successfully inhibited cell proliferation, this study lacks the comparison between MTX and MTX-loaded bi-HNTs. As an FDA approved anti-cancer drug, MTX would inhibit cell proliferation for sure. As a drug delivery system, bi-HNTs could extend the drug release time. We hypothesis MTX-loaded bi-HNTs would limit cell proliferation for a longer time compared to pure MTX treatment.

5. Conclusions

bi-HNTs were cytocompatible in an appropriate dosage range, permitting a decrease in MTX dose when used with size reduced bi-HNTs. The results further showed that caveolae-mediated endocytosis is the main uptake pathway of bi-HNTs, and multi-photon images confirmed cellular uptake of bi-HNTs. This modified nanocarrier also showed excellent MTX drug loading capability. Most importantly, drug-loaded MTX-bi-HNTs exhibited an excellent selectively targeting ability in vitro, as both colon carcinoma and osteosarcomas cells demonstrated bi-HNT uptake. Due to the drug specificity, the inhibition of cell proliferation was restricted to osteosarcomas, while murine colon carcinoma cells and pre-osteoblasts were not affected. Surface modification of HNTs with two ligands—FA and FITC—provided a selective targeting ability for osteosarcoma cells and an imaging vehicle for tracking bi-HNTs, and may have potential as an alternative treatment for osteosarcoma.

Author Contributions: The authors all contributed to the writing of the manuscript. Y.L. conducted the experiments under the direction of D.K.M. Both authors reviewed and analyzed the data. All authors have read and agreed to the published version of the manuscript.

Acknowledgments: The authors also wish to acknowledge the support of the College of Applied and Natural Sciences (Louisiana Tech University) Matching Grant Program. In addition, the authors appreciate Mengcheng Liu and William Clower for thier help in this study.

References

1. Global Burden of Disease Cancer Collaboration. Global, regional, and national cancer incidence, mortality, years of life lost, years lived with disability, and disability-adjusted life-years for 29 cancer groups, 1990 to 2017: A systematic analysis for the global burden of disease study. *JAMA Oncol.* **2019**, *5*, 1749–1768. [CrossRef] [PubMed]
2. Seigel, R.; Jemal, A. *American Cancer Society: Cancer Facts and Figures 2015*; American Cancer Society: Atlanta, GA, USA, 2015.
3. Caraglia, M.; De Rosa, G.; Abbruzzese, A.; Leonetti, C. Nanotechnologies: New Opportunities for Old Drugs. The Case of Aminobisphosphonates. *J. Nanomed. Biother. Discov.* **2011**, *1*, 1–2. [CrossRef]
4. Yoon, S.-A.; Choi, J.R.; Kim, J.-O.; Shin, J.-Y.; Zhang, X.; Kang, J.-H. Influence of Reduced Folate Carrier and Dihydrofolate Reductase Genes on Methotrexate-Induced Cytotoxicity. *Cancer Res. Treat.* **2010**, *42*, 163–171. [CrossRef] [PubMed]
5. Lima, S.A.C.; Gaspar, A.; Reis, S.; Durães, L. Multifunctional nanospheres for co-delivery of methotrexate and mild hyperthermia to colon cancer cells. *Mater. Sci. Eng. C* **2017**, *75*, 1420–1426. [CrossRef] [PubMed]
6. Jang, J.-H.; Jeong, S.-H.; Lee, Y.-B. Preparation and In Vitro/In Vivo Characterization of Polymeric Nanoparticles Containing Methotrexate to Improve Lymphatic Delivery. *Int. J. Mol. Sci.* **2019**, *20*, 3312. [CrossRef] [PubMed]
7. Harila-Saari, A.H.; Vainionpää, L.K.; Kovala, T.T.; Tolonen, E.U.; Marjatta Lanning, M.D.B. Nerve lesions after therapy for childhood acute lymphoblastic leukemia. *Cancer* **1998**, *82*, 200–207. [CrossRef]
8. Gaïes, E.; Jebabli, N.; Trabelsi, S.; Salouage, I.; Charfi, R.; Klouz, M.L.A.A. Methotrexate Side Effects: Review Article. *J. Drug Metab. Toxicol.* **2012**, *3*, 125. [CrossRef]
9. Darrat, Y.; Naumenko, E.; Cavallaro, G.; Lazzara, G.; Lvov, Y.; Fakhrullin, R.F. Tubular Nanocontainers for Drug Delivery. In *Materials Nanoarchitectonics*; Wiley: Hoboken, NJ, USA, 2018; pp. 85–108.
10. Dionisi, C.; Hanafy, N.A.; Nobile, C.; De Giorgi, M.; Rinaldi, R.; Casciaro, S.; Lvov, Y.M.; Leporatti, S. Halloysite Clay Nanotubes as Carriers for Curcumin: Characterization and Application. *IEEE Trans. Nanotechnol.* **2016**, *15*, 720–724. [CrossRef]
11. Hu, Y.; Chen, J.; Li, X.; Sun, Y.; Huang, S.; Li, Y.; Liu, H.; Xu, J.; Zhong, S. Multifunctional halloysite nanotubes for targeted delivery and controlled release of doxorubicin in-vitro and in-vivo studies. *Nanotechnology* **2017**, *28*, 375101. [CrossRef]

12. Gianni, E.; Avgoustakis, K.; Pšenička, M.; Pospíšil, M.; Papoulis, D. Halloysite nanotubes as carriers for irinotecan: Synthesis and characterization by experimental and molecular simulation methods. *J. Drug Deliv. Sci. Technol.* **2019**, *52*, 568–576. [CrossRef]
13. Vergaro, V.; Lvov, Y.M.; Leporatti, S. Halloysite Clay Nanotubes for Resveratrol Delivery to Cancer Cells. *Macromol. Biosci.* **2012**, *12*, 1265–1271. [CrossRef] [PubMed]
14. Ramasamy, T.; Ruttala, H.B.; Gupta, B.; Poudel, B.K.; Choi, H.-G.; Yong, C.S.; Kim, J.O. Smart chemistry-based nanosized drug delivery systems for systemic applications: A comprehensive review. *J. Control. Release* **2017**, *258*, 226–253. [CrossRef] [PubMed]
15. Leamon, C. Folate-targeted chemotherapy. *Adv. Drug Deliv. Rev.* **2004**, *56*, 1127–1141. [CrossRef] [PubMed]
16. Grimes, W.R.; Luo, Y.; McFarland, J.A.W.; Mills, D.K. Bi-Functionalized Clay Nanotubes for Anti-Cancer Therapy. *Appl. Sci.* **2018**, *8*, 281. [CrossRef]
17. Lee, S.A.; Holly, K.S.; Voziyanov, V.; Villalba, S.L.; Tong, R.; Grigsby, H.E.; Glasscock, E.; Szele, F.G.; Vlachos, I.; Murray, T.A. Gradient Index Microlens Implanted in Prefrontal Cortex of Mouse Does Not Affect Behavioral Test Performance over Time. *PLoS ONE* **2016**, *11*, e0146533. [CrossRef]
18. Pernici, C.D.; Kemp, B.S.; Murray, T.A. Time course images of cellular injury and recovery in murine brain with high-resolution GRIN lens system. *Sci. Rep.* **2019**, *9*, 7946. [CrossRef] [PubMed]
19. Riela, S.; Massaro, M.; Colletti, C.G.; Bommarito, A.; Giordano, C.; Milioto, S.; Noto, R.; Poma, P.; Lazzara, G. Development and characterization of co-loaded curcumin/triazole-halloysite systems and evaluation of their potential anticancer activity. *Int. J. Pharm.* **2014**, *475*, 613–623. [CrossRef] [PubMed]
20. Guo, M.; Wang, A.; Muhammad, F.; Qi, W.; Ren, H.; Guo, Y.-J.; Zhu, G. Halloysite Nanotubes, a Multifunctional Nanovehicle for Anticancer Drug Delivery. *Chin. J. Chem.* **2012**, *30*, 2115–2120. [CrossRef]
21. Vikulina, A.; Voronin, D.; Fakhrullin, R.; Vinokurov, V.; Volodkin, D. Naturally derived nano- and micro-drug delivery vehicles: Halloysite, vaterite and nanocellulose. *New J. Chem.* **2020**, *44*, 5638–5655. [CrossRef]
22. Bediako, E.G.; Nyankson, E.; Dodoo-Arhin, D.; Agyei-Tuffour, B.; Łukowiec, D.; Tomiczek, B.; Yaya, A.; Efavi, J.K. Modified halloysite nanoclay as a vehicle for sustained drug delivery. *Heliyon* **2018**, *4*, E00869. [CrossRef] [PubMed]
23. Yang, J.; Wu, Y.; Shen, Y.; Zhou, C.; Li, Y.-F.; He, R.-R.; Liu, M. Enhanced Therapeutic Efficacy of Doxorubicin for Breast Cancer Using Chitosan Oligosaccharide-Modified Halloysite Nanotubes. *ACS Appl. Mater. Interfaces* **2016**, *8*, 26578–26590. [CrossRef] [PubMed]
24. Shi, Y.-F.; Tian, Z.; Zhang, Y.; Shen, H.-B.; Jia, N.-Q. Functionalized halloysite nanotube-based carrier for intracellular delivery of antisense oligonucleotides. *Nanoscale Res. Lett.* **2011**, *6*, 608. [CrossRef] [PubMed]
25. Massaro, M.; Piana, S.; Colletti, C.G.; Noto, R.; Riela, S.; Baiamonte, C.; Giordano, C.; Pizzolanti, G.; Cavallaro, G.; Milioto, S.; et al. Multicavity halloysite–amphiphilic cyclodextrin hybrids for co-delivery of natural drugs into thyroid cancer cells. *J. Mater. Chem. B* **2015**, *3*, 4074–4081. [CrossRef] [PubMed]
26. Rao, K.M.; Kumar, A.; Suneetha, M.; Han, S.S. pH and near-infrared active; chitosan-coated halloysite nanotubes loaded with curcumin-Au hybrid nanoparticles for cancer drug delivery. *Int. J. Biol. Macromol.* **2018**, *112*, 119–125. [CrossRef] [PubMed]
27. Liu, M.; Chang, Y.; Yang, J.; You, Y.; He, R.; Chen, T.; Zhou, C. Functionalized halloysite nanotube by chitosan grafting for drug delivery of curcumin to achieve enhanced anticancer efficacy. *J. Mater. Chem. B* **2016**, *4*, 2253–2263. [CrossRef] [PubMed]
28. Dzamukova, M.R.; Naumenko, E.A.; Lvov, Y.M.; Fakhrullin, R.F. Enzyme-activated intracellular drug delivery with tubule clay nanoformulation. *Sci. Rep.* **2015**, *5*, 10560. [CrossRef] [PubMed]
29. Saleh, M.; Prajapati, N.; DeCoster, M.; Lvov, Y. Tagged halloysite nanotubes as a carrier for intercellular delivery in brain microvascular endothelium. *Front. Bioeng. Biotechnol.* **2020**, *8*, 451. [CrossRef]
30. Kamalieva, R.F.; Ishmukhametov, I.R.; Batasheva, S.N.; Rozhina, E.V.; Fakhrullin, R.F. Uptake of halloysite clay nanotubes by human cells: Colourimetric viability tests and microscopy study. *Nano-Struct. Nano-Objects* **2018**, *15*, 54–60. [CrossRef]
31. Sun, L.; Boyer, C.; Grimes, R.; Mills, D. Drug Coated Clay Nanoparticles for Delivery of Chemotherapeutics. *Curr. Nanosci.* **2016**, *12*, 207–214. [CrossRef]
32. Rahimi, M.; Shojaei, S.; Safa, K.D.; Ghasemi, Z.; Salehi, R.; Yousefi, B.; Shafiei-Irannejad, V. Biocompatible magnetic tris(2-aminoethyl)amine functionalized nanocrystalline cellulose as a novel nanocarrier for anticancer drug delivery of methotrexate. *New J. Chem.* **2017**, *41*, 2160–2168. [CrossRef]

33. Lu, S.; Neoh, K.G.; Huang, C.; Shi, Z.; Kang, E.-T. Polyacrylamide hybrid nanogels for targeted cancer chemotherapy via co-delivery of gold nanoparticles and MTX. *J. Colloid Interface Sci.* **2013**, *412*, 46–55. [CrossRef] [PubMed]
34. Shin, J.M.; Kim, S.-H.; Thambi, T.; Gil You, D.; Jeon, J.; Lee, J.O.; Chung, B.Y.; Jo, D.-G.; Park, J.H. A hyaluronic acid–methotrexate conjugate for targeted therapy of rheumatoid arthritis. *Chem. Commun.* **2014**, *50*, 7632–7635. [CrossRef] [PubMed]
35. Parker, N.; Turk, M.J.; Westrick, E.; Lewis, J.D.; Low, P.S.; Leamon, C.P. Folate receptor expression in carcinomas and normal tissues determined by a quantitative radioligand binding assay. *Anal. Biochem.* **2005**, *338*, 284–293. [CrossRef] [PubMed]
36. Dramou, P.; Fizir, M.; Taleb, A.; Itatahine, A.; Dahiru, N.S.; Mehdi, Y.A.; Wei, L.; Zhang, J.; He, H. Folic acid-conjugated chitosan oligosaccharide-magnetic halloysite nanotubes as a delivery system for camptothecin. *Carbohydr. Polym.* **2018**, *197*, 117–127. [CrossRef] [PubMed]
37. Chen, J.; Huang, L.; Lai, H.; Lu, C.; Fang, M.; Zhang, Q.; Luo, X. Methotrexate-loaded PEGylated chitosan nanoparticles: Synthesis, characterization, and in vitro and in vivo antitumoral activity. *Mol. Pharm.* **2014**, *11*, 2213–2223. [CrossRef] [PubMed]
38. Wu, Y.-P.; Yang, J.; Gao, H.-Y.; Shen, Y.; Jiang, L.; Zhou, C.; Li, Y.-F.; He, R.-R.; Liu, M. Folate-Conjugated Halloysite Nanotubes, an Efficient Drug Carrier, Deliver Doxorubicin for Targeted Therapy of Breast Cancer. *ACS Appl. Nano Mater.* **2018**, *1*, 595–608. [CrossRef]
39. Li, L.-Y.; Zhou, Y.-M.; Gao, R.-Y.; Liu, X.-C.; Du, H.-H.; Zhang, J.-L.; Ai, X.-C.; Zhang, J.-P.; Fu, L.-M.; Skibsted, L.H. Naturally occurring nanotube with surface modification as biocompatible, target-specific nanocarrier for cancer phototherapy. *Biomaterials* **2019**, *190*, 86–96. [CrossRef]
40. Liu, H.; Wang, Z.-G.; Liu, S.-L.; Yao, X.; Chen, Y.; Shen, S.; Wu, Y.; Tian, W. Intracellular pathway of halloysite nanotubes: Potential application for antitumor drug delivery. *J. Mater. Sci.* **2018**, *54*, 693–704. [CrossRef]

9

Development and Characterization of Liquisolid Tablets Based on Mesoporous Clays or Silicas for Improving Glyburide Dissolution

Marzia Cirri [1], Paola Mura [1,*], Maurizio Valleri [2] and Letizia Brunetti [1]

1 Department of Chemistry, University of Florence, via Schiff 6, Sesto Fiorentino, 50019 Florence, Italy; marzia.cirri@unifi.it (M.C.); letizia.brunetti@stud.unifi.it (L.B.)
2 Menarini Manufacturing Logistics and Services, s.r.l. (AMMLS), 50019 Florence, Italy; mvalleri@menarini.it
* Correspondence: paola.mura@unifi.it

Abstract: The aim of this work was to evaluate the effectiveness of mesoporous clays or silicas to develop fast-dissolving glyburide tablets based on a liquisolid approach. Selected clay (Neusilin®US2) and silica (Aeroperl®300) allowed preparation of innovative drug liquisolid systems containing dimethylacetamide or 2-pyrrolidone as drug solvents, without using coating materials which are necessary in conventional systems. The obtained liquisolid powders were characterized for solid-state properties, flowability, compressibility, morphology, granulometry, and then used for directly compressed tablet preparation. The developed liquisolid tablets provided a marked drug dissolution increase, reaching 98% dissolved drug after 60 min, compared to 40% and 50% obtained from a reference tablet containing the plain drug, and a commercial tablet. The improved glyburide dissolution was attributed to its increased wetting properties and surface area, due to its amorphization/solubilization within the liquisolid matrix, as confirmed by DSC and PXRD studies. Mesoporous clay and silica, owing to their excellent adsorbent, flow, and compressibility properties, avoided use of coating materials and considerably improved liquid-loading capacity, reducing the carrier amount necessary to obtain freely flowing powders. Neusilin®US2 showed a superior performance than Aeroperl®300 in terms of the tablet's technological properties. Finally, simplicity and cost-effectiveness of the proposed approach make it particularly advantageous for industrial scale-up.

Keywords: mesoporous clay; Neusilin; aeroperl; liquisolid technique; glyburide; dissolution improvement

1. Introduction

Glyburide (GLY) belongs to the second generation of sulfonylurea antidiabetic drugs, and it is one of the most widely utilized oral hypoglycemic agents [1]. Moreover, its ability to prevent cerebral ischemia and hemorrhagic stroke has been recently proved [2,3], and from 2015 it has been included in the model list of Essential Medicines of World Health Organization [4]. Due to its high permeability but very low aqueous solubility [5], GLY is classified as a class II drug according to the biopharmaceutical classification system [6]. As known, the dissolution rate of poorly water-soluble drugs often represents the main limiting factor in their absorption rate [6,7]. Clinical studies evidenced a variable in vitro dissolution, in vivo bioavailability, and the hypoglycaemic effect of GLY from different commercial tablets [8]. Problems of bio-inequivalence among pharmaceutically equivalent dosage forms of the drug were confirmed by a multinational post-market comparative study of various marketed products of the drug [9]. Such findings were found to be related to the unsatisfactory and variable dissolution behavior of GLY, further supporting the previously reported problems of formulation-dependent oral absorption of the drug [10].

Despite the fact that several strategies have been investigated in an effort to improve the dissolution performance of GLY, including complexation with cyclodextrins [11–13], solid dispersions in hydrophilic carriers [14–16], micellar solubilization [17], and formulation of self-micro-emulsifying drug delivery systems (SMEDDS) [18–20], at present, there are no commercial GLY products arising from such approaches. As a result, the development of effective GLY tablets with optimized dissolution behavior and ease of manufacture with industrial scale-up feasibility still remains a challenge and would be an important and useful result.

The liquisolid technique is a recent and promising alternative approach for improving the dissolution properties of poorly soluble drugs. This technique was initially used to transform liquid or semi-solid drugs into free-flowing, non-adherent, and readily compressible powders by simple mixing with suitable solid excipients [21]. Subsequently, the possibility of preparing liquisolid systems of solid poorly soluble drugs by dissolving them in a non-volatile water-miscible solvent, and then converting the liquid system in an apparently dry, well flowable powder, suitable for tableting, by mixing with proper solid excipients referred as carrier and coating materials [22,23] has been considered. The non-volatile solvents would remain on the carrier surface, so that the drug is kept within the powder substrate in a solubilized, almost molecularly dispersed state, with a great increase in both its wetting properties and surface area available for dissolution, and thus a consequent improvement in release rate and bioavailability is expected [22,24,25]. The actual effectiveness of this technique in improving the dissolution performance [26–30] and, consequently, the bioavailability [31–33] of several poorly-soluble drugs has been shown. Moreover, in addition to its drug release enhancement ability, the liquisolid strategy is particularly interesting and attractive because of the manufacturing process simplicity, low production costs, and ease of scale-up to industrial tablet production. Compounds such as various grades of cellulose derivatives, starch, and lactose are mainly used as carrier materials, while Aerosil is the most used coating material [26–29,31].

Mesoporous clays and silicas represent interesting and versatile pharmaceutical excipients, due to their numerous attractive features, such as large surface area and great loading ability, good flow and tableting properties, joined to very low toxicity, and low cost [34–36]. The multifaceted applications of clay materials in the pharmaceutical field have been carefully reviewed [37,38]. In particular, their effective use as drug delivery systems to modulate, extend, and/or target drug release has been widely described [39–43]. Furthermore, they also proved their effectiveness in enhancing the dissolution behavior, and then the bioavailability of scarcely water-soluble drugs [44–46]. Mesoporous clays and silicas can thus be considered as potentially suitable materials for liquisolid systems preparation.

Therefore, based on all these premises, we considered it worthy of interest to investigate the effectiveness of the liquisolid approach in the development of fast dissolving tablets of GLY with improved drug dissolution performance, by replacing the mixture of carrier and coating materials commonly used for their formulation with suitable mesoporous silicas or clays which would be able to simultaneously perform both such functions.

This novel strategy should enhance the applicability of the liquisolid technique in the pharmaceutical field, making it possible to decrease the necessary amount of adsorbent material, and, consequently, reducing the tablet final weight, known as the main limiting factor of this approach [47]. At the same time, it should facilitate the formulation scale-up from laboratory to industrial production, enabling the simplification of liquisolid tablet development by decreasing the number of formulation components (and the problems of their proper choice and of their relative w/w ratios).

With this aim, after selection of the most suitable non-volatile water-miscible solvent, based on its better solubilizing power towards GLY, the efficacy as carrier-coating materials of two different mesoporous silicas (i.e., Aeroperl®300/30 and Zeopharm®5170) and a mesoporous clay (Neusilin®US2) was investigated. Various liquisolid systems were then prepared and fully characterized for solid-state properties, flowability, compressibility, morphology, particle size, specific surface area, and then used for the preparation of directly compressed tablets. The obtained liquisolid tablets were tested for technological properties (mean weight, crushing strength, disintegration time) and their drug dissolution profile was compared to those of a reference conventional tablet formulation containing the drug as such and of a commercial tablet (Gliboral®).

2. Materials and Methods

2.1. Materials

Micronized glyburide (mean particle size 1.66 μm) (GLY) was from Laboratori Guidotti S.p.A. (Pisa, Italy). Glyburide has a pH-dependent solubility; its saturation solubility at 37 ± 0.5 °C was determined at pH 1.1 (0.93 ± 0.3 mg/L), pH 6.8 (4.0 ± 0.2mg/L), pH 7.4 (14.9 ± 1.1 mg/L) and pH 8.5 (108.9 ± 10.1 mg/L) (n = 3).

Neusilin®US2 (synthetic magnesium alumino-metasilicate) was from Fuji Chemicals, Toyama, Japan), Aeroperl®300 (colloidal silica) from Degussa (Munich, Germany), and Zeopharm®5170 (silicon dioxide) from Huber Engineering Materials (Atlanta, GA, USA). Labrasol® (caprylocaproyl macrogol-8 glycerides) and Transcutol® (diethylene glycol monoethyl ether) were kindly donated by Gattefossé Italia s.r.l. (Milano, Italy). Kollisolv® PYR (2-pyrrolidone, 2-PYR), Kolliphor®HS15 (macrogol 15 hydroxy-stearate), Kollisolv® PEG 400, Kollidon®CL (crospovidone) and Kollidon®VA 64F (copolymer 1vinyl-2-pyrrolidone vinylacetate 60/40) were from BASF Co. Ltd. (Ludwigshafen, Germany). Glycofurol was from Alchymars (Milano, Italy), N,N-dimethylacetamide (DMA) from Carlo Erba (Milano, Italy), Solketal® (1,2-Isopropylidene-*rac*-glycerol), benzyl benzoate and 1,3-butandiole from Merck (Kenilworth, NJ, USA). Avicel®PH102 (microcrystalline cellulose) was from FMC Biopolymer (Philadelphia, PA, USA), Explotab® (sodium starch glycolate) was from Penwest Pharmaceuticals (Patterson, NY, USA), and Ceolus®KG802 (microcrystalline cellulose) from Asahi Kasei (Tokyo, Japan). Mg stearate was from Peter Greven Fett Chemie (Bad Munsterefeil, Germany). Water was obtained from a Milli-Q water purification system (Millipore, MA, USA). All other chemicals and reagents were of analytical grade.

2.2. Solubility Studies

To select the most effective drug solvent for liquisolid systems formulation, the GLY solubility in different non-volatile water-miscible solvents, namely Labrasol®, Transcutol®, Kolliphor®HS15, PEG 400, Kollisolv®, Solketal®, Kollisolv®PYR (2-pyrrolidone, 2-PYR), N,N-dimethylacetamide (DMA), benzyl benzoate and 1,3-butandiole, was evaluated. The minimum amount necessary to solubilize 5 mg GLY (drug therapeutic dose) was determined by adding progressive aliquots of each solvent to the exactly weighed drug amount, at room temperature. Only in the case of Kolliphor®HS15, solid at room temperature, it was necessary to heat to 40 °C for obtaining its fusion. The stability of GLY dissolved in the various solvents was checked by UV assay (UV/Vis 1601 Shimadzu, Tokyo, Japan) at 300 nm of its concentration immediately after the solution preparation, and then every 30 days for 6 months.

2.3. Characterization of the Mesoporous Silicas and Clays

2.3.1. Apparent and Tapped Density

Apparent density (D_A) and tapped density (D_T) were evaluated according to the USP method, using a PT-TD 300 instrument (Pharma Test, Hainburg, Germany) endowed with a standard 100 mL graduated cylinder. Carr's Index (CI) and Hausner Ratio (HR), indicative of the powder compressibility and flowability, were determined by the following equations:

$$CI(\%) = 100\frac{D_{T1250} - D_A}{D_{T1250}};\ HR = DT_{1250}/D_A \tag{1}$$

where D_{T1250} is the tapped density value obtained after 1250 taps of the cylinder.

2.3.2. Powder Flowability

Powder flowability was determined by the Copley flow-test (Copley Scientific Ltd., Nottingham, UK), evaluating the powder ability to freely flow through a circular orifice of known diameter. The flowability index is given by the diameter (ranged from 4 to 26 mm) of the smallest hole through which the powder falls freely (mean of three determinations).

2.3.3. Powder Compactability

Powder compactability was evaluated according to the Wells method [48]. Briefly, 3 samples were prepared for each carrier, by weighing each time aliquots of 5 g of powder, adding 50 mg of Mg stearate as a lubricant, and mixing in a V-mixer 3 min (samples A and B) or 30 min (sample C). From each sample blend, five tablets (13 mm diameter) were then obtained, by compacting with a hydraulic press 500 mg powder, under 1 ton of pressure for 5 s (A and C) or 30 s (B). After 24 h, the tablets' crushing force (N) was measured (Schleuniger Hardness Tester model 6D, JB Pharmatron, Northampton, UK).

2.3.4. Specific Surface Area

Specific surface area measurements were performed according to the BET (Brunauer-Hemmet-Teller) method using an automated ASAP (Accelerated Surface Area and Pore) 2010 adsorption analyzer (Micromeritics, Norcross, GA, USA) at −196 °C. Before analysis, samples were degassed 24 h at room temperature using a VacPrep apparatus (Micromeritics, Norcross, GA, USA).

2.4. Preparation of Liquisolid Systems

The drug was completely dissolved in the minimum necessary amount of solvent; then the drug solution was put in a mortar, where the mesoporous silica (or clay) powder was gradually added, under mixing, up to obtain an apparently dry powder.

2.5. Characterization of Liquisolid Systems

2.5.1. Particle Size Distribution

Granulometric analysis of the various liquisolid systems was performed using a Mastersizer 3000 Laser Particle Size (LPS) analyzer (Malvern Instruments, Malvern, UK). The particle size distribution curves were obtained, and Dv_{10}, Dv_{90}, and Dv_{50} were evaluated, indicating, respectively, 10% or 90% of the cumulative percent distribution and the median of the powder distribution curve. The SPAN value, i.e., the curve distribution width around the median, was determined as an index of the powder particle size homogeneity, by the following equation [49]:

$$\text{SPAN} = (Dv_{90} - Dv_{10})/Dv_{50} \tag{2}$$

2.5.2. Differential Scanning Calorimetry (DSC)

Exactly weighed samples (5–10 mg, M3 microbalance, Mettler Toledo, Greifensee, Switzerland) of pure drug and mesoporous silica or clay, and of the corresponding liquisolid systems were put in pierced Al pans and scanned under static air at 10 °C/min from 30 to 300 °C using a TA4000 Star^e system (Mettler Toledo, Greifensee, Switzerland) equipped with a DSC 25 cell.

2.5.3. Powder X-Ray Diffractometry (PXRD)

Powder X-ray diffraction patterns of pure drug and mesoporous silica and clay and of the corresponding liquisolid systems were recorded by a Bruker D8 Advance apparatus (Brucker, Billerica, MA, USA), using a Cu Kα radiation and a graphite monochromator, under the following experimental conditions: 40 mV voltage, 40 mA current, scan rate 0.05°/s in the 2.5–50° 2Θ range, room temperature.

2.5.4. Environmental Scanning Electron Microscopy (ESEM)

The morphological properties of the different liquisolid systems as well as of the final tablet formulations were investigated using a Fei ESEM Quanta 200 Apparatus. Before performing the analyses, samples were sputter-coated with gold-palladium under argon atmosphere, to make them electrically conductive.

2.5.5. Dissolution Test

Dissolution rate experiments were performed according to the dispersed amount method. A sample of each liquisolid system, equivalent to 5 mg drug, was added to 350 mL of pH 7.4 phosphate buffer solution thermostated at 37 ± 0.5 °C, in a 400 mL beaker. A three-blade paddle was centrally put in the beaker and rotated at 100 rpm. At given times, aliquots were withdrawn (syringe-filter, pore size 0.45 μm), spectrometrically assayed at 300 nm (UV-Vis 1600 Shimadzu, Tokyo, Japan) for drug content, and replaced with an equal fresh medium volume. A correction fort the cumulative dilution was made. Each test was repeated four times (C.V. < 3.5%). Values of percent of drug dissolved at 10, 30, and 60 min were analyzed by one-way analysis of variance (ANOVA) followed by the Student-Newman-Keuls multiple comparison post-test (Graph Pad Prism 4.0 program, San Diego, CA, USA). Differences were considered statistically significant when $p < 0.05$.

2.6. Tablets Preparation

Tablets containing 5 mg GLY as liquisolid system, accurately mixed with suitable excipients for direct compression and Mg stearate as a lubricant, were prepared using a Manesty 2 alternative tableting machine. A reference conventional tablet formulation containing the plain drug was also prepared.

2.7. Tablets Characterization

Appearance and morphologic analysis: the regularity of the tablets' appearance was checked by visual inspection. The morphology of the tablets' surface was examined more in detail by ESEM analysis.

Weight uniformity: 20 tablets randomly taken from the batch were individually weighed (Mettler XP2003S balance, Mettler Toledo, Greifensee, Switzerland). The mean tablet weight, and the relative CV percentage values were then determined.

Hardness: determined using a Schleuniger Hardness Tester mod 6D as crushing force (N). Tensile strength was also calculated to eliminate the possible effects of variations in tablet thickness on the measured crushing force;

Disintegration time: evaluated using the T2 221 Erweka disintegration apparatus (Erweka GmbH, Langen, Germany) at 37 ± 0.5 °C in pH 7.4 phosphate buffer;

Dissolution test: performed using a USP Paddle apparatus (Sotax AT7, Sotax, Thun, Switzerland). Tablets were added to 900 mL of pH 7.4 phosphate buffer solution thermostated at 37 ± 0.5 °C, at a stirring rate of 75 rpm. The concentration of dissolved drug was UV-monitored at 300 nm (Lambda 2 spectrophotometer, Perkin Elmer, Waltham, MA, USA). Each test was simultaneously carried out on six samples. Dissolution efficiency (DE) was calculated from the area under the dissolution curve at time t and expressed as a percentage of the area of the rectangle described by 100% dissolution in the same time [50]. Percent of drug dissolved and DE values were analyzed by one-way analysis of variance (ANOVA) followed by the Student–Newman–Keuls multiple comparison post-test (Graph Pad Prism 4.0 program, San Diego, CA, USA). Differences were considered statistically significant when $p < 0.05$.

3. Results and Discussion

3.1. Selection of the Solvents

The proper selection of the best solvent for the development of a liquisolid system, mainly based on its solubilizing power towards the drug, is of critical importance to reduce the amount of solid adsorbent excipient, and, consequently, the final total weight of the dosage form. Then, as the first step of this study, the solubilizing effect towards GLY of a wide variety of non-volatile, water-miscible solvents (Labrasol®, Transcutol®, Solketal®, Kolliphor®HS15, 2-PYR, PEG 400, glycofurol, DMA, benzyl benzoate and 1,3-butandiole), was evaluated. With this purpose, the minimal amount of each solvent necessary to solubilize 5 mg GLY (therapeutic drug dosage) was determined. As shown in Figure 1, DMA and 2-PYR emerged as the most effective solvents, requiring, respectively, only 0.025 or 0.050 mL to solubilize 5 mg drug, and then were chosen as the liquid vehicles for GLY liquisolid systems preparation. The safe and effective use of 2-PYR as a solvent for drug solubilization has been reported, in virtue of its lack of mutagenic or genotoxic activity [51], and its low developmental toxicity, and high oral LD_{50} (5g/kg body weight in rats) (www.epa.gov/chemical-under-tsca). On the other hand, DMA is approved by FDA as an excipient in parenteral and nasal spray products (www.accessdata.fda.gov) and its safe use as a solubilizer, included also in intravenous pediatric formulations, has been proved [52–54].

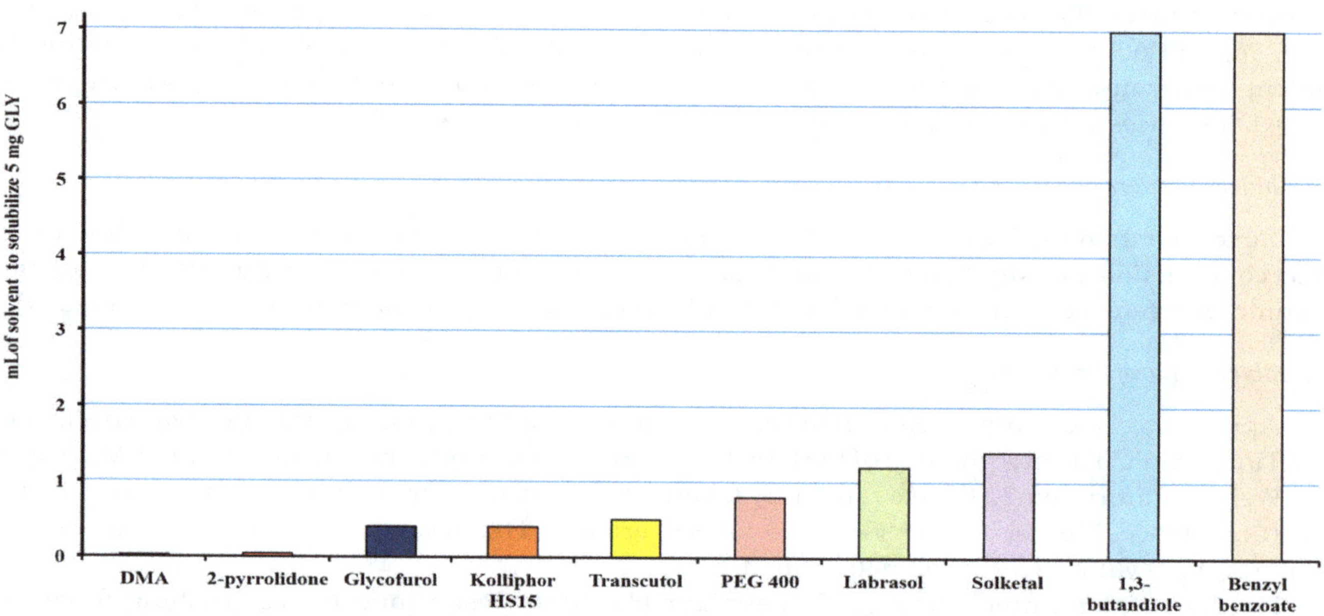

Figure 1. Solubility of glyburide (GLY) in the different solvent examined, expressed as mL of solvent necessary to solubilize 5 mg drug (therapeutic single dose).

GLY stability in the selected solvents was verified, by checking its concentration at interval times up to six months by spectrophotometric assay. No variations of drug concentration, and no modifications of its UV curve were observed, indicative of drug stability and absence of degradation phenomena.

3.2. *Characterization and Selection of Mesoporous Carriers as Adsorbent Carrier*

The powder materials used as a carrier for preparation of liquisolid systems should have high liquid adsorbent power, and, at the same time, good flow and compaction properties, to allow uniform feed and reproducible filling of tablet dies and good tableting. Then, the flow and compaction properties of the mesoporous silicas and clay materials considered as potential adsorbent carriers for preparation of liquisolid systems, namely Aeroperl®300, Zeopharm®5170 and Neusilin®US2, were firstly investigated. The results of these studies, in terms of apparent and tapped density, Carr's Index and Hausner ratio, flowability (Copley test) and compactability (Wells test) are presented in Table 1.

Table 1. Apparent (D_A) and tapped (D_T) Density, Carr Index % (CI), Hausner Ratio (HR), flowability (as flow through an orifice), and compactability (determined by Wells test A, B and C) of Aeroperl®300, Neusilin®US2, Zeoparm®5170.

Sample	Da (g/cm³)	D_T (g/cm³)	CI %	HR	Flow (∅, mm)	Wells A (N)	Wells B (N)	Wells C (N)
Aeroperl®300	0.23	0.28	17.8	1.22	4	30	32	30
Neusilin®US2	0.17	0.20	16.5	1.19	4	390	400	400
Zeopharm®5170	0.32	0.34	6.2	1.07	4	15	16	16

Based on Carr's Index and Hausner Ratio values, Zeopharm®5170 showed the best fluidity level, followed by Neusilin®US2 and then by Aeroperl®300. However, according to the flow Copley test, all powders presented excellent flowability, freely falling through the smallest apparatus hole (4 mm diameter). As for the compaction properties, the results of the Wells test showed that all powders samples exhibited a fragmenting behavior since similar crushing strength values were obtained in the different conditions of the test (A≈B≈C). This is considered a desirable characteristic of powders to be compressed, since the crushing strength of tablets made with fragmenting materials should be less negatively affected by the presence of hydrophobic lubricant, such as Mg stearate, with respect to plastic-deforming materials [55,56]. Neusilin®US2 gave rise to the tablets with the highest hardness, but acceptable breaking strength values (around 30 N) were obtained also with Aeroperl®300. On the contrary, the crushing strength values of Zeopharm®5170 tablets were very low, probably due to its poor binding properties, and then this excipient was discarded in subsequent studies.

The selected mesoporous clay and silica were then further characterized by BET analysis. Both compounds showed a very extended specific surface area, which confirmed their highly porous nature. However, the chosen clay Neusilin®US2 showed a clearly greater surface area (355.5 vs. 268.4 m²/g) and also a significantly higher volume (1.0 vs. 0.5 cm³/g) of mesopores (i.e., pores in the 2.0–50 nm range) compared to the chosen silica Aeroperl®300.

3.3. Preparation and Characterization of Liquisolid Systems

Liquisolid systems were then prepared by dissolving 5 mg GLY (drug therapeutic single dose) in 0.05 mL of the selected solvents (DMA or 2-PYR), and then gradually adding, under continuous mixing, Neusilin®US2 or Aeroperl®300, selected as carrier-coating materials. The strong adsorptive power of the selected mesoporous clay and silica allowed to use a liquid load factor (i.e., the w/w ratio of liquid medication to the carrier powder) of 1.1, clearly higher than the values commonly used in conventional liquisolid systems [22,27,29,47], and obtain dry-looking powders, with practically unchanged flow properties (measured according to the Copley flow test) compared to the respective pure carriers.

The obtained liquisolid systems were then characterized by LPS for granulometric distribution and compared with the corresponding pure carriers. As can be observed in Figure 2, both Aeroperl®300 and Neusilin®US2 exhibited a satisfactorily homogeneous distribution curve, with a mean volumetric diameter of 31 μm and 76 μm, respectively. The formation of liquisolid systems did not substantially change the original granulometric distribution of the corresponding carriers, irrespective of the type of solvent used, indicating in all cases the absence of appreciable aggregation phenomena and the obtainment of homogeneous systems looking as dry powders.

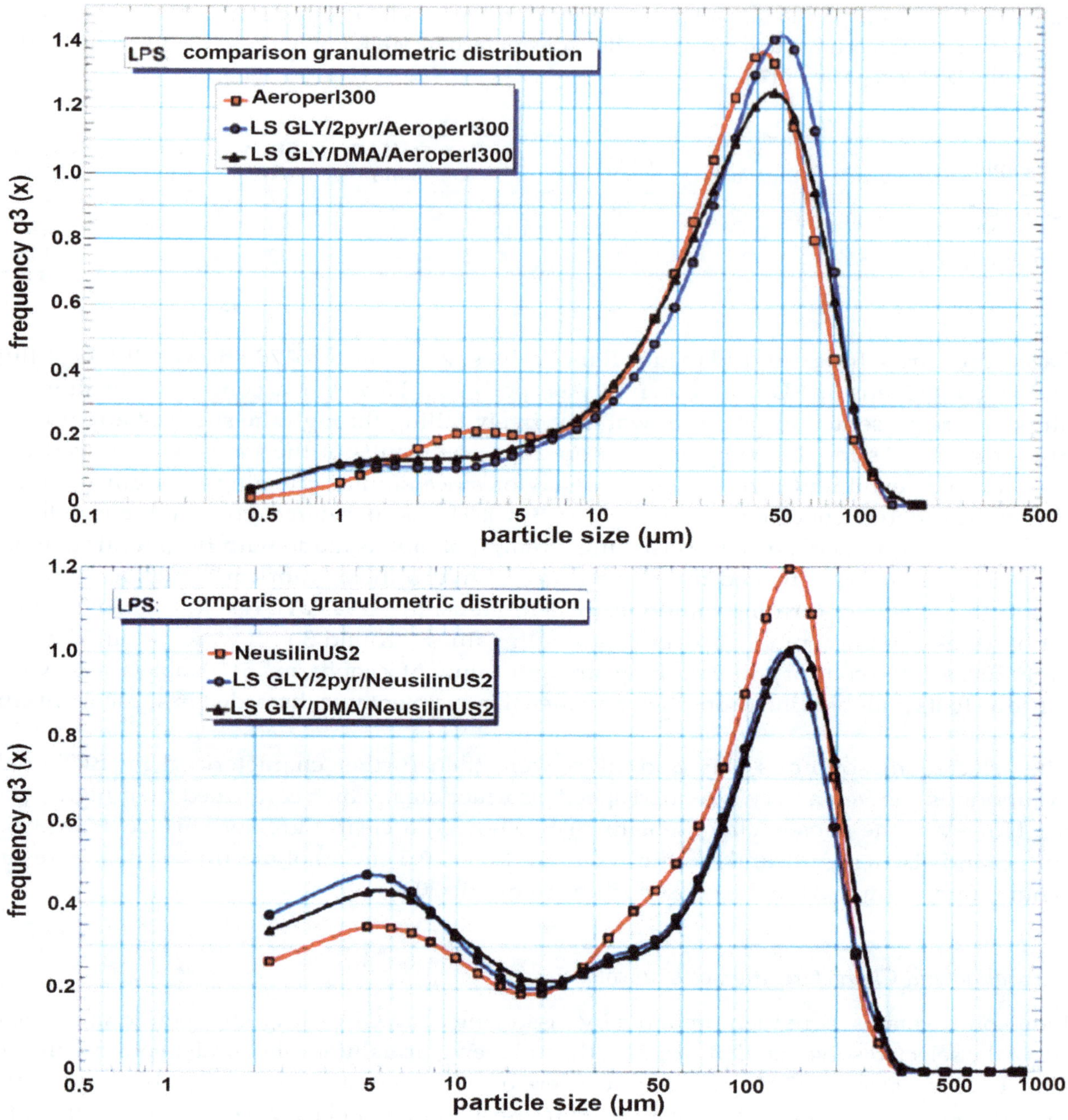

Figure 2. Granulometric analysis, by Laser Particle Size (LPS), of pure Aeroperl®300 and Neusilin®US2, and of the corresponding liquisolid systems with glyburide (GLY) containing 2-pyrrolidone (2-PYR) or dimetylacetamide (DMA) as non-volatile water miscible solvent.

DSC analyses were performed on pure drug and mesoporous clay and silica and on the corresponding liquisolid systems, in order to evaluate possible solid-state modifications or interactions between the components (Figure 3). The DSC curve of GLY was typical of a crystalline, pure, anhydrous compound, showing a flat profile before the sharp endothermic peak at 175 °C (ΔH 180 J/g) due to the drug melting. On the contrary, the thermal curves of both carriers indicated their amorphous nature, being characterized by a broad endothermal band in the range 70–140 °C, due to evaporation of associated water molecules, followed, in the case of Neusilin®US2, by another endothermic effect at a higher temperature (240 °C), due to decomposition phenomena.

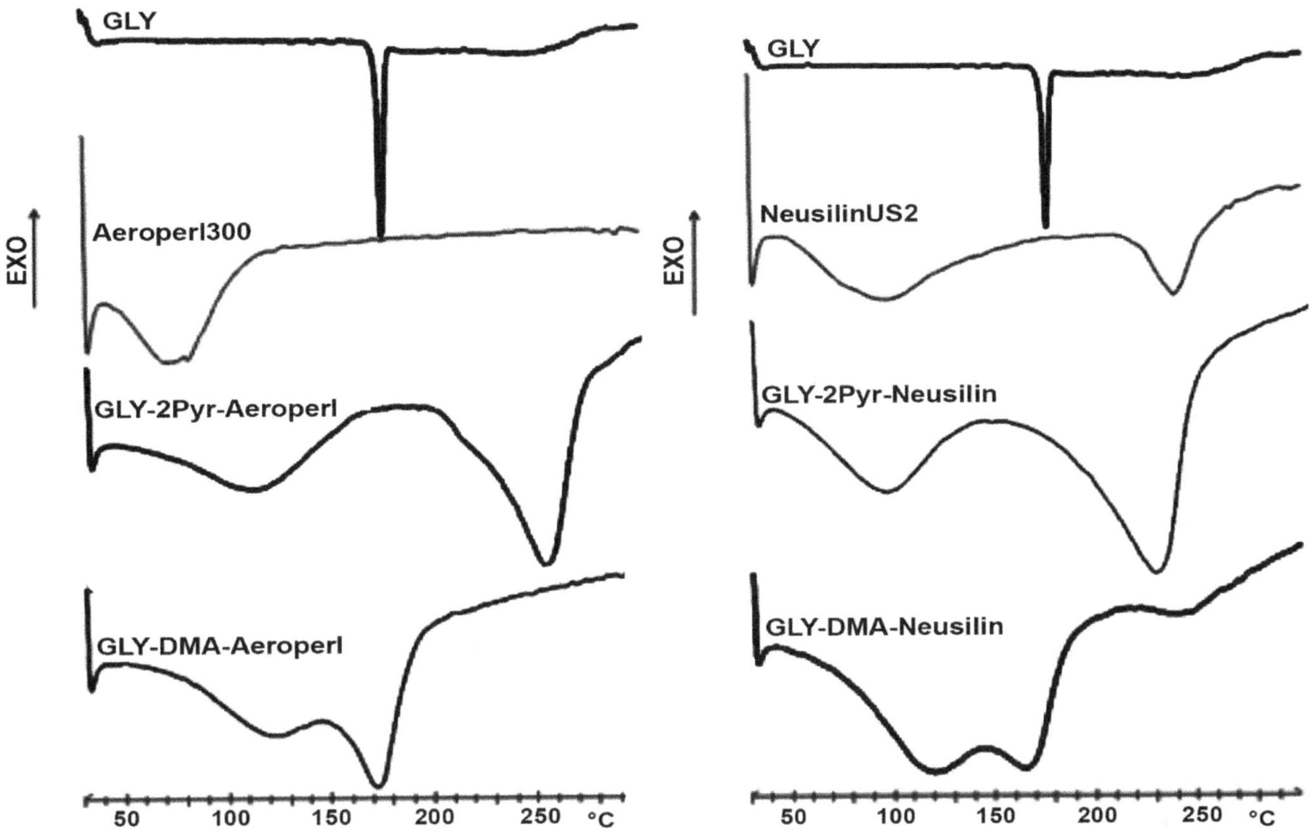

Figure 3. Differential Scanning Calorimetry (DSC) curves of pure glyburide (GLY), Aeroperl®300 and Neusilin®US2 and of the corresponding liquisolid systems with 2-pyrrolidone (2-PYR) or dimetylacetamide (DMA) as non-volatile water miscible solvent.

DSC curves of liquisolid systems containing 2-PYR as a solvent showed two broad endothermic effects: the first, which peaked around 100 °C, was due to the carrier (Neusilin®US2 or Aeroperl®300) dehydration, while the second one, which peaked around 240 °C, was due to the solvent evaporation (boiling point 245 °C), partially superimposed, in the case of Neusilin®US2, to the carrier decomposition phenomena. An analogous thermal behavior was displayed by liquisolid systems prepared with DMA as a solvent; however, in this case, due to the lower boiling point of this solvent (165 °C), a partial superimposition of the carrier dehydration band to that of solvent evaporation happened. Interestingly, in all cases the complete disappearance of the drug melting peak was observed, which can be considered indicative of drug amorphization and/or solubilization in the liquisolid system, i.e., its almost molecular dispersion within the liquisolid matrix [26,27].

The results of PXRD studies were substantially in agreement with those of DSC analysis. In fact, as can be observed in Figure 4, the diffraction pattern of pure GLY exhibited the presence of numerous sharp peaks, in particular at 18.8, 19.4, 20.8 and 22.9° 2Θ, indicative of its crystalline nature, while a diffuse halo pattern, characteristic of amorphous powders, was shown by both mesoporous clay and silica.

The typical diffraction peaks of the drug were no more detectable in the X-ray spectra of all the liquisolid formulations, thus confirming the conversion of the drug in an amorphous or solubilized form within the liquisolid matrix, as suggested by DSC analysis, and allowing to exclude any possible artifact of this last technique, due to the sample heating during the scan.

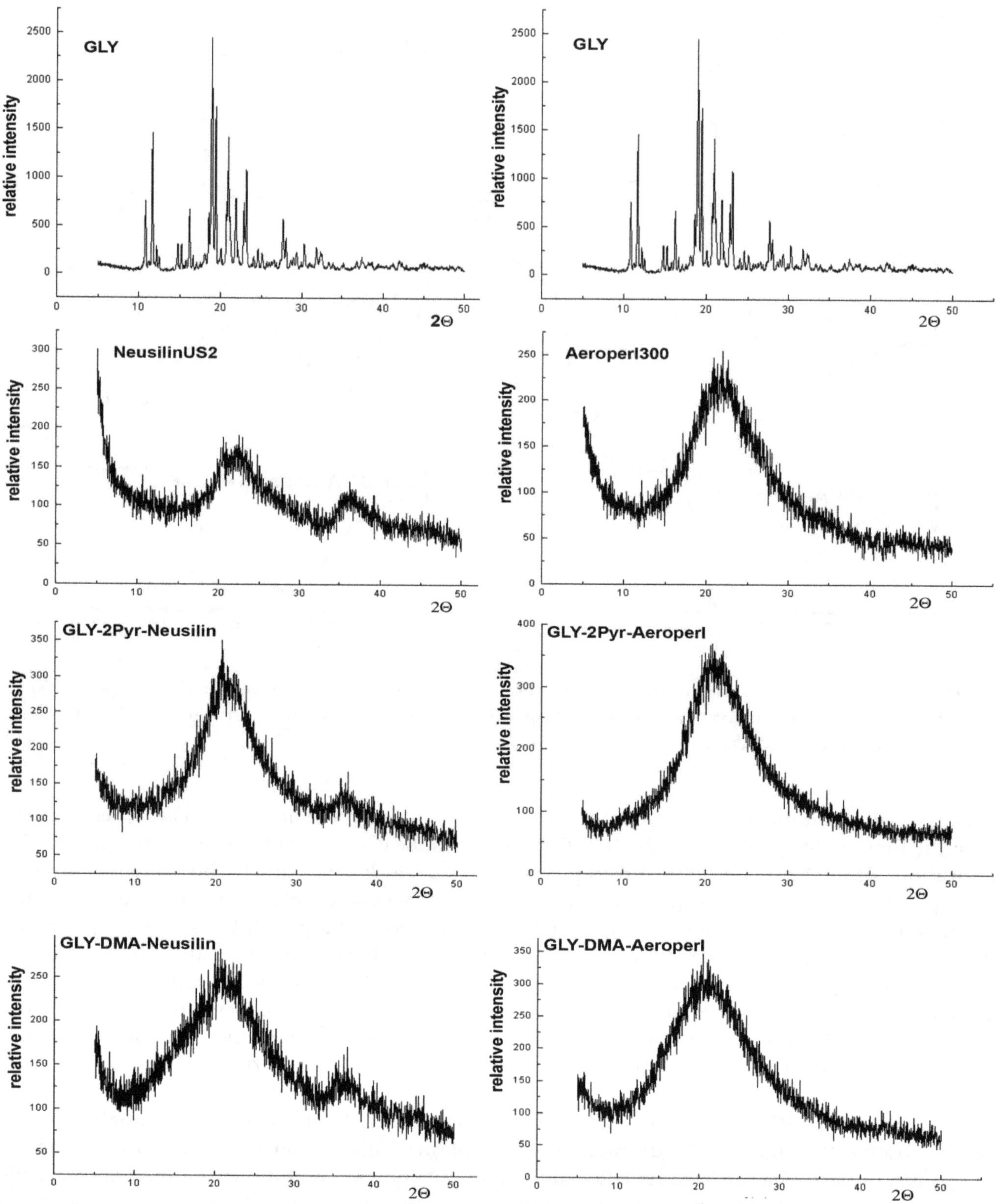

Figure 4. X-Ray powder diffraction patterns of pure glyburide (GLY), Neusilin®US2 and Aeroperl®300 and of the corresponding liquisolid systems with 2-pyrrolidone (2-PYR) or dimetylacetamide (DMA) as non-volatile water miscible solvent.

The ESEM outcomes (Figure 5) further supported the results of DSC and XRPD analyses. The ESEM image of pure micronized GLY showed its crystalline nature and its very homogeneous particle size. Neusilin®US2 appeared instead as particles of almost spherical form, with a highly porous surface, and Aeroperl®300 as spherical particles, many of which characterized by the presence of an internal cavity. The morphology of liquisolid systems obtained with both Neusilin®US2 or Aeroperl®300 as carrier-coating material was very similar to that of the corresponding pure samples, thus confirming their excellent adsorbent power and the absence of agglomeration phenomena.

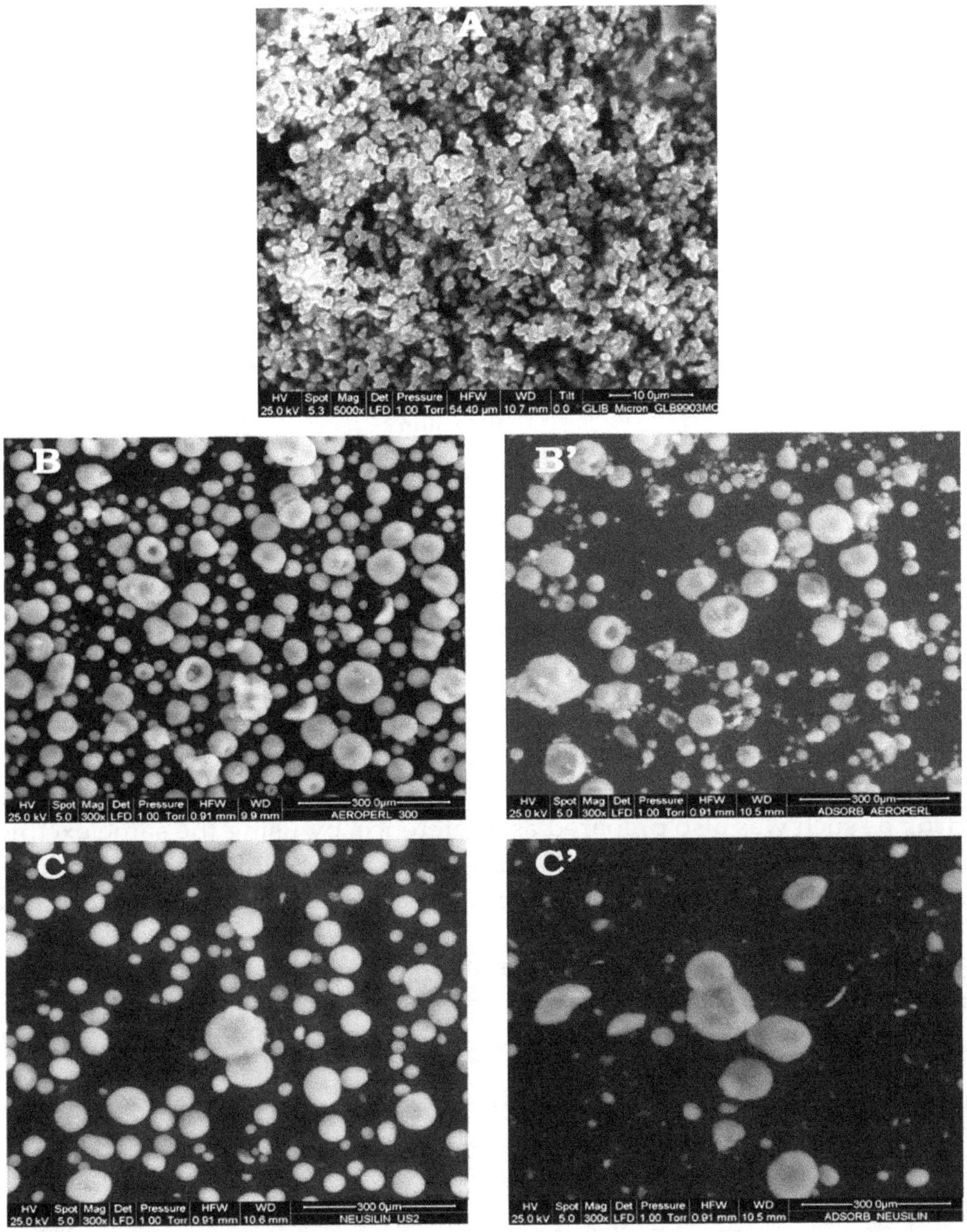

Figure 5. ESEM images of pure glyburide (**A**), Aeroperl®300 (**B**) and Neusilin®US2 (**C**) and of the corresponding liquisolid systems (**B′** and **C′**).

Dissolution studies were then performed to evaluate the ability of the various liquisolid systems to improve the GLY dissolution rate and select the more effective ones for the preparation of liquisolid tablets. As can be seen in Figure 6, all the developed liquisolid systems showed a very marked improvement of GLY dissolution rate compared to the plain GLY, with an about 27 times increase of percent drug dissolved after only 2 min, and an about 4 times increase at the end of the test (60 min). No statistically significant ($p > 0.05$) differences were found among the different kinds of liquisolid systems and then they were all employed for tablet preparation.

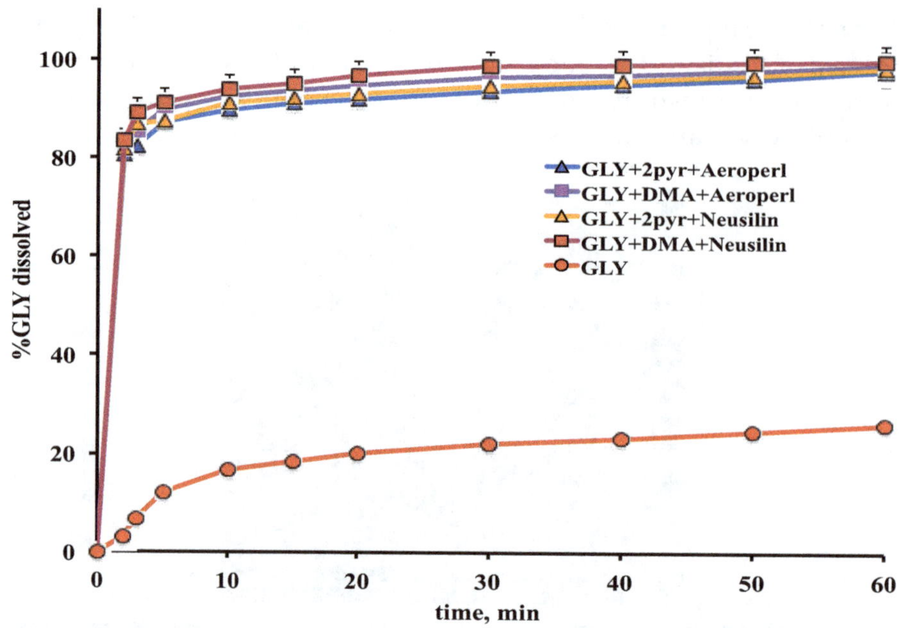

Figure 6. Dissolution profiles of glyburide (GLY) as such or from the different liquisolid systems.

3.4. Preparation and Characterization of Liquisolid-Tablets

Preformulation studies, performed to select the most suitable excipients to use, in mixture with the liquisolid systems, for obtaining direct-compressed tablets with the proper characteristics of hardness and disintegration time, enabled the selection of two kinds of microcrystalline cellulose (Avicel®PH102 and Ceolus®KG802) as binders, in virtue of their high flowability and compressibility, and of Explotab® (sodium starch glycolate) as super-disintegrant. The composition and properties of the examined tablets are reported in Table 2. For each tablet formulation, the lowest compression force allowing to obtain tablets with suitable hardness and tensile strength was used (Table 2). A conventional tablet containing the drug as such was also prepared as a reference, by using the same excipients present in liquisolid tablets, except the solvent, replaced by an equivalent quantity by weight of Avicel®PH102. A GLY commercial tablet at the same drug dosage (Gliboral®) was also used as a further reference.

Table 2. Composition and properties of glyburide (GLY) liquisolid tablets.

Tablet Code	Ingredients (mg)									Properties			
	GLY	2pyr	DMA	Neusilin	Aeroperl	Avicel	Ceolus	Explotab	Mg st	Compr. Force (kN)	Crush. Force (N)	Tens str (MPa)	Disin. Time (s)
LS1	5	55	–	55	–	44	20	10	0.5	3.4	62	1.42	50
LS2	5	55	–	–	55	44	20	10	0.5	15	50	1.28	90
LS3	5	–	47	47	–	44	20	10	0.5	3.4	32	0.85	60
LS4	5	–	47	–	47	44	20	10	0.5	15	29	0.79	85

All tablets complied with the USP friability test (weight loss in all cases less than 0.2%) and weight uniformity and showed short disintegration times, always less than 2 min.

Dissolution test was performed under the same experimental conditions (900 mL of pH 7.4 buffer solution) used in our previous studies aimed at the development of GLY fast-dissolving tablets [12,15,16,20], in order to obtain comparable results. Moreover, these conditions of medium volume and pH are those indicated by FDA and USP (test 5, Revision Bulletin 2010, 1st Supplement USP 34-NF 29) for the dissolution test of GLY (micronized) tablets. The dissolution profiles of GLY from liquisolid-tablets are shown in Figure 7, in comparison with those from the conventional reference and the marketed tablets, while their dissolution parameters, in terms of percentage drug dissolved and Dissolution Efficiency (DE) at 10 min and 60 min, indicative, respectively, of the rate and of the totality of the process, are collected in Table 3.

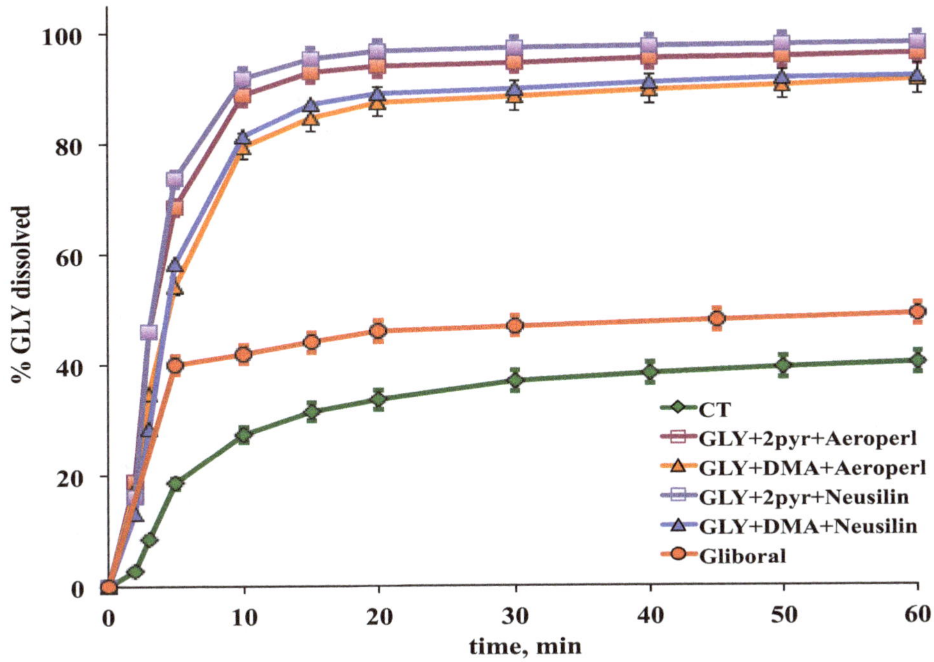

Figure 7. Dissolution profiles of glyburide (GLY) from liquisolid tablets (LS 1–4) and from the commercial tablet (Gliboral®) and the reference conventional tablet (CT).

Table 3. Dissolution parameters of glyburide from liquisolid (LS) and conventional (CT) tablets in terms of percent dissolved (PD) and dissolution efficiency (D.E.) at 10 and 60 min.

Tablet Code *	PD10	PD60	DE10	DE60
LS1	91.8	98.1	58.1	90.4
LS2	88.6	96.3	55.9	88.1
LS3	81.3	92.1	47.1	82.7
LS4	79.6	91.4	46.8	81.5
CT	27.5	40.7	15.1	33.4

* For the composition of tablet batches, see Table 2.

As is evident, all liquisolid tablets exhibited a marked enhancement of the GLY dissolution performance, with respect to both the reference tablet containing the plain drug and the commercial tablet. In fact, the percentage of drug dissolved at 60 min from the conventional reference and from the commercial tablets reached only 40% and 50%, respectively, while it exceeded 90% for all liquisolid systems. The observed improvement in dissolution rate can be attributed to the increased wetting properties and to the larger surface area of drug particles exposed to the dissolution medium, in virtue of its almost molecular dispersion within the liquisolid matrix [26–28]. However, interestingly, tablets with liquisolid systems containing 2-PYR as solvent showed a slightly better dissolution profile, particularly in terms of percentage dissolved at 10 min ($p < 0.05$), than those containing DMA, despite the slightly higher solubility of GLY in DMA than in 2-PYR (see Figure 1). Nevertheless, this result may be somehow connected to the tablet formulation and/or compression process. In fact, dissolution experiments performed directly on the plain liquisolid systems as powders, exhibited an inverted behavior, with a slight, even not significant, better performance of those containing DMA as solvent (see Figure 6).

On the other hand, no significant differences ($p > 0.05$) in the drug dissolution behavior were instead observed between systems with Neusilin®US2 or Aeroperl®300. However, as can be seen in

Table 2, when comparing liquisolid formulations containing the same solvent (LS1 vs. LS2, or LS3 vs. LS4), Neusilin®US2 allowed to obtain tablets with similar or even better hardness, than those with Aeroperl®300, but using lower compression force. This is considered a desirable property, since tablets of suitable hardness, necessary to avoid breakage problems, should be ideally obtained without applying excessive compression force, in order to can be easily disintegrated when in contact with the dissolution medium. In fact, tablets prepared under large compression force will have a reduced porosity and will require more time for water penetration into the compact, thus resulting in prolonged disintegration times [27].

A comparison between the drug dissolution properties from the new liquisolid tablets and those from the previously developed GLY fast-dissolving tablets based on other different formulation approaches, showed that the new technology was actually more effective in enhancing the GLY dissolution properties than the formation of binary or ternary solid dispersions [15,16], cyclodextrin complexation [12] or simple adsorption on mesoporous silicas [46]. The performance of the new GLY liquisolid tablets resulted comparable only to that of fast-dissolving tablets based on solid-self-microemulsifying systems (SMEDDS) [20]. However, the new liquisolid-tablets presented the strong advantage of a simpler and faster formulation development and of a lower production cost. In fact, they did not require the time-consuming construction of pseudo-ternary phase diagrams to select the best surfactant and co-surfactant and to define the zone of microemulsion existence, which are instead necessary for the SMEDDS development. On the contrary, their very basic preparation procedure should assure an easy and economic industrial scale-up feasibility.

Finally, ESEM analyses were performed on final liquisolid tablets (Figure 8). The results further confirmed the better technological performance of tablets containing Neusilin®US2, whose whole surface appeared highly porous but perfectly homogeneous (Figure 8A); on the contrary, some horizontal fracture lines and thin fissures were observed on the surface of tablets containing Aeroperl®300, indicative of not optimal technological properties of the formulation and of a potential tablet delamination process (Figure 8B).

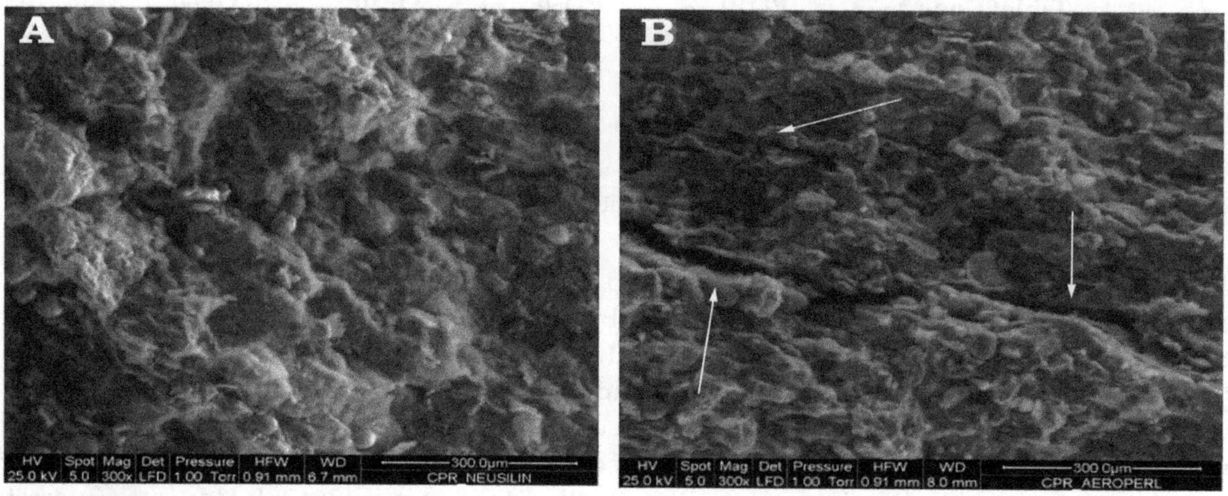

Figure 8. ESEM images of the surface of glyburide liquisolid tablets LS1 (**A**) and LS2 (**B**).

4. Conclusions

New liquisolid-tablet formulations of GLY, based on the use of a mesoporous clay (Neusilin®US2) or silica (Aeroperl®300), were successfully developed.

Both the selected mesoporous clay and silica, in virtue of their very marked adsorbent power joined to excellent flow and compactability properties, allowed to replace the use of combinations of carrier and coating materials, which are instead commonly employed for the preparation of conventional liquisolid systems.

The use of 2-PYR and DMA as very powerful solvents towards GLY (never employed before, to the best of our knowledge, in liquisolid formulations), enabled to strongly reduce the solvent volume necessary (0.05 mL) to completely dissolve the drug therapeutic dose (5 mg). Moreover, the selected highly-porous clay (Neusilin®US2) and silica (Aeroperl®300) enabled a high liquid load factor (1.1), because of their small amount necessary to convert drug solutions into well-flowable powders.

All the obtained liquisolid-tablets exhibited satisfying technological properties and exhibited a marked improvement of GLY dissolution properties, allowing in all cases to overcome 90% of dissolved drug after 60 min, with respect to only 40% obtained with the reference formulation containing the plain drug. However, the mesoporous clay Neusilin®US2 showed a superior performance with respect to the mesoporous silica Aeroperl®300 since it allowed to obtain tablets with more suitable technological properties.

The improved GLY dissolution behavior was attributed to its increased wetting properties and surface area, in virtue of its solubilization or almost molecular dispersion within the liquisolid matrix, as confirmed by DSC and PXRD studies.

In conclusion, the proposed strategy offers the benefits not only of simplifying the liquisolid formulation development, reducing the number of components, but also, and above all, of considerably increasing the liquid loading capacity, thus strongly reducing the amount of adsorbent material necessary to obtain dry-looking, freely-flowing powders, and ultimately decreasing the final tablet weight. Finally, simplicity, ease of handling, high cost-effectiveness of the proposed approach, make it particularly advisable for a possible industrial scale-up.

Author Contributions: Conceptualization, M.C., P.M. and M.V.; methodology, M.V.; formal analysis, M.C., P.M., and L.B.; investigation, L.B.; resources, M.V.; data curation, M.C., P.M., and L.B.; writing–original draft preparation, P.M.; writing–review and editing, P.M. and M.C.; supervision, M.V.; project administration, M.V.; All authors have read and agreed to the published version of the manuscript.

References

1. Pearson, J.G. Pharmacokinetics of glyburide. *Am. J. Med.* **1985**, *79*, 67–71. [CrossRef]
2. Simard, J.M.; Sheth, K.N.; Kimberly, W.T.; Stern, B.J.; del Zoppo, G.J.; Jacobson, S.; Gerzanich, V. Glibenclamide in cerebral ischemia and stroke. *Neurocrit. Care* **2014**, *20*, 319–333. [CrossRef]
3. Caffes, N.; Urland, D.B.; Gerzanich, V.; Simard, J.M. Glibenclamide for the treatment of ischemic and hemorrhagic stroke. *Int. J. Mol. Sci.* **2015**, *16*, 4973–4984. [CrossRef] [PubMed]
4. World Health Organization (WHO). Model List of Essential Medicines. 2015. Available online: http://www.who.int/medicines/publications/essentialmedicines/en/index.html (accessed on 24 April 2020).
5. Lobenberg, R.; Kramer, J.; Shah, V.P.; Amidon, G.L.; Dressman, J.B. Dissolution testing as prognostic tool for oral drug absorption dissolution behavior of glibenclamide. *Pharm. Res.* **2000**, *17*, 439–444. [CrossRef] [PubMed]
6. Lobenberg, R.; Amidon, G.L. Modern bioavailability, bioequivalence and biopharmaceutics classification system. New scientific approaches to international regulatory standards. *Eur. J. Pharm. Biopharm.* **2000**, *50*, 3–12. [CrossRef]
7. Galia, E.; Nicolaides, E.; Hörter, D.; Lobenberg, R.; Reppas, C.; Dressman, J.B. Evaluation of various dissolution media for predicting in vivo performance of class I and II drugs. *Pharm. Res.* **1998**, *15*, 698–705. [CrossRef]
8. Chalk, J.B.; Patterson, M.; Smith, M.T.; Eadie, M.J. Correlations between in vitro dissolution, in vivo bioavailability and hypoglycaemic effect of oral glibenclamide. *Eur. J. Clin. Pharmacol.* **1986**, *31*, 177–187. [CrossRef]
9. Blume, H.; Ali, S.L.; Siewert, M. Pharmaceutical quality of glibenclamide products: A multinational postmarket comparative study. *Drug Dev. Ind. Pharm.* **1993**, *19*, 2713–2741. [CrossRef]

10. Neugebauer, G.; Betzien, G.; Hrstka, V.; Kaufmann, B.; von Mollendorff, E.; Abshagen, U. Absolute bioavailability and bioequivalence of glibenclamide. *Int. J. Clin. Pharmacol. Ther. Toxicol.* **1985**, *23*, 453–460.
11. Mitrevej, A.; Sinchaipanid, N.; Juniaprasert, V.; Warintornuwat, L. Effect of grinding of β-cyclodextrin and glibenclamide on tablet properties. *Drug Dev. Ind. Pharm.* **1996**, *22*, 1237–1241. [CrossRef]
12. Cirri, M.; Righi, F.; Maestrelli, F.; Mura, P. Development of glyburide fast-dissolving tablets base on the combined use of cyclodextrins and polymers. *Drug Dev. Ind. Pharm.* **2009**, *35*, 73–82. [CrossRef] [PubMed]
13. Klein, S.; Wempe, M.F.; Zoeller, T.; Buchanan, N.L.; Lambert, J.L.; Ramsey, M.G.; Edgar, K.J.; Buchanan, C.M. Improving glyburide solubility and dissolution by complexation with hydroxybutyl-beta-cyclodextrin. *J. Pharm. Pharmacol.* **2009**, *61*, 23–30. [CrossRef] [PubMed]
14. Tashtoush, B.M.; Al-Oashi, Z.S.; Najib, N.M. In vitro and in vivo evaluation of glibenclamide in solid dispersion systems. *Drug Dev. Ind. Pharm.* **2004**, *30*, 601–607. [CrossRef] [PubMed]
15. Valleri, M.; Mura, P.; Maestrell, F.; Cirri, M.; Ballerini, R. Development and evaluation of glyburide fast dissolving tablets using solid dispersion technique. *Drug Dev. Ind. Pharm.* **2004**, *30*, 525–534. [CrossRef]
16. Cirri, M.; Valleri, M.; Maestrelli, F.; Corti, G.; Mura, P. Fast-dissolving tablets of glyburide based on ternary solid dispersions with PEG 6000 and surfactants. *Drug Deliv.* **2007**, *14*, 247–255. [CrossRef]
17. Seedher, N.; Kanojia, M. Micellar solubilization of some poorly soluble antidiabetic drugs. *AAPS PharmSciTech* **2008**, *9*, 431–436. [CrossRef]
18. Bachhav, Y.G.; Patravale, V.B. SMEDDS of glyburide: Formulation, in vitro evaluation, and stability studies. *AAPS PharmSciTech* **2009**, *10*, 482–487. [CrossRef]
19. Albertini, B.; Sabatino, M.D.; Melegari, C.; Passerini, N. Formulation of spray-congealed microparticles with self-emulsifying ability for enhanced glibenclamide dissolution performance. *J. Microencapsul.* **2015**, *32*, 181–192. [CrossRef]
20. Cirri, M.; Roghi, A.; Valleri, M.; Mura, P. Development and characterization of fast-dissolving tablet formulations of glyburide based on solid self-microemulsifying systems. *Eur. J. Pharm. Biopharm.* **2016**, *104*, 19–29. [CrossRef]
21. Spireas, S. Liquisolid Systems and Methods of Preparing Same. U.S. Patent 6,423,339 B1, 19 August 1998.
22. Spireas, S.; Sadu, S. Enhancement of prednisolone dissolution properties using liquisolid compacts. *Int. J. Pharm.* **1998**, *166*, 177–188. [CrossRef]
23. Spireas, S.; Wang, T.; Grover, R. Effect of powder substrate on the dissolution properties of methychlothiazide liquisolid compacts. *Drug Dev. Ind. Pharm.* **1999**, *25*, 163–168. [CrossRef] [PubMed]
24. Nokhodchi, A.; Hentzschel, C.M.; Leopold, C.S. Drug release from liquisolid systems: Speed it up, slow it down. *Expert Opin. Drug Deliv.* **2011**, *8*, 1–15. [CrossRef] [PubMed]
25. Vraníková, B.; Niederquell, A.; Ditzingerb, F.; Šklubalová, Z.; Kuentz, M. Mechanistic aspects of drug loading in liquisolid systems with hydrophilic lipid-based. *Int. J. Pharm.* **2020**, *578*, 110999. [CrossRef] [PubMed]
26. Fahmy, R.H.; Kassem, M.A. Enhancement of famotidine dissolution rate through liquisolid tablets formulation: In vitro and in vivo evaluation. *Eur. J. Pharm. Biopharm.* **2008**, *69*, 993–1003. [CrossRef]
27. Tiong, N.; Elkordy, A.A. Effects of liquisolid formulations on dissolution of naproxen. *Eur. J. Pharm. Biopharm.* **2009**, *73*, 373–384. [CrossRef] [PubMed]
28. Hentzschel, C.M.; Alnaief, M.; Smirnova, I.; Sakmann, A.; Leopold, C.S. Enhancement of griseofulvin release from liquisolid compacts. *Eur. J. Pharm. Biopharm.* **2012**, *80*, 130–135. [CrossRef]
29. Chella, N.; Narra, N.; Rao, T.R. Preparation and characterization of liquisolid compacts for improved dissolution of telmisartan. *J. Drug Deliv.* **2014**. [CrossRef]
30. Azharshekoufeh, L.; Shokri, J.; Adibkiac, K.; Javadzadeh, Y. Liquisolid technology: What it can do for NSAIDs delivery? *Colloids Surf. B* **2015**, *136*, 185–191. [CrossRef]
31. Khaled, K.A.; Asiri, Y.A.; El-Sayed, Y.M. In vivo evaluation of hydrochlorothiazide liquisolid tablets in beagle dogs. *Int. J. Pharm.* **2007**, *222*, 1–6. [CrossRef]
32. El-Houssieny, B.M.; Wahman, L.F.; Arafa, N.M.S. Bioavailability and biological activity of liquisolid compact formula of repaglinide and its effect on glucose tolerance in rabbits. *Biosci. Trends* **2010**, *4*, 17–24.

33. Sanka, K.; Poienti, S.; Bari Mohd, A.; Diwan, P.V. Improved oral delivery of clonazepam through liquisolid powder compact formulations: In-vitro and ex-vivo characterization. *Powder Technol.* **2014**, *256*, 336–344. [CrossRef]
34. Manzano, M.; Colilla, M.; Vallet-Regí, M. Drug delivery from ordered mesoporous matrices. *Expert Opin. Drug Deliv.* **2009**, *6*, 1383–1400. [CrossRef] [PubMed]
35. Mazanoab, M.; Vallet-Regí, M. New developments in ordered mesoporous materials for drug delivery. *J. Mater. Chem.* **2010**, *20*, 5593–5604.
36. Huang, X.; Young, N.P.; Townley, H.E. Characterization and comparison of mesoporous silica particles for optimized drug delivery. *Nanomater. Nanotechnol.* **2014**, *4*. [CrossRef]
37. Carretero, M.I.; Pozo, M. Clay and non-clay minerals in the pharmaceutical industry: Part I. Excipients and medical applications. *Appl. Clay Sci.* **2009**, *46*, 73–80. [CrossRef]
38. Kim, M.H.; Choi, G.; Elzatahry, A.; Vinu, A.; Choy, Y.B.; Choy, J.H. Review of clay-drug hybrid materials for biomedical applications. *Clays Clay Miner.* **2016**, *64*, 115–130. [CrossRef]
39. Aguzzi, C.; Cerezo, P.; Viseras, C.; Caramella, C. Use of clays as drug delivery systems: Possibilities and limitations. *Appl. Clay Sci.* **2007**, *36*, 22–36. [CrossRef]
40. Viseras, C.; Cerezo, P.; Sanchez, R.; Salcedo, I.; Aguzzi, C. Current challenges in clay minerals for drug delivery. *Appl. Clay Sci.* **2010**, *48*, 291–295. [CrossRef]
41. Hua, S.; Yang, H.; Wang, W.; Wang, A. Controlled release of ofloxacin from chitosan_montmorillonite hydrogel. *Appl. Clay Sci.* **2010**, *50*, 112–117. [CrossRef]
42. Salcedo, I.; Aguzzi, C.; Sandri, G.; Bonferoni, M.C.; Mori, M.; Cerezo, P.; Sanchez, R.; Viseras, C.; Caramella, C. In vitro biocompatibility and mucoadhesion of montmorillonite chitosan nanocomposite: A new drug delivery. *Appl. Clay Sci.* **2012**, *55*, 131–137. [CrossRef]
43. De Sousa Rodrigues, L.A.; Figueiras, A.; Veiga, F.; de Freitas, R.M.; Nunes, L.C.C.; da Silva Filho, E.C.; da Silva Filho, E.C.; da Silva Leite, C.M. The systems containing clays and clay minerals from modified drug release: A review. *Colloids Surf. B* **2013**, *103*, 642–651. [CrossRef]
44. Choudhari, Y.; Hoefer, H.; Libanati, C.; Monsuur, F.; McCarthy, W. Mesoporous silica drug delivery systems. In *Amorphous Solid Dispersions*; Shah, N., Sandhu, H., Choi, D.S., Chokshi, H., Malick, A.W., Eds.; Springer: New York, NY, USA, 2014; pp. 665–693.
45. Le, T.T.; Elyafi, A.K.E.; Mohammed, A.R.; Al-Khattawi, A. Delivery of poorly soluble drugs via mesoporous silica: Impact of drug overloading on release and thermal profile. *Pharmaceutics* **2019**, *11*, 269. [CrossRef]
46. Mura, P.; Valleri, M.; Fabianelli, E.; Maestrelli, F.; Cirri, M. Characterization and evaluation of different mesoporous silica kinds as carriers for the development of effective oral dosage forms of glibenclamide. *Int. J. Pharm.* **2019**, *563*, 43–52. [CrossRef] [PubMed]
47. Javadzadeh, Y.; Jafari-Navimipour, B.; Nokhodchi, A. Liquisolid technique for dissolution rate enhancement of a high-dose water-insoluble drug (carbamazepine). *Int. J. Pharm.* **2007**, *341*, 26–34. [CrossRef] [PubMed]
48. Wells, J.I. Powder flow properties: Compression properties. In *Pharmaceutical Preformulation: The Physicochemical Properties of Drug Substances*; Wiley, J., Ed.; Ellis Horwood: Chichester, UK, 1988; pp. 211–214.
49. Washington, C. *Particle Size Analysis in Pharmaceuticals and Other Industries*; Taylor & Francis e-Library: Chichester, UK, 2005; pp. 1–19.
50. Khan, K.A. The concept of dissolution efficiency. *J. Pharm. Pharmacol.* **1975**, *27*, 48–49. [CrossRef] [PubMed]
51. Jain, P.; Yalkowsky, S.H. Solubilization of poorly soluble compounds using 2-pyrrolidone. *Int. J. Pharm.* **2007**, *342*, 1–5. [CrossRef]
52. Kawakami, K.; Oda, N.; Miyoshi, K.; Funaki, T.; Ida, Y. Solubilization behavior of a poorly soluble drug under combined use of surfactants and cosolvents. *Eur. J. Pharm. Sci.* **2006**, *28*, 7–14. [CrossRef]
53. Oechtering, D.; Boos, J.; Hempel, G. Monitoring of N,N-dimethylacetamide in children during i.v.-busulfan therapy by liquid chromatography-mass spectrometry. *J. Chromatogr. B* **2006**, *838*, 129–134. [CrossRef]
54. Trame, M.N.; Bartelink, I.H.; Boos, J.; Boelens, J.J.; Hempel, G. Population pharmacokinetics of dimethylacetamide in children during standard and once-daily IV busulfan administration. *Cancer Chemother. Pharmacol.* **2013**, *72*, 1149–1155. [CrossRef]
55. Bolhuis, G.K.; Van Der Voort, M.K.; Zuurman, K. Effect of magnesium stearate on bonding and porosity expansion of tablets produced from materials with different consolidation properties. *Int. J. Pharm.* **1999**, *179*, 107–115.
56. Rojas, J.; Aristozabal, J.; Henao, M. Screening of several excipients for direct compression of tablets: A new perspective based on functional properties. *J. Bas. Appl. Pharm. Sci.* **2013**, *34*, 17–23.

10

Norfloxacin-Loaded Electrospun Scaffolds: Montmorillonite Nanocomposite vs. Free Drug

Angela Faccendini [1], Marco Ruggeri [1], Dalila Miele [1], Silvia Rossi [1], Maria Cristina Bonferoni [1], Carola Aguzzi [2], Pietro Grisoli [1], Cesar Viseras [2], Barbara Vigani [1], Giuseppina Sandri [1,*] and Franca Ferrari [1]

1 Department of Drug Sciences, University of Pavia, Viale Taramelli 12, 27100 Pavia, Italy; angela.faccendini@gmail.com (A.F.); marco.ruggeri02@universitadipavia.it (M.R.); dalila.miele@gmail.com (D.M.); silvia.rossi@unipv.it (S.R.); cbonferoni@unipv.it (M.C.B.); pietro.grisoli@unipv.it (P.G.); barbara.vigani@unipv.it (B.V.); franca.ferrari@unipv.it (F.F.)

2 Department of Pharmacy and Pharmaceutical Technology, Faculty of Pharmacy, University of Granada, Campus of Cartuja, 18071 Granada, Spain; carola@ugr.es (C.A.); cviseras@ugr.es (C.V.)

* Correspondence: giuseppina.sandri@unipv.it

Abstract: Infections in nonhealing wounds remain one of the major challenges. Recently, nanomedicine approach seems a valid option to overcome the antibiotic resistance mechanisms. The aim of this study was the development of three types of polysaccharide-based scaffolds (chitosan-based (CH), chitosan/chondroitin sulfate-based (CH/CS), chitosan/hyaluronic acid-based (CH/HA)), as dermal substitutes, to be loaded with norfloxacin, intended for the treatment of infected wounds. The scaffolds have been loaded with norfloxacin as a free drug (N scaffolds) or in montmorillonite nanocomposite (H—hybrid-scaffolds). Chitosan/glycosaminoglycan (chondroitin sulfate or hyaluronic acid) scaffolds were prepared by means of electrospinning with a simple, one-step process. The scaffolds were characterized by 500 nm diameter fibers with homogeneous structures when norfloxacin was loaded as a free drug. On the contrary, the presence of nanocomposite caused a certain degree of surface roughness, with fibers having 1000 nm diameters. The presence of norfloxacin–montmorillonite nanocomposite (1%) caused higher deformability (90–120%) and lower elasticity (5–10 mN/cm^2), decreasing the mechanical resistance of the systems. All the scaffolds were proven to be degraded via lysozyme (this should ensure scaffold resorption) and this sustained the drug release (from 50% to 100% in 3 days, depending on system composition), especially when the drug was loaded in the scaffolds as a nanocomposite. Moreover, the scaffolds were able to decrease the bioburden at least 100-fold, proving that drug loading in the scaffolds did not impair the antimicrobial activity of norfloxacin. Chondroitin sulfate and montmorillonite in the scaffolds are proven to possess a synergic performance, enhancing the fibroblast proliferation without impairing norfloxacin's antimicrobial properties. The scaffold based on chondroitin sulfate, containing 1% norfloxacin in the nanocomposite, demonstrated adequate stiffness to sustain fibroblast proliferation and the capability to sustain antimicrobial properties to prevent/treat nonhealing wound infection during the healing process.

Keywords: electrospinning; chitosan; glycosaminoglycans; scaffolds; fibroblasts proliferation; antimicrobial properties

---

1. Introduction

The skin is the major protective barrier against the environment and the loss its integrity, as a result of injury or illness, may lead to morbidity or even death.

Wound healing is a complex event, based on overlapping but well-orchestrated cellular and molecular processes, to repair damaged tissue and restore skin function [1,2]. The process of healing proceeds through different phases (hemostasis, inflammatory, proliferative and remodeling) and involves extracellular matrix (ECM) molecules, soluble mediators, as cytokines and growth factors, various resident cells, and infiltrating leucocytes. In nonhealing wounds, the healing process stops at the inflammatory state, and chronic wounds, such as venous leg ulcers, arterial ulcers, diabetic ulcers, and pressure ulcers, i.e., bed sores, fail to proceed through an orderly and timely process to restore skin anatomical and functional integrity [1,2]. Moreover, all of these wounds are contaminated by proliferating bacteria from the surrounding skin, the local environment, and the endogenous patient sources, resulting in wound colonization [3,4]. This could enhance or impair wound healing, depending on the bacterial load. In the absence of an effective immune response, impeded by underlying morbidity, as venous and arterial insufficiency, diabetes, or ageing, bacterial colonization becomes critical and an unavoidable transition towards infection occurs [3,4]. In fact, the exposed subcutaneous tissue provides a favorable substrate for the microbial growth of a wide variety of microorganisms. Moreover, a longer healing time could dramatically increase the possible occurrence of infection and biofilm formation [4,5].

Infections in nonhealing wounds remain one of the major challenges. Although appropriate systemic antibiotics are considered essential for the treatment of clinically infected wounds, topical antibiotics are not recommended since they could promote bacterial resistance. Recently, a nanomedicine approach, creating antimicrobial nanotherapeutics, has appeared to be a valid option to eliminate bacterial infections, since nanomaterials can overcome antibiotic resistance mechanisms, owing to their unique and advantageous physico-chemical properties [6,7]. In fact, several studies report that nanosystems interact with microorganisms upon multiple mechanisms, including electrostatic attraction, hydrophobic and Van der Waals forces through surface interactions, and this makes them promising candidates to achieve enhanced therapeutic efficacy against multidrug resistant (MDR) infections [6,7]. Considering this evidence, in this work, a norfloxacin–montmorillonite nanocomposite (VHS-N), previously prepared by an intercalation solution procedure, was encapsulated in nanofibrous scaffolds, since it proved to increase drug potency against both *Pseudomonas aeruginosa* and *Staphylococcus aureus* (probably due to the high surface area to volume ratio, which increases the contact area with target organisms), maintaining cytocompatibility towards fibroblasts in vitro [8].

Given this premise, the aim of this study was the loading of montmorillonite norfloxacin nanocomposite (VHS-N) in three types of biopolymer–polysaccharide-based scaffolds (chitosan-based (CH), chitosan/chondroitin sulfate-based (CH/CS), chitosan/hyaluronic acid-based (CH/HA) (H hybrid scaffolds) to obtain dermal substitutes, intended for the treatment of wounds prone to infection, such as chronic ulcers (diabetic foot, venous leg ulcers) and burns.

The hybrid scaffolds were compared with scaffolds with the same compositions in polysaccharides, but loaded with norfloxacin as a free drug (N scaffolds).

The unloaded scaffolds were previously designed and developed [9,10]. Briefly, chitosan and chitosan/glycosaminoglycan electrospun scaffolds were manufactured using electrospinning by means of a simple/single-step process. Polymeric blends in water/acetic acid mixture were electrospun and the resulting random scaffolds were crosslinked by heating to obtain water resistant systems. The scaffolds proved their effectiveness in enhancing cell growth in vitro (fibroblasts and endothelial cells) and wound healing in vivo in a murine, burn/excisional model [9]. Moreover, lysozyme, normally secreted by macrophages and polymorphonuclear neutrophilis during the inflammatory phase of the healing process, proved to degrade the scaffolds in vitro [10].

Chitosan, glycosaminoglycans and pullulan were selected since they are polysaccharide biopolymers (organic molecules synthesized by the living organisms [11]), and biopolymers are recognized as the most promising materials in wound healing since they are characterized by having many advantages over synthetic materials because of their biocompatibility, biodegradability, lower antigenicity and renewability [11]. Therefore, although there are some examples in the literature focused on the enhancement of wound healing using antimicrobial loaded electrospun scaffolds/

dressings [12–15], those were in large part based on synthetic polymers, as polycaprolactone [12–14] or polyethylene glycol [15], and produced using critical solvents such as formic acid [12], or chloroform [15].

Furthermore, biomaterial-based complex nanostructures developed by electrospinning could lead to great advancements in the drug delivery and bioengineering/biomedical panorama [16]. In fact, electrospinning is a robust and on-demand process with high-throughput capable of making available broadly used drugs, such as antibiotics/chemotherapeutics, and enhancing their activities thanks to the nanostructure. Moreover, the electrospun materials are characterized by high mimicry and mechanical properties capable of modulating biological processes and determining cell fate, as the case of biochemical signals [17].

2. Materials and Methods

2.1. Materials

Chitosan (CH) (β-(1-4)-linked *D*-glucosamine and *N*-acetyl-D-glucosamine) with a low molecular weight of 251 kDa, deacetylation degree 98%, (ChitoClear, Giusto Faravelli, Milan, Italy); chondroitin sodium sulfate (CS) (β-1,4-linked d-glucuronic acid and β-1,3-linked N-acetyl galactosamine) bovine 100 EP, with a low molecular weight of 14 kDa, mixture of chondroitin A (chondroitin 4 sulfate) and chondroitin C (chondroitin 6 sulfate) (Bioiberica, Barcellona, Spain); hyaluronic acid (HA) (based on β -1,3-linked N-acetylglucosamine and β-(1,4)-D-glucuronic acid) with a low molecular weight of 212 kDa (Bioiberica, Barcellona, Spain); and pullulan (PUL) (based on maltotriose repeating units, linear α 1-4 and α 1-6 glucan, produced by *Aureobasidium pullulans*) with a low molecular weight of ~200–300 kDa (food grade, Hayashibara, Japan, Giusto Faravelli, Milan, Italy) were used for the scaffold preparations. Citric acid (CA) (monohydrated citric acid, European Pharmacopeia grade, Carlo Erba, Milan, Italy) was used as a crosslinking agent. Norfloxacin (N) (Sigma-Aldrich, Milan, Italy) was used as an antimicrobial drug.

2.2. Methods

2.2.1. Preparation of the Polymer Blends

All the polymeric blends were based on: PUL, CH and CA; PUL, CH and CA containing CS or HA. PUL solution was prepared in distilled water and CS or HA were added to PUL, thus preparing three different solutions: PUL; PUL/CS and PUL/HA. N, as a free drug, or loaded in a hybrid system (H) (nanocomposite based on VHS and N [8]), was mixed with PUL, PUL/CS or PUL/HA. Then, CH was hydrated in acetic acid and CA was added. Three different polymeric blends were prepared by mixing each PUL, PUL/CS, and PUL/HA with CH solution at 1:1 weight ratio and norfloxacin concentration was 0.15% or 0.30% *w/w*, respectively, corresponding to 1% or 2% *w/w* in dry systems, after electrospinning. The composition of the blends prepared is reported in Table 1.

Table 1. Quali-quantitative composition of polymeric blends.

% *w/w*	PUL	CH	CA	CS	HA	N	VHS	H_2O/CH_3COOH
CH-N1				–	–	0.15	–	
CH-N2				–	–	0.30	–	
CH-H1				–	–	0.15	0.94	
CH-H2				–	–	0.30	1.88	
CH/CS-N1				0.5	–	0.15	–	
CH/CS-N2				0.5	–	0.30	–	
CH/CS-H1	10	2.5	2.5	0.5	–	0.15	0.94	55/45
CH/CS-H2				0.5	–	0.30	1.88	
CH/HA-N1				–	0.5	0.15	–	
CH/HA-N2				–	0.5	0.30	–	
CH/HA-H1				–	0.5	0.15	0.94	
CH/HA-H2				–	0.5	0.30	1.88	

2.2.2. Electrospinning Process

The polymer blends were electrospun using an electrospinning apparatus (STKIT-40, Linari Engineering, Pisa, Italy), equipped with a high voltage generator (5–40 kV), a glass syringe of 10 mL with a stainless steel needle (0.8 mm), a volumetric pump (Razel R99-E) and a planar collector. The following parameters were used to obtain N loaded scaffolds: DV (voltage) = 22 kV, needle-to-collector distance = 24 cm, flow = 0.379 mL/h, to obtain H loaded scaffolds: DV (voltage) = 24 kV, needle-to-collector distance = 22 cm, flow = 0.379 mL/h, relative humidity: 40%, environmental temperature: 25 °C. All the scaffolds were then crosslinked by heating at 150 °C for 1 h in a tight container protected from light; the process was also reported as being able to dry sterilize the products [18]. Preliminarily, N stability in the heating process was assessed using a diode array detector (DAD) HPLC (see Section 2.2.5.1). For this purpose, the active ingredient was subjected to the heating treatment in the same conditions as the scaffolds (150 °C for 1 h) (in a tight container protected from light). Chromatograms and UV/visible spectra (200–700 nm) at the maximum of the corresponding chromatographic peaks were compared.

2.2.3. Chemico-Physical Characterization

Scaffold morphology was analyzed using scanning electron microscopy (SEM, Tescan, Mira3XMU, Brno, Czechia, CISRIC, University of Pavia, Pavia, Italy) after graphite sputtering in a vacuum. Nanofiber diameters were measured (Image J, ICY, Institute Pasteur, Paris, France). The presence of nanocomposite (VHS-Ns) loaded into the hybrid scaffolds was investigated by ultra-high-resolution transmission electron microscope (HR-TEM, FEI Titan G2 60–300, Thermo Fisher, Barcellona, Spain), coupled with analytical electron microscopy (AEM), with a SUPER-X silicon-drift windowless energy-dispersive X-ray spectroscopy detector. X-ray chemical element maps were collected. The samples were directly deposited onto copper grids (300 mesh coated by formvar/carbon film, Agar Scientific, Rome, Italy).

X-ray powder diffraction (XRPD) analysis was carried out using a diffractometer (X-Pert Pro model, Malven Panalytical, Monza, Italy) equipped with a solid-state detector (X-Celerator) and a spinning sample holder. The diffractogram patterns were recorded using random oriented mounts with CuKα radiation, operating at 45 kV and 40 mA, in the range 4°–60° 2θ. The diffraction data were analyzed using the XPOWDER® software (Version 2017).

Fourier transform infrared spectroscopy (FTIR) spectra of the samples were recorded using spectrophotometer (Spectrum BX FTIR, PerkinElmer, Milan, Italy). All analyses were performed from 400 to 4000 cm^{-1} with a resolution of 0.25 cm^{-1}. The results were processed with a software package (Spectrum, Perkin Elmer, I). In the Supplementary Materials, the spectra of the pristine components are reported (Figure S1).

2.2.4. Mechanical Properties

Mechanical properties were assessed using a texture analyzer (TA-XT plus, Stable Microsystems, Enco, Spinea, Italy) equipped with a 1 kg load cell and A/TG tensile grips [19]. Rectangular portions (3 × 1 cm) of each scaffold (thickness ~100 µm) were kept vertical by means of two grips, the lower one fixed and the upper one movable at a constant rate of 0.5 mm/s. Dry or hydrated scaffolds were stretched up to break and the force was recorded as a function of the movable grip displacement.

The force at break was recorded and elongation % was calculated as follows:

$$E\% = 100 \times (L_{\text{break}} - L_0)/L_{\text{break}}, \quad (1)$$

where L_{break} = the distance of the two grips at scaffold breaking and L_0 = the initial distance of the two grips.

Moreover, the Young's modulus (mN/cm^2) was calculated as the slope of the initial linear portion of force vs. grip displacement.

2.2.5. Norfloxacin Release Measurements

All the release measurements were performed in sink conditions to study drug liberation from the systems independent of the concentration of the drug released during the test [20]. Two different approaches were considered: in the first one, the drug release was studied using saline solution to simulate the lesion exudates, while in the second one, the effect of lysozyme on drug release was analyzed. Each scaffold was placed in 3 mL of dissolution medium to simulate the small number of exudates generally present in the wound, and the scaffold was completely dipped in the dissolution medium to simulate the implant of the system in the lesion bed. For this purpose, two different media were considered: saline solution (NaCl 0.9% w/v) or phosphate buffer 0.05 M (pH 6.2) containing 3.3 mg/mL of lysozyme (120.530 IU/mg, Sigma-Aldrich, Milan, Italy). As for saline solution, at prefixed times, 500 μL of dissolution medium was collected and replaced with fresh medium to keep the volume constant. The samples were analyzed by means of the DAD–HPLC method (Section 2.2.5.1) [21]. When lysozyme was present, the dissolution medium was totally collected and completely substituted with fresh medium every 24 h to avoid a loss of the enzyme activity over time. Each sample was divided in two aliquots. One aliquot was assayed to quantify the norfloxacin released from each scaffold (Section 2.2.5.1) and, for this purpose, each sample was pre-processed by diluting 1:1 with 1 N perchloric acid and by centrifugation (5000 rpm for 15 min), to precipitate the lysozyme in the solution. The second aliquot was assayed to quantify the glucosamine release, as product of lysozyme activity (Section 2.2.5.2). Moreover, the morphology of scaffolds subjected to lysozyme degradation (after 10 days) was analyzed using SEM as previously described.

2.2.5.1. Norfloxacin Assay

Norfloxacin released from each scaffold was determined by DAD–HPLC (Series 200 system, PerkinElmer, Milan, Italy). A Zorbax Eclipse XDB-C8 column (4.6 mm × 150 mm, silica particle size 5 μm, Agilent, Milan, Italy) was used as the stationary phase. The mobile phase was based on acetonitrile/methanol/citric acid 0.4 M, 7:15:78 (% *v/v*) at a flow rate of 1.0 mL/min, using 275 nm wavelength detection [21,22]. The injection volume was 10 μL. Calibration curves were obtained using norfloxacin standard solution in the mobile phase, in saline solution or processed as the samples subjected to lysozyme degradation. In every case, the method was linear from 0.08 to 200 μg/mL with an R^2 value that was always higher than 0.995.

2.2.5.2. Glucosamine Assay

Glucosamine released due to the lysozyme degradation of the scaffolds was quantified by means of ninhydrin assay [23].

All samples were diluted 1:1 ratio (*v/v*) with 400 μL of ninhydrin reagent (ninhydrin 2% *w/v*, hydrindantin 6.8 mg/L in 3:1 *v/v* dimethylsulfoxide: lithium acetate buffer 4 M, pH 5.2; Sigma-Aldrich, Milan, Italy) under a nitrogen blanket. Each sample was stirred at 100 °C for 8 min, and vortexed until cooling, then the samples were diluted 1:10 (*v/v*) with a 1:1 ethanol:water mixture and quantified by a colorimetric test at λ = 570 nm using an ELISA Plate Reader (iMARK Microplate Absorbance Reader, BioRad, Milan, Italy). The calibration curve (glucosamine in phosphate buffer 0.05 M at pH 6.2) was linear in the range from 0.0125 to 0.1 μg/mL with a $R^2 > 0.995$.

2.2.6. Biopharmaceutical Characterizations

Adhesion and proliferation assay was carried out using normal human dermal fibroblasts (NHDF) from juvenile foreskin (PromoCell, VWR, Milan, Italy) [9,10]. Fibroblasts were grown in the presence of 150 μL Dulbecco's modified Eagle medium (DMEM, Sigma-Aldrich, Milan, Italy) supplemented with 10% *v/v* fetal bovine serum (Euroclone, Milan, Italy), and with penicillin/streptomycin solution (pen/strep, 100 UI/100 μg/mL, Sigma-Aldrich, Merck, Milan, Italy), at 37 °C in a 5% CO_2 atmosphere with 95% relative humidity. The 0.36 cm^2 circular portion scaffolds were placed at the bottom of the wells in a 96-well plate (flat bottom, Cellstar©, Greiner bio-one, Frickenhausen, Germany). Fibroblasts were seeded onto the scaffolds at a seeding density of 35,000 cells/well and grown for 3 or 6 days. The cell growth without scaffolds (35,000 cells/well) was considered the standard growth (growth medium (GM)). After 3 or 6 days, the MTT [3-(4,5-dimethylthiazol-2-yl)-2,5-diphenyltetrazolium bromide] assays were performed. The fibroblasts that adhered and grew onto the scaffolds (growth for 6 days) were fixed for 2 h at 4 °C, using 3% *w/v* of glutaraldehyde in Dulbecco's phosphate buffered saline (PBS, Sigma-Aldrich, Milan, Italy) and analyzed by SEM and confocal laser scanning microscopy (CLSM), as described in the following paragraphs.

MTT Assay

The biocompatibility was performed by MTT test (tetrazolium salt, [3-(4,5-dimethylthiazol-2-yl)-2,5-diphenyltetrazolium bromide]; Sigma-Aldrich, Milan, Italy). Briefly, MTT was solubilized at 2.5 mg/mL in PBS (phosphate buffer solution, Sigma-Aldrich, Milan, Italy). At prefixed days, the medium in each well was removed and 50 µL of MTT solution plus 100 µL of PBS were added and subsequently put in contact with the cell substrates at 37 °C for 3 h in the incubator. Then, MTT solution was removed from each well and 100 µL of dimethylsulfoxide (DMSO, Sigma-Aldrich, Milan, Italy) was added. The absorbance was read using an ELISA Plate Reader at λ = 570 nm (with reference λ = 690 nm).

SEM Analysis

The substrates were then washed three times with PBS and dehydrated with ethanol solutions at increasing concentrations (50–75–100% *v/v*). The scaffolds were then removed from culture wells, applied onto stubs, sputtered with graphite and analyzed by SEM, as previously described.

CLSM Analysis

The substrates were then washed three times with PBS. Then cell actin cytoskeleton was stained with phalloidin FITC Atto 488 (50 µL at 20 µg/mL in PBS in each well, contact time 30 min) (Sigma-Aldrich, Milan, Italy). Subsequently, after three PBS washes, the cell nuclei were stained with Hoechst 33258 (100 µL of solution at 1:10,000 dilution in PBS per each well, contact time 10 min in the dark) (Sigma-Aldrich, Milan, Italy), for 10 min. After three further PBS washes, the scaffolds were mounted on glass slides, covered using coverslips and analyzed using CLSM (Leica TCS SP2, Leica Microsystems, Milan, Italy) at λ_{ex} = 346 nm and λ_{em} = 460 nm for Hoechst 33258 and λ_{ex} = 501 nm and λ_{em} = 523 nm for phalloidin FITC. The acquired images were processed by means of Leica software (Leica Microsystem, Milan, Italy).

2.2.7. In Vitro Antimicrobial Assay

The antimicrobial activity of norfloxacin-loaded scaffolds, either as free drug, N, or in nanocomposite, H, was evaluated against two bacteria strains—*Staphylococcus aureus* ATCC 6538 and *Pseudomonas aeruginosa* ATCC 15442. In particular, killing time was determined as the exposure time required to kill a standardized microbial inoculum [8,10,23]. Bacteria used for killing time evaluation were grown overnight in Tryptone Soya Broth (Oxoid, Basingstoke, Hampshire, UK) at 37 °C. The bacteria cultures were centrifuged at 2000 rpm for 20 min to separate the cells from the broth and then suspended in phosphate buffer saline (PBS, pH 7.3). The suspension was diluted to adjust the number of cells to 10^7–10^8 CFU/mL (CFU = colony forming unit).

For each microorganism strain, a suspension was prepared in PBS without scaffolds and used as the control. Unloaded scaffolds were also tested for comparison. Bacterial suspensions were incubated at 37 °C. Viable microbial counts were evaluated after contact for 0, 5, and 24 h with scaffolds and in control suspensions; bacterial colonies were enumerated in Tryptone Soya Agar (Oxoid, Basingstoke, Hampshire, UK) after incubation at 37 °C for 24 h. The microbiocidal effect (ME value) was calculated for each test organism and contact times were calculated according to the following equation [10,23]:

$$ME = \log Nc - \log Nd, \quad (2)$$

where Nc is the number of CFUs in the control microbial suspension and Nd is the number of CFUs in the microbial suspension in the presence of the scaffold.

2.2.8. Statistical Analysis

Statistical differences were evaluated by means of a one-way ANOVA post-hoc Fisher's Least Significant Difference (LSD) or Mann–Whitney (Wilcoxon) W test (Statgraphics Centurion XV, Statistical Graphics Corporation, Statgraphics Technologies, Inc., The Plains, Virginia, USA). Differences were considered significant at $p < 0.05$.

3. Results and Discussion

3.1. *Chemico-Physical Characterization*

Preliminarily, to scaffold preparation and cross-linking by heating, the drug stability in the heating process was assessed. For this purpose, the drug was subjected to a heating treatment in the same conditions used for the scaffold cross-linking (1 h at 150 °C). The heating treatment did not cause the drug degradation; in fact, after the process, the N content was 99.21% *w/w* (SD = 2.04) compared to the active ingredient in standard storage conditions. Figure 1 reports the UV spectra of N, and N subjected to the heating treatment at the maximum of the chromatographic peak (N retention time).

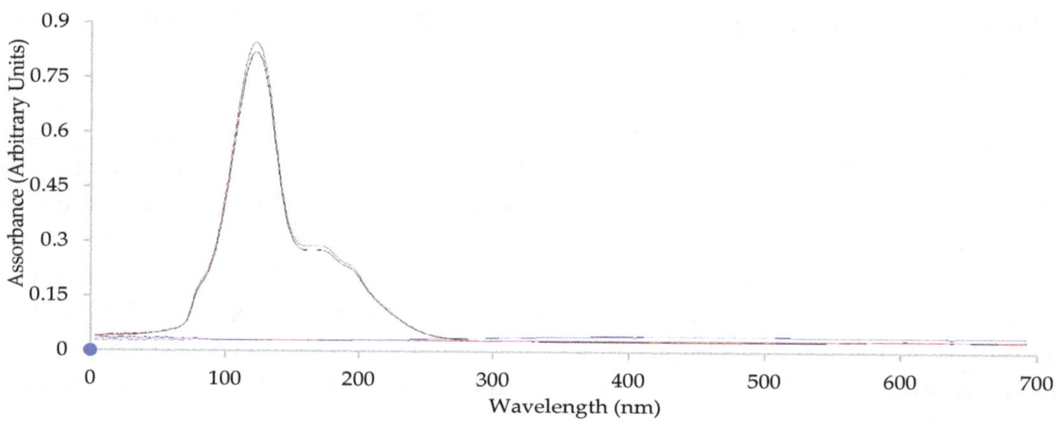

Figure 1. UV spectra of N (red line) and N subjected to heat treatment (1 h at 150 °C) (black line) obtained from the HPLC analysis at N peak maximum.

The complete overlapping of the spectra supported the stability of the drug in the heating treatment.

In a previous work [8], norfloxacin was loaded in montmorillonite, a phyllosilicate widely used in pharmaceutical field, to obtain a nanocomposite. This was prepared by means of the adsorption mechanism, as one single process, and the clay–drug adsorption isotherm was calculated. The solid-state analysis (XRPD, FTIR, thermal analysis—differential scanning calorimetry/ thermogravimetric analysis DSC/TGA, HRTEM) evidenced that protonated norfloxacin molecules interact with the active sites of montmorillonite located at its edges and within its interlayer space, thus forming a drug monolayer onto the clay mineral interlayer surface. Norfloxacin in the nanocomposite was proved in an amorphous state, and its loading (16% *w/w* of total nanocomposite weight) is homogeneous and causes an expansion of montmorillonite interlayer spaces. Moreover, the nanocomposite causes a prolonged norfloxacin release over time. Moreover, the nanocomposite was characterized by good biocompatibility in vitro toward fibroblasts, and it was able to increase the antimicrobial potency of the free drug against *P. aeruginosa* and *S. aureus*, Gram-negative and Gram-positive bacteria, respectively, both of which are often concurrent causes of wound chronicization, leading to the possible impairment of the healing path and, finally, to nonhealing wounds. Montmorillonite norfloxacin nanocomposite was loaded into scaffolds and their performance was compared to those loaded with the free drug scaffolds.

Figure 2 reports SEM microphotographs of CH, CH/CS or CH/HA scaffolds loaded with 1% or 2% norfloxacin, as a free drug (1% N or 2% N), or loaded with VHS-N nanocomposite (1% H or 2% H).

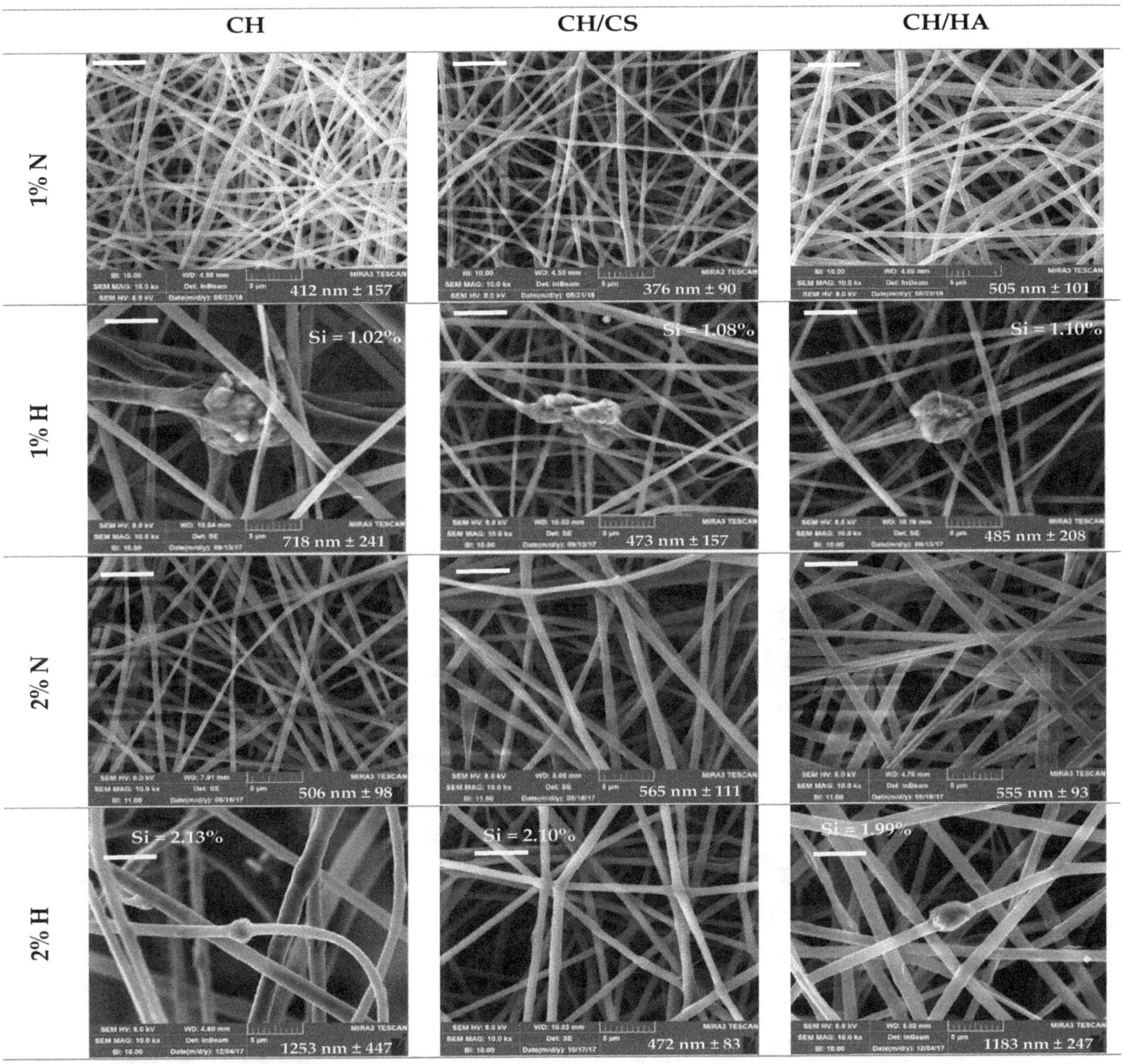

Figure 2. SEM microphotographs of chitosan-based (CH), chitosan/chondroitin sulfate-based (CH/CS) and chitosan/hyaluronic acid-based (CH/HA) scaffolds loaded with 1% or 2% norfloxacin, as a free drug (1% N or 2% N), or in VHS-N nanocomposite. In each image, the nanofiber diameters (nm, mean values ± SD; n = 30) and Si content for hybrid scaffolds are reported. Statistics: Mann–Whitney (Wilcoxon) W test $p < 0.05$: CH2H vs. CH/CS2H; CH/CS2H vs. CH/HA2H; CH/HA1H vs. CH/HA2H; CH/HA2H vs. CH/HA2N (scale bar 5 μm).

The N scaffolds, loaded with N as a free drug, were characterized by a regular structure with a smooth surface where no ribbon could be detected, independent of drug concentration. The H scaffolds, loaded with N in nanocomposite, presented nanofiber portions with a regular, smooth surface spaced out in broadened parts, with knots and a scattered structure. These conceivably could be related to the montmorillonite–norfloxacin (VHS-N) nanocomposite. Moreover, the presence of glycosaminoglycans (CS or HA) in the scaffolds caused a certain degree of surface roughness (probably due to chitosan and glycosaminoglycan interaction [9]) and this was more evident due to the increasing drug concentration in the fibers.

Nanofiber diameters were generally smaller when norfloxacin was loaded as a free drug (around 500 nm), independent of the drug concentration, although the differences were not statistically significant. On the contrary, H scaffolds were characterized by nanofibers with higher diameters (around 500 nm for 1% scaffold and around 1000 nm for 2% scaffolds) compared to those containing 1% of the drug, although this was significant only for the CH/HA scaffold; in this case, HA's high molecular weight was ten folds greater than that of CS and could cause the formation of fibers with greater diameters. On the contrary, H scaffold containing chondroitin sulfate and loaded with 2% of the drug showed similar nanofiber diameters to those loaded with the free drug. The content of Si, an element characteristic of montmorillonite, was consistent with the nanocomposite concentration in each scaffold [23].

The analysis of system viscosity previously performed on the blank systems [9], stated that chondroitin sulfate (negatively charged) conceivably interacted with chitosan (positively charged) and this could be due to the high charge density of sulfate groups greater than those of the carboxylic moieties of hyaluronic acid. However, the presence of particles in suspension, as was the case in nanocomposite, could cause unbalanced particle charge density that generally increases the conductivity, influencing fiber diameter during electrospinning [24]. Moreover, the acid environment of the polymer blends, due to the 45% *v/v* acetic acid in the medium, conceivably prevented the interactions between the various moieties and drug precipitation [25,26].

Figure 3 reports the HR-TEM microphotographs and EDX spectra obtained for CH (A–C), CH/CS (G–I) and CH/HA (D–F) H scaffolds, loaded with N in the nanocomposite at 2%.

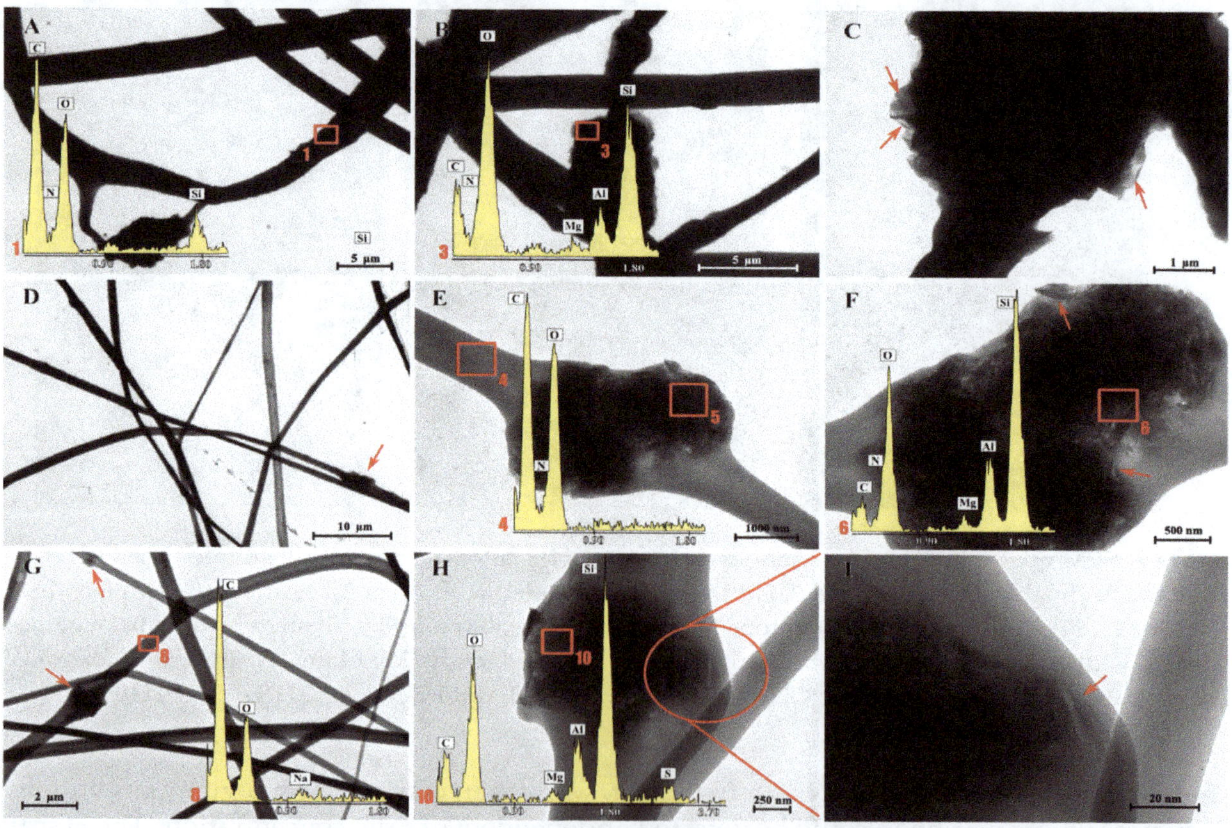

Figure 3. Transmission electron microscope (TEM) microphotographs and EDX spectra for CH, CH/CS and CH/HA scaffolds loaded with 2% norfloxacin in nanocomposite CH (**A–C**), CH/CS (**G–I**) and CH/HA (**D–F**).

The EDX analysis performed in the marked zone (red square) confirms that there was the presence of C, O and N (typical of organic elements) and characteristic elements of montmorillonite (Si, Al, Mg) in the broad, interwoven knots. This was observed for all the scaffolds, independent of their polymeric composition. At a higher magnification (Figure 3C,F,I), it was possible to identify the typical lamellar structure of montmorillonite (red arrows).

Figure 4 reports FTIR spectra evaluated for norfloxacin-loaded scaffolds (CH-N2, CH/CS-N2, CH/HA-N2) and VHS-N loaded scaffolds (CH-H2, CH/CS-H2, CH/HA-H2), both types containing 2% *w/w* norfloxacin.

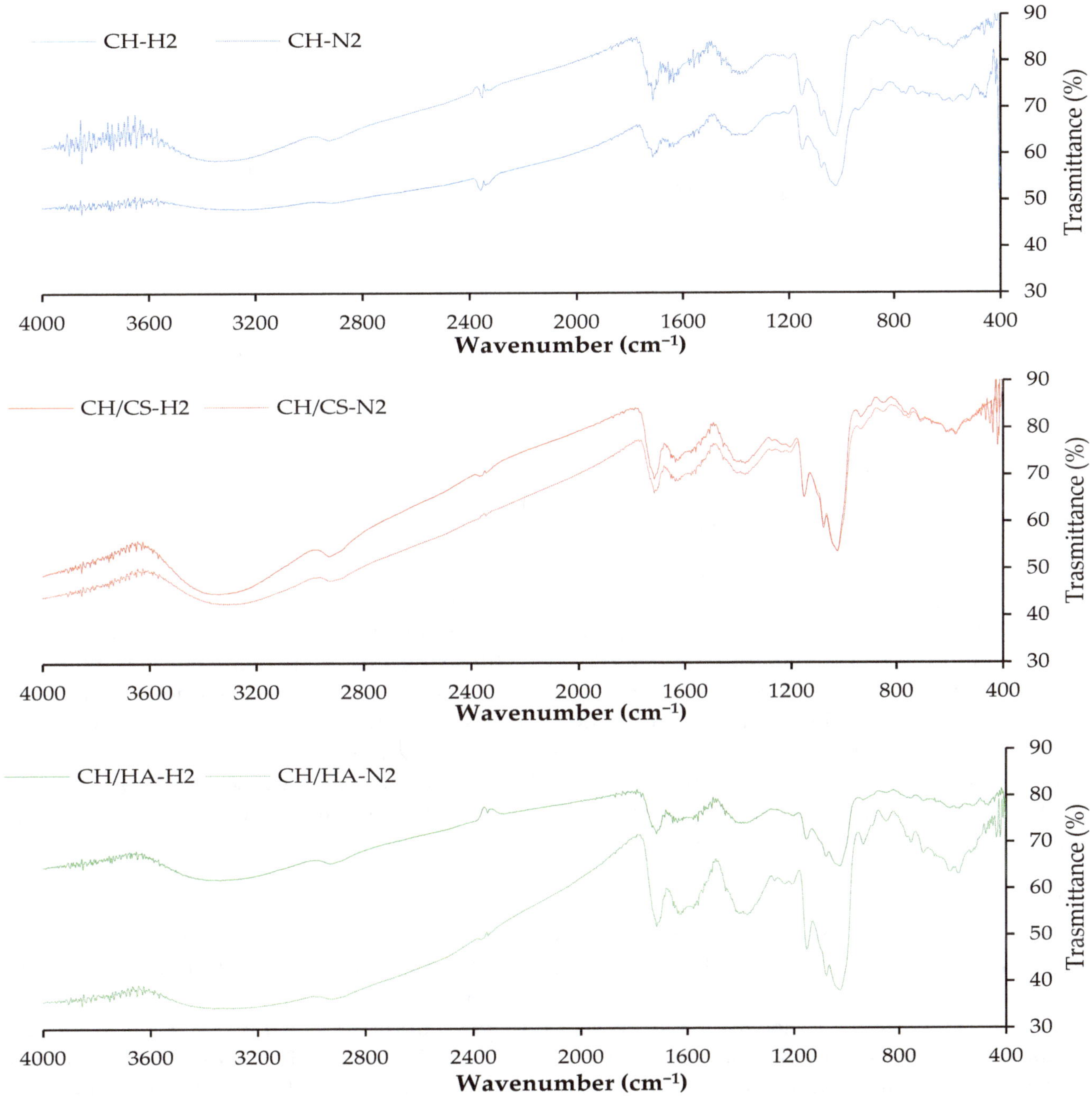

Figure 4. Fourier transform infrared spectroscopy (FTIR) spectra evaluated for norfloxacin-loaded scaffolds (CH-N2, CH/CS-N2, CH/HA-N2) and VHS-N loaded scaffolds (CH-H2, CH/CS-H2, CH/HA-H2), both types containing 2% *w/w* norfloxacin in norfloxacin–montmorillonite nanocomposite (VHS-N).

Independent of the polysaccharide composition and loading type, either with N (free drug, norfloxacin) or H (VHS-N nanocomposite), the typical polysaccharide signals (hydrogen bonds of –OH and $-NH_2$ groups) (pullulan: 3331 cm^{-1} and chitosan: 3355 cm^{-1}) hid the drug and nanocomposite-related peaks [27]. In fact, the VHS spectrum should present a band around 1017 cm^{-1} due to the vibrational band of the silicates.

Figure 5 reports the XRPD patters of the scaffolds loaded with VHS-N nanocomposite containing norfloxacin at 2% compared to VHS-N, the nanocomposite and the unloaded CH scaffold.

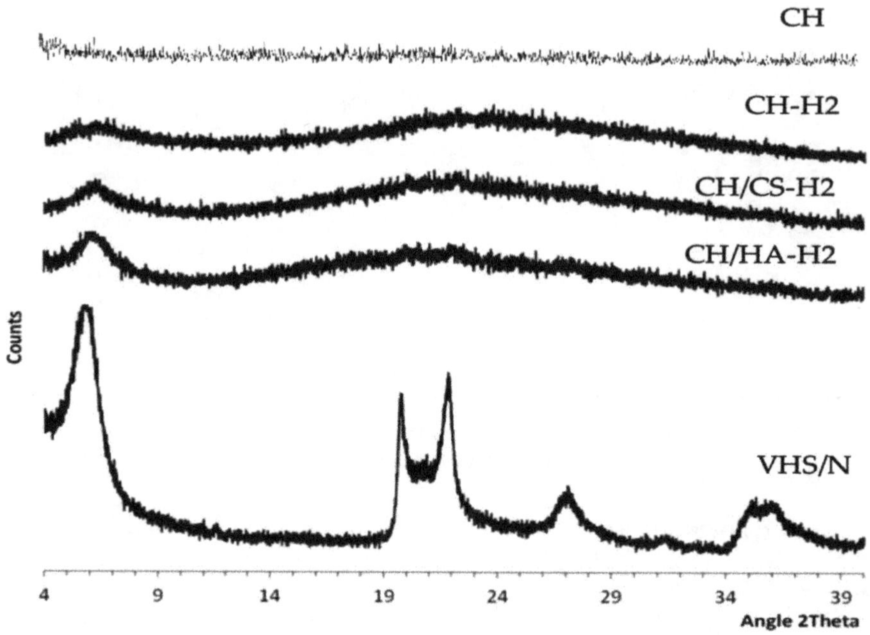

Figure 5. X-ray powder diffraction (XRPD) diffractograms of the scaffolds loaded with VHS-N at 2% norfloxacin (CH-H2, CH/CS-H2, CH/HA-H2) compared to unloaded CH scaffolds (CH) and VHS-N.

All the unloaded scaffolds were characterized by amorphous behavior (CH pattern is reported in Figure 5 as example) and no paracrystallinity could be detected. This was probably related to the electrospinning process. For all the scaffolds, the diffractograms were characterized by a hump between 20° and 29° 2θ, which was probably due to the presence of the polysaccharides. The reflection peak centered at 6° 2θ, which was probably due to the nanocomposite (VHS-NF) since it coincided with the d001 of montmorillonite once NF located in the interlayer space (5.94° 2θ). Similar XRD results were obtained by Rabbani et al. (2016) [28]. Moreover, there was an absence of other intense peaks that could be attributable to the nanocomposite (VHS-N), probably due to the nanocomposite concentration in the scaffolds, which was too low.

3.2. Mechanical Properties

Figure 6 reports the mechanical properties (force at break mN, a–b; elongation %, c–d; Young's modulus mN·cm^2, e–f) of scaffolds loaded with 1% or 2% of norfloxacin as a free drug (N) or as a nanocomposite (H), in dry (a, c, e) or wet (b, d, f) conditions.

In a dry state, the increase in N concentration in the scaffolds caused an increase in the force at break, except for the scaffold containing hyaluronic acid (Figure 3a). This was less evident when norfloxacin was loaded as a nanocomposite: it is conceivable that the effect of montmorillonite, which altered the entanglement of polymer chains in the scaffolds, causing lower resistance to break, prevailed over the effect attributable to the free drug, which seems to reinforce the structure. In this condition, the N scaffolds were less deformable than H scaffolds and the N concentration at 1% in H scaffolds was responsible for a higher deformability (Figure 3c). Moreover, the free drug seems to increase scaffold elasticity, especially for scaffolds containing chondroitin sulfate (Figure 3e). The hydration of the scaffolds, which simulates the application/implant in the lesion, dramatically changed the scaffold mechanical properties. N scaffolds, loaded with N as a free drug, were characterized by slightly higher resistance to break with respect to H scaffolds, confirming the behavior of the dry state (Figure 3b), while the scaffolds were simultaneously characterized by a higher degree of deformability (Figure 3d), which could be advantageous for wound bed application, and low elasticity (Figure 3f). The hydration caused a remarkable decrease in resistance to break, an increase in deformability and a loss of elasticity.

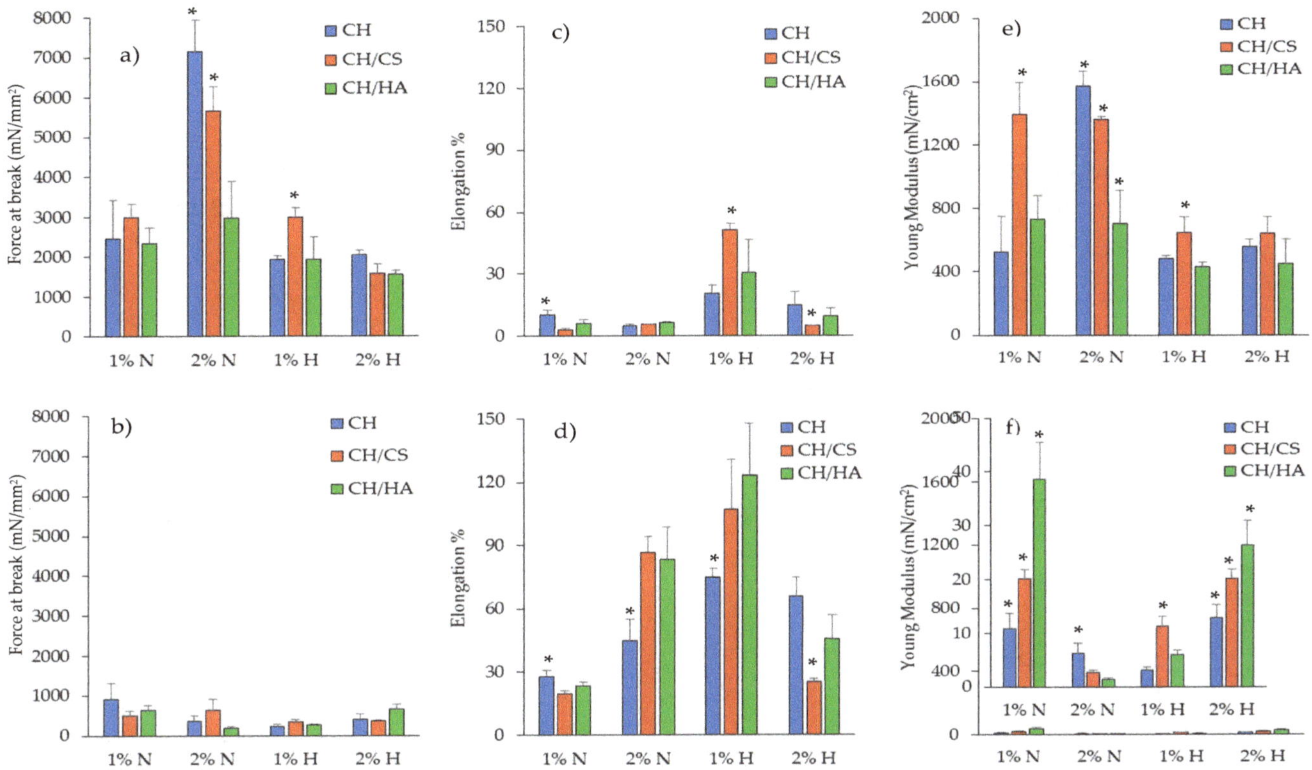

Figure 6. Mechanical properties (force at break mN, a-b; elongation %, c-d; Young's modulus mN.cm^2, e-f) for dry (**a**,**c**,**e**) and wet (**b**,**d**,**f**) scaffolds loaded with 1% (**a**) or 2% (**b**) of norfloxacin as a free drug (N) or as nanocomposite (H) (mean values ± SD; $n = 3$). Statistics: * = Mann–Whitney (Wilcoxon) W test $p < 0.05$.

The presence of montmorillonite in the hybrid scaffolds seems to weaken the scaffold structure, and this was probably due to the presence of particles embedded into the polymeric matrix that could disrupt the polymer chain entanglements, causing a significant decrease in the scaffold elasticity, and mechanical resistance, and a directly related increase in the deformability: this was more evident when 2% of drug in the nanocomposite was loaded in the scaffolds compared to scaffolds loaded with the free drug.

The mechanical properties are key features for the success of scaffold implants and their integration with the surrounding tissue. In fact, the native skin is characterized by tensile strength values approximately between 5.0 and 30.0 MPa (5000–30,000 mN/mm^2), the Young's modulus in the range of 4.6–20.0 MPa (46–200 mN/cm^2) and the elongation at break of about 35.0–115.0% [29]. Clearly, the ranges of the reference values are wide since the mechanical properties of the skin are strictly related to age and body lines (static lines, as described by Langer, Kraissl's lines or Borge's lines) [30]. In particular, force at break (mechanical strength) is related to the scaffold's capability to maintain its integrity during implantation, which should occur in the dry state, while the elongation and the Young's modulus are mainly related to the scaffold performance upon implantation. The scaffolds developed in the present work were characterized by force at break in the dry state close to the skin, especially for CH and CH/CS scaffolds, when loaded with norfloxacin at 2% as a free drug. Moreover, upon hydration, all the scaffolds were characterized by elongation superimposable to that of native skin. Furthermore, as for the Young's modulus, the scaffolds were characterized by the stiffness/elasticity closest to that of the skin, both in dry and hydrated states. Moreover, there is evidence in the literature that correlates the fibroblast adhesion and proliferation to substrate stiffness [31]; stiff matrices with a 2 MPa Young's modulus enhanced fibroblast proliferation much more than an elastic substrate (0,042 MPa). In fact, in the literature, there is evidence that the fibroblasts of granulation tissue are proliferative and motile, while those of the dermis are in a quiescent and stationary state [32]. Moreover, stiff substrates were demonstrated to sustain cell spreading and to facilitate guiding the pro-angiogenic signaling of fibroblasts [33].

3.3. *Norfloxacin Release Properties*

Figure 7 reports the release profiles of norfloxacin in saline solution. As for H scaffolds (N loaded as nanocomposite), independent of the drug loading, the profiles reached plateau values at 20% of the drug released after 3 h.

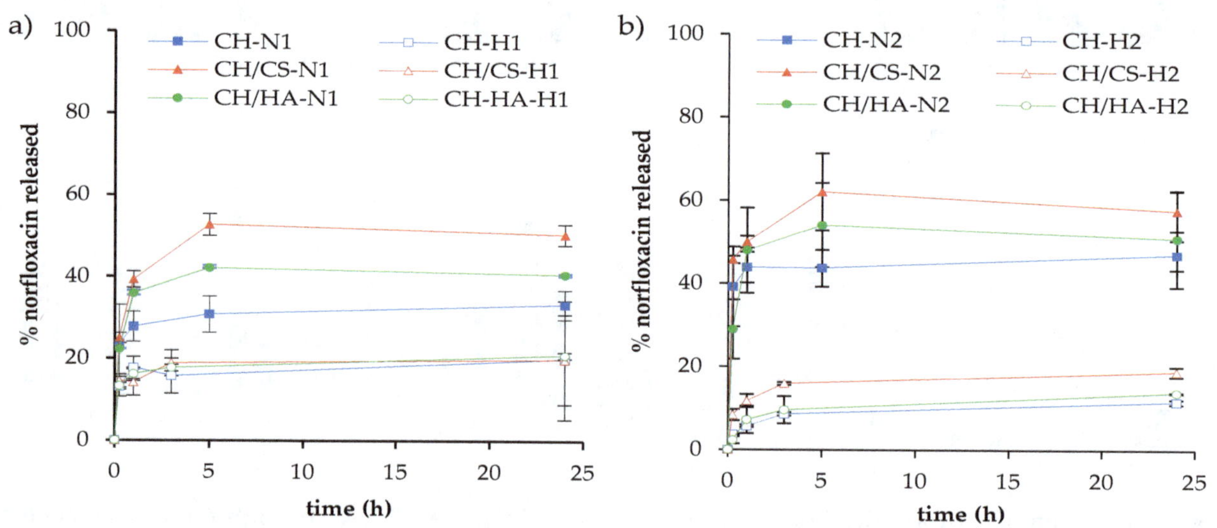

Figure 7. Release profiles (%) of norfloxacin from the N or H scaffolds loaded with 1% (**a**) or 2% (**b**) as a free drug (N) or as nanocomposite (H), in saline solution (mean values ± SD; $n = 3$).

As for N scaffolds (N loaded as a free drug), independent of the drug loading, the release profiles reached plateau values after 5 h; CH/CS scaffolds were characterized by their higher profile (50% and 57% for 1% and 2% N loading, respectively) followed by CH/HA scaffolds (about 40% and 50% for 1% and 2% N loading, respectively) and finally by CH scaffolds (33% and 50% for 1% and 2% N loading, respectively). When norfloxacin was loaded in the scaffolds as a nanocomposite (H scaffolds), the release was lower than when the scaffolds contained the free drug, and this seems to be independent of scaffold polymer composition. On the contrary, when norfloxacin was loaded as a free drug (N scaffolds), the presence of glycosaminoglycans markedly influenced norfloxacin release. This could be due to an interaction between anionic glycosaminoglycans and cationic chitosan forming a polyelectrolyte complex, which could make the fibrous structure less entangled and, therefore, more available to interact with the dissolution medium and to allow drug diffusion through the polymer matrix and, consequently, its release. In fact, scaffolds containing chondroitin sulfate, characterized by a charge density greater than hyaluronic acid, were characterized by a higher release profile. Chondroitin sulfate is characterized by the sulfate groups having an acid behavior greater than the carboxylic groups of hyaluronic acid. Consequently, the interaction between chondroitin sulfate and chitosan could cause a coiled structure less prone to polymer chain entanglements [34].

In any case, in the scaffolds loaded with higher concentrations of the drug, this difference was less evident with respect to those with lower drug loadings.

Figure 8 reports the norfloxacin release profiles (a and b) and glucosamine release profiles (c and d) of scaffolds subjected to lysozyme degradation.

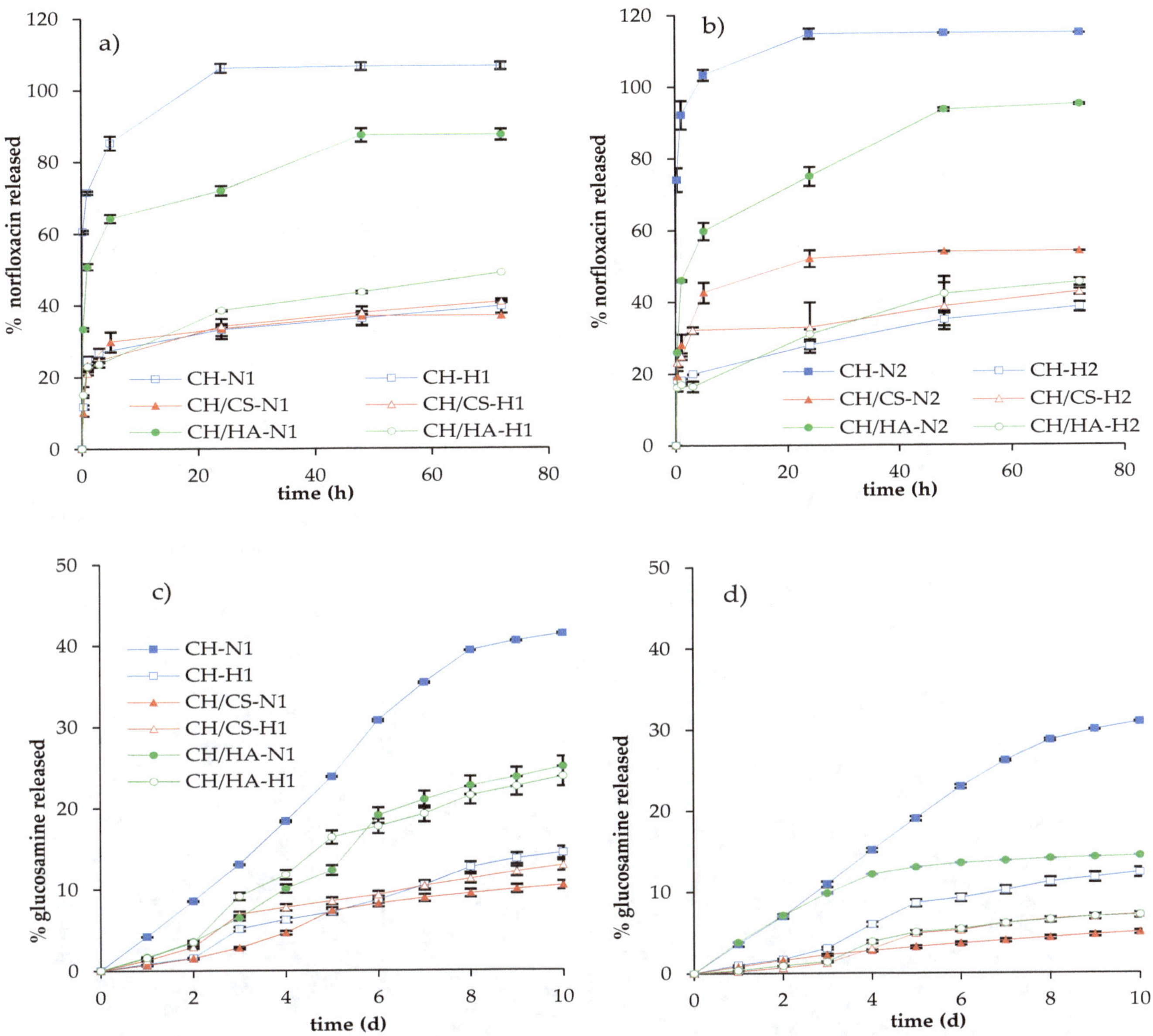

Figure 8. Norfloxacin released (%) in lysozyme from the scaffolds loaded with 1% (**a**) or 2% (**b**) of norfloxacin as a free drug (N) or as nanocomposite (H) and glucosamine released (%) from the scaffolds loaded with 1% (**c**) or 2% (**d**) of norfloxacin as a free drug (N) or as nanocomposite (H) subjected to lysozyme activity (mean values ± SD; n = 3)

Independent of norfloxacin concentration in the N scaffolds (free drug loading), the activity of lysozyme markedly increased the drug release: CH scaffolds containing chitosan, without glycosaminoglycans, showed higher release profiles, reaching, in almost 24 h, 100% of the drug being released; scaffolds based on CH/HA showed 80% of the drug being released in 48 h, while CH/CS scaffolds were characterized by a lower release close to 40–50% of the drug being released in 72 h, for 1% or 2% norfloxacin loading, and these profiles were similar to those obtained in saline solution. These behaviors could be explained considering that the activity of lysozyme on the scaffold matrices:

CH scaffolds completely lost their nanofibrous structure in contact with lysozyme (Figure 9). On the contrary, after 10 days of lysozyme activity, the CH/CS scaffold and, mainly, the CH/HA scaffold showed a residual of nanofibrous structure, submerged in a non-structured material. It is conceivable that the interaction of chitosan amino groups (positively charged) with either sulfate groups of chondroitin sulfate or the carboxylic ones of hyaluronic acid (both negatively charged) conferred a higher resistance against enzyme degradation, probably hindering interaction with the substrate. Moreover, chitosan/glycosaminoglycan interactions could partially prevent the loss of the system morphology, decreasing drug release.

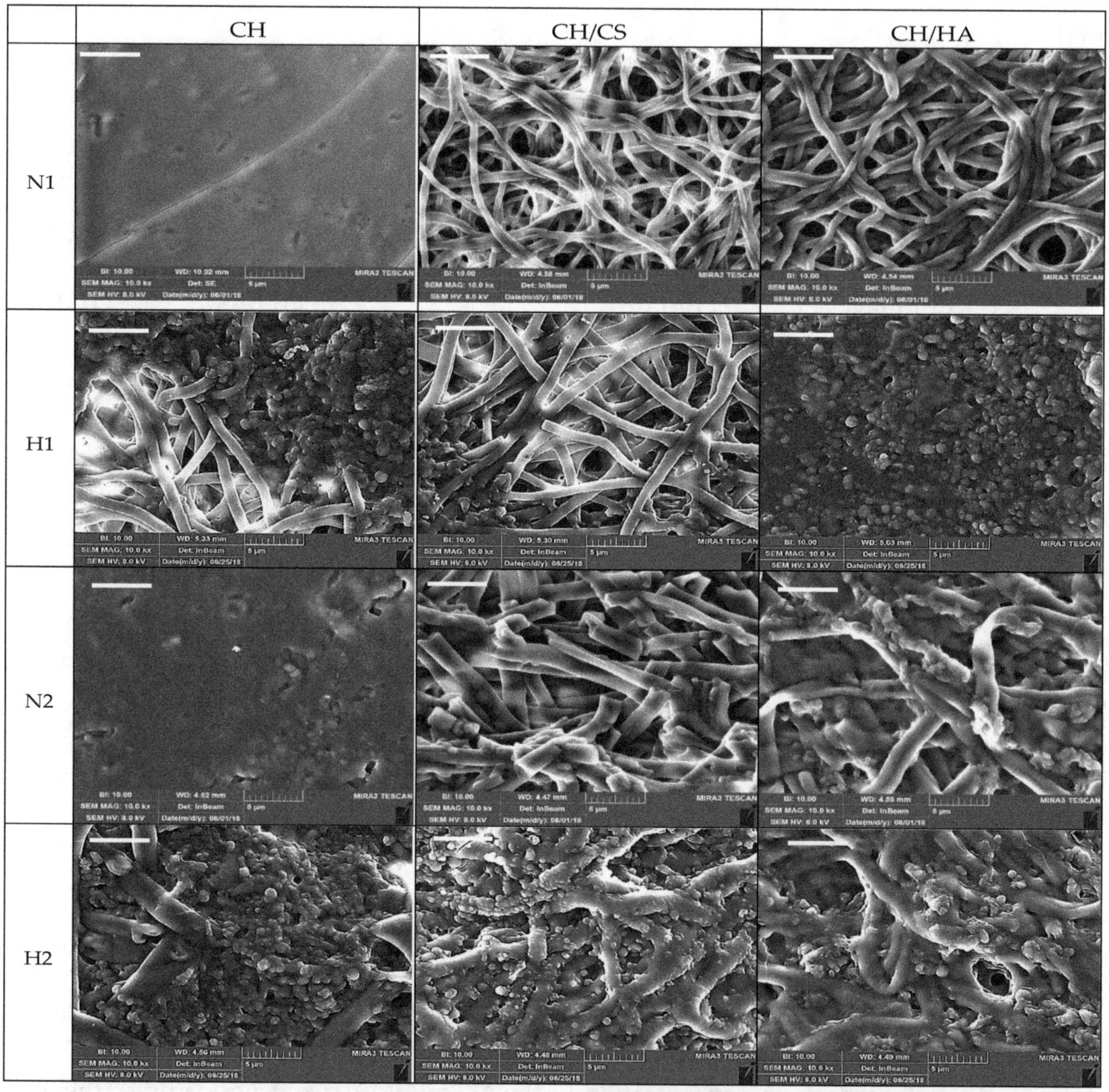

Figure 9. SEM microphotographs of the scaffolds loaded with 1% or 2% of norfloxacin as a free drug (N) or as nanocomposite (H) subjected to lysozyme activity for 10 days (scale bar: 5 μm).

In hybrid H scaffolds, loaded with norfloxacin in the montmorillonite nanocomposite, the profiles of norfloxacin released in the presence of the lysozyme were higher than those obtained in saline solution, although no difference could be evidenced, considering both the scaffold composition and the percentage of drug loaded, and all the scaffolds were characterized by release profiles reaching drug loading of 50% in 72 h.

However, in all cases, the glucosamine release profiles suggest that the enzymatic degradation of chitosan occurred, independent of system composition and percentage of drug loaded. CH scaffolds were characterized by their higher profiles, followed by H/HA scaffolds and CH/CS ones. Generally, the presence of norfloxacin–montmorillonite nanocomposite seems to decrease the lysozyme activity and the profiles of glucosamine (degradation product) were consistent with the norfloxacin release ones. Furthermore, the drug loading seems to have a negative impact on enzymatic activity and the glucosamine release profiles were higher in 1% loaded systems than in 2% ones. It is reported in the literature that lysozyme interacts with quinolones and this supports that there is a competition between norfloxacin and chitosan, as enzyme substrates, decreasing the enzymatic activity towards chitosan degradation when norfloxacin is at higher concentrations [35]. Moreover, the presence of montmorillonite in the scaffolds could impair lysozyme activity, probably due to a certain degree of interaction between montmorillonite and chitosan, which could prevent chitosan interaction with the enzyme. Furthermore, the interaction between chitosan and either chondroitin sulfate or hyaluronic acid could render chitosan, as lysozyme substrate, less prone to interaction with lysozyme, resulting in less efficient degradation activity towards chitosan [36].

Similar norfloxacin release profiles were observed by Dua et al. [37] for semisolid systems loaded with 1% norfloxacin. Dependent of the type of system, drug release ranged from 70% to 41% in 7 h. The highest drug release was observed for Carbopol-based gel (about 70%) followed by polyethylene glycol-based formulation (66%), HPMC-based gel (45%) and, finally, the slowest release was evidenced in the case of an ointment. Analogous behavior was observed by Denkbaş et al. [38] and Mahmoud and Salama [21] for chitosan and chitosan collagen sponge-like dressings loaded with norfloxacin. In those cases, the norfloxacin release was mainly related to system swelling that controlled the drug diffusion for an extended time of up to 4 days.

However comparing the features of the nanofibrous scaffolds presented in this work with those of the systems in the literature, the capability of the scaffolds based on chitosan or glycosaminoglycan (either chondroitin sulfate or hyaluronic acid) associated with chitosan (CH, CH/CS and CH/HA) to possess minimal swelling (as shown by SEM images after 6 days of hydration in aqueous environment) and controlled norfloxacin release, tuned up by both the hydration and the activity of lysozyme (secreted during the inflammatory phase of wound healing), confer the ideal properties of these systems. Indeed, as soon as the systems can be implanted, norfloxacin release should occur due to the hydration of exudate from the lesions; subsequently, the inflammatory phase, preceding the proliferative one, should lead to a further release of the drug to support the whole healing process.

Figure 9 reports SEM microphotographs of all the scaffolds subjected to 10 days of enzymatic degradation by lysozyme. These images are in agreement with the glucosamine release profiles (Figure 8c,d). In fact, the higher degree of scaffold degradation (loss of nanofibrous structure) was associated with a higher glucosamine release profile. Independent of drug concentrations in CH scaffolds containing chitosan, without glycosaminoglycans, and loaded with norfloxacin as a free drug, the nanofibrous structure was no longer visible, while CH scaffolds loaded with norfloxacin in nanocomposite were characterized by a nanofibrous structure, partially covered by spherical particles, reported in the literature as lysozyme molecules attached to the biopolymer matrix [36]. The presence of glycosaminoglycans in the scaffolds determined a higher resistance against enzymatic activity. In some cases, as for the CH/CS-N2 scaffold, nanofibers were partially broken, swollen, and partially fused. Long-lasting scaffold degradation could be advantageous, especially in deep/cavity wounds, since this should allow the gradual replacement of the scaffold matrix with native tissue, due to the production of the extracellular matrix by fibroblasts.

3.4. Cytocompatibility: Fibroblast Adhesion and Proliferation

Figure 10 reports the cytocompatibility (optical density (OD)) of the scaffolds towards fibroblasts after 3 or 6 days of growth. Fibroblast adhesion and proliferation onto the scaffolds were compared to those of the control (GM and cell growth in standard conditions).

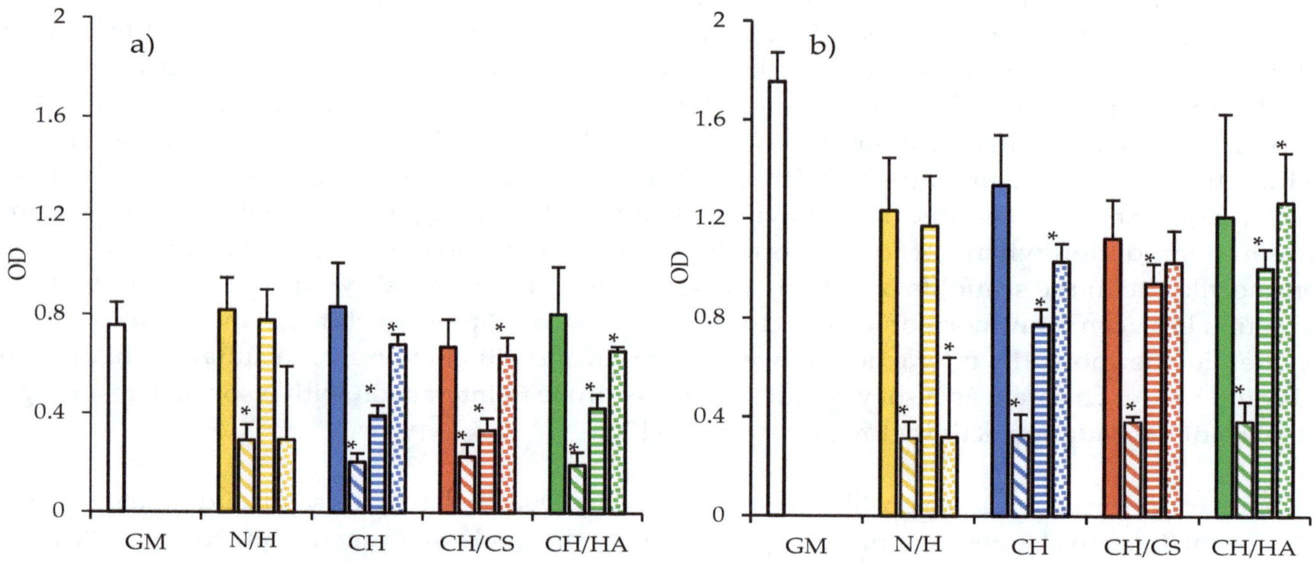

Figure 10. Cytocompatibility (optical density (OD)) of fibroblasts grown for 3 days (**a**) and 6 days (**b**) onto CH (blue), CH/CS (red), CH/HA (green) loaded with norfloxacin at 1% (plain color) and 2% (oblique lines), and with norfloxacin–montmorillonite nanocomposite (N-VHS) at 1% (horizontal lines) and 2% (dots) in norfloxacin. N norfloxacin as a free drug and H (N-VHS nanocomposite) at the same concentrations of the scaffolds are evaluated (mean values ± SD; n = 8). Statistics: * = Mann–Whitney (Wilcoxon) W test $p < 0.05$.

The cytocompatibility of the scaffolds loaded either with norfloxacin as a free drug or with the nanocomposite VHS-N at 1% or 2% were evaluated and N or H at the same concentrations as in the scaffolds were considered for comparison. After 6 days of growth, all the samples were characterized by higher OD than those after 3 days of growth, suggesting that the cells were in proliferation. Considering the scaffolds loaded with N as a free drug, the increase in drug concentration caused a significant decrease in cell viability with respect to the control. These results were similar to those obtained for N. This indicates that the decrease in cytocompatibility could be completely attributed to the drug and not to the scaffolds.

On the contrary, for the scaffolds loaded with the nanocomposite, the drug loading increased the cytocompatibility, suggesting that the nanocomposite in the scaffolds was able to prevent the negative effect of norfloxacin towards the fibroblasts (this was also evident considering the cytocompatibility of the nanocomposite, which was higher for the 1% solution than the 2% solution). Such an increase in cytocompatibility could be due to montmorillonite, which was able to control the drug release and could enhance fibroblast proliferation [39].

Figures 11 and 12 report CLSM and SEM microphotographs of fibroblasts grown for 6 days onto CH, CH/CS, CH/HA loaded with norfloxacin at 1% or 2%, either as a free drug or in the nanocomposite. The complementary information from the SEM and CLSM analyses suggests that in the scaffolds loaded with N as a free drug, the fibroblasts were not homogeneously distributed on the scaffolds and mainly formed aggregates as cell clusters. This behavior was dramatically influenced by drug concentration, in agreement with the cytocompatibility. However, both the scaffolds containing glycosaminoglycans allowed the fibroblasts to maintain their fusiform structure and cytoskeletons based on aligned and elongated filaments. However, norfloxacin concentration did not alter nuclei morphology. In the hybrid scaffolds, loaded with norfloxacin nanocomposite, fibroblasts were spread out all over the scaffolds and, in some areas, confluence could be reached and, although all the scaffolds were effective to allow cell adhesion and proliferation, the scaffolds containing chondroitin sulfate were characterized by their better performance.

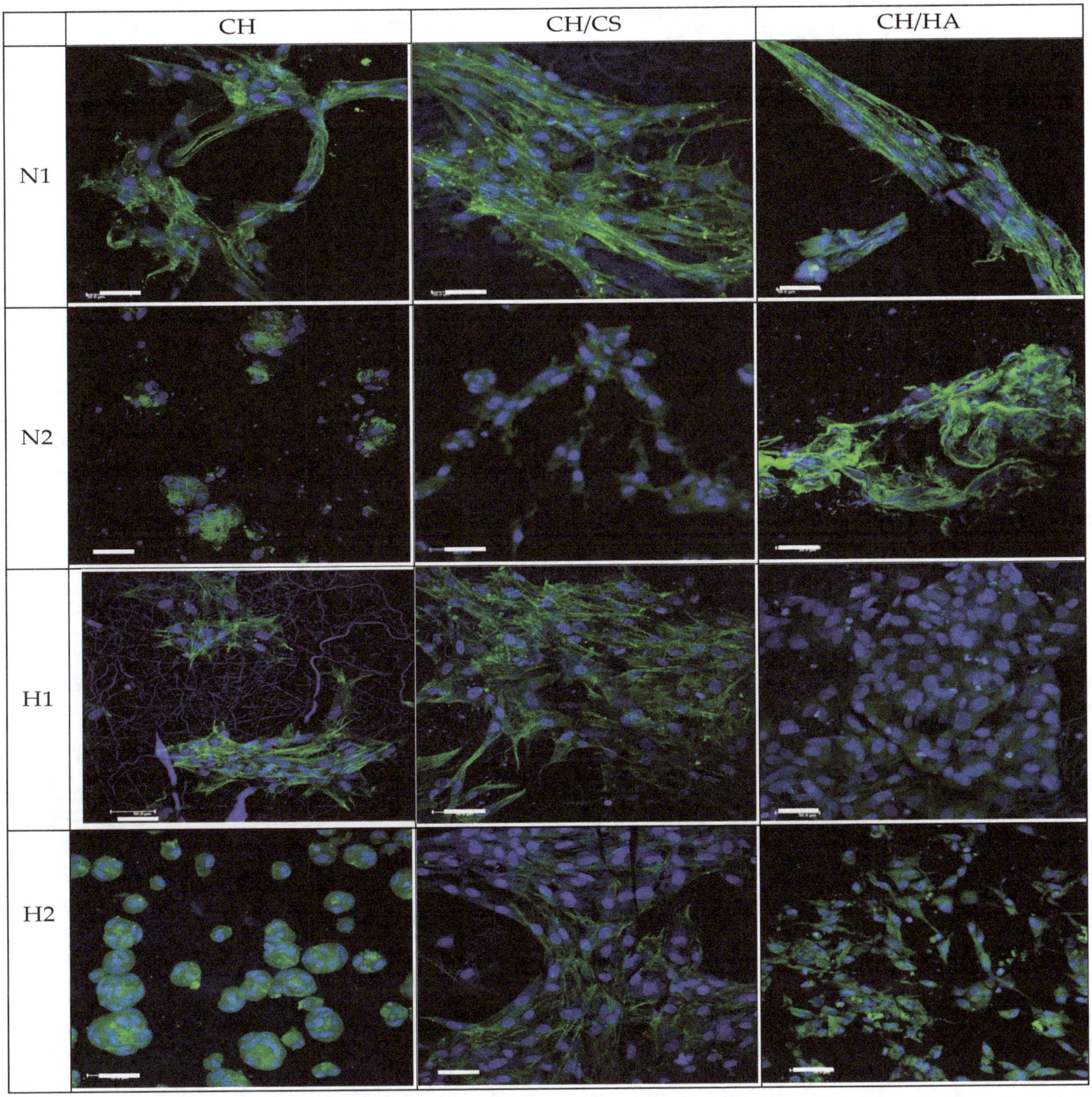

Figure 11. Confocal laser scanning microscopy (CLSM) microphotographs of fibroblasts grown for 6 days onto CH, CH/CS, CH/HA loaded with norfloxacin as a free drug (N) or norfloxacin–montmorillonite nanocomposite (H, N-VHS) at 1% or 2% (in blue: nuclei; in green: cytoskeleton) (scale bar: 50 μm).

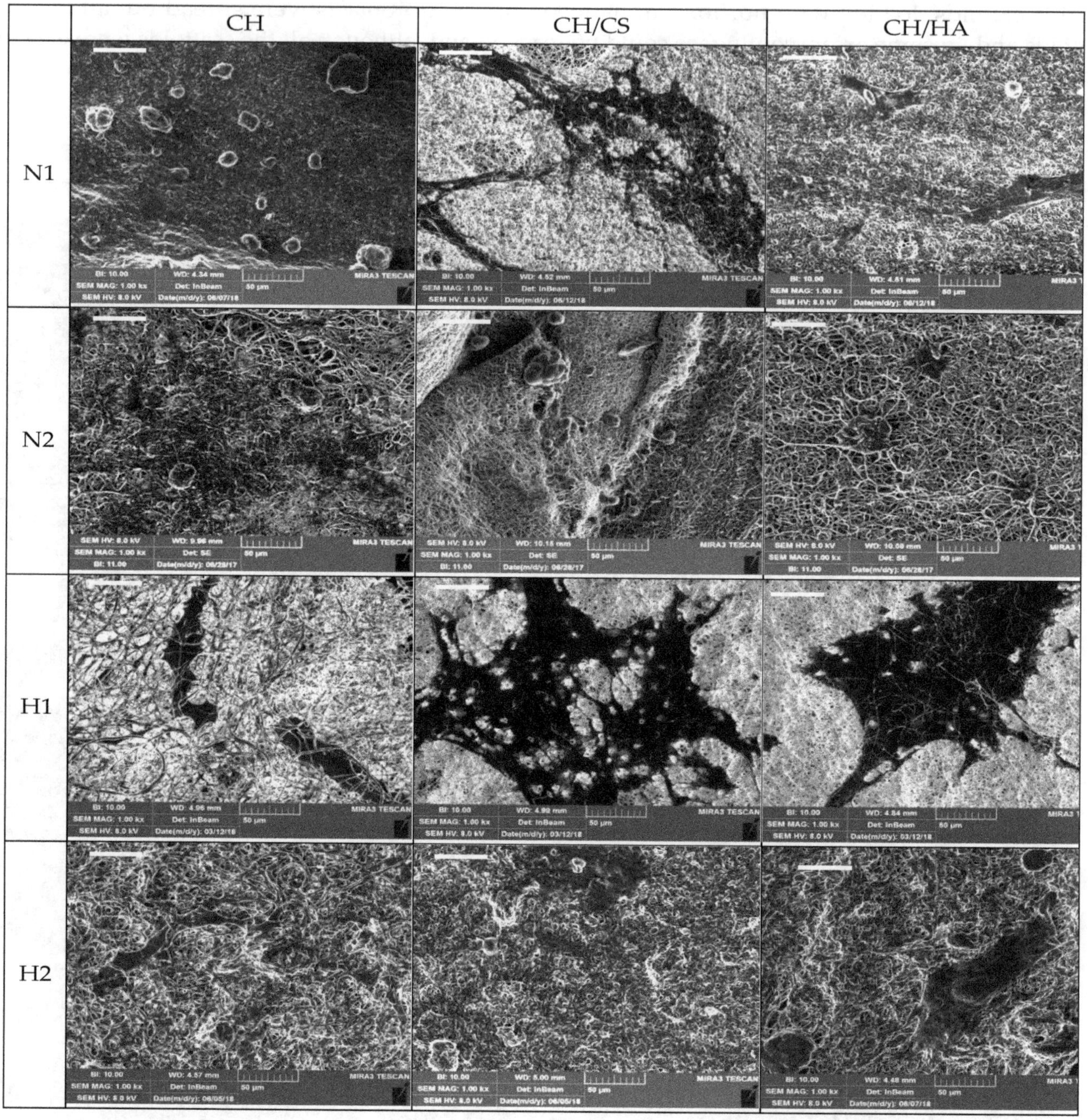

Figure 12. SEM microphotographs of fibroblasts grown for 6 days onto CH, CH/CS, CH/HA loaded with norfloxacin as a free drug (N) or norfloxacin–montmorillonite nanocomposite (H, N-VHS) at 1% or 2% (scale bar: 50 μm).

These results are in agreement with others in the literature stating the biocompatibility and the proliferation enhancement properties of montmorillonite and halloysite, both phyllosilicates with a planar and rolled structure, respectively [40–42]. Moreover, the polymer matrix of the scaffolds had a synergic effect with montmorillonite, leading to effectiveness in enhancing cell growth in the presence of norfloxacin [43].

Moreover, the mechanical properties combined with norfloxacin release could better support fibroblast adhesion, proliferation and spreading all over the scaffold when the norfloxacin is loaded in the scaffolds as a nanocomposite, at 1% concentration, and chondroitin sulfate or hyaluronic acid are present in the composition.

3.5. Antimicrobial Properties

Figure 13 reports the microbicidal effect vs. time profiles evaluated for CH, CH/CS and CH/HA scaffolds loaded with norfloxacin as a free drug (a, c) and (b, d) as nanocomposite at 1% against Pseudomonas aeruginosa and Staphylococcus aureus.

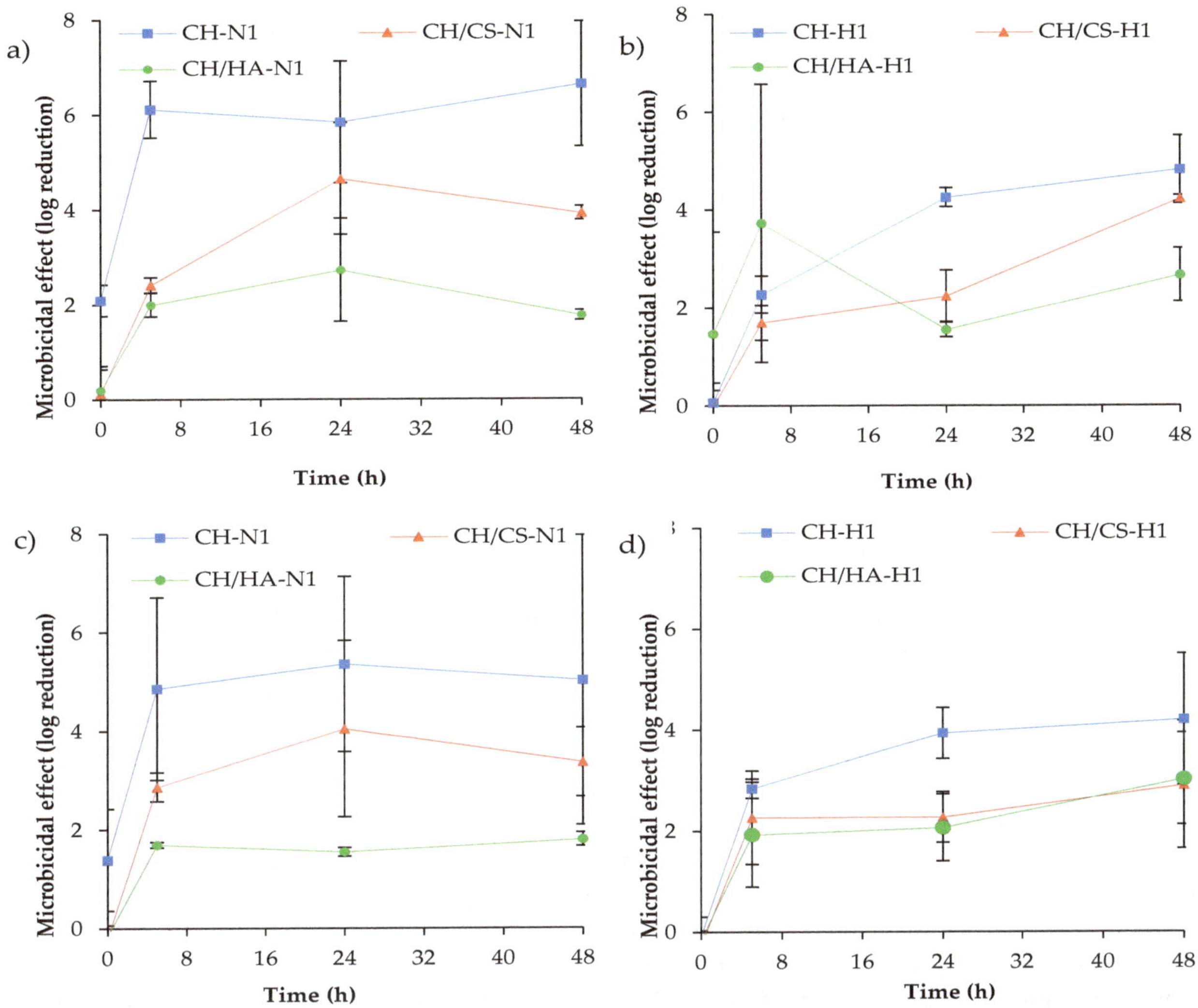

Figure 13. Microbicidal effect evaluated for 1% norfloxacin as a free drug (**a**,**c**) and (**b**,**d**) as nanocomposite loaded into CH, CH/CS and CH/HA scaffolds against Pseudomonas aeruginosa (**a** and **b**) and Staphylococcus aureus (**c** and **d**), in comparison to norfloxacin as a free drug and as nanocomposite, with the same concentration as in the scaffolds (mean values ± SD; n = 3).

Pseudomonas aeruginosa is a facultative Gram-negative anaerobe bacterium. It is recognized as a multidrug-resistant pathogen for its intrinsically advanced antibiotic resistance mechanisms since it causes infections of considerable medical importance, among them hospital-acquired infections such as sepsis syndromes. *Staphylococcus aureus* is facultative Gram-positive anaerobe bacterium. It is part of the skin microbiota; however, as an opportunistic pathogen, it could cause skin infections. Moreover, *S. aureus* could become resistant to antibiotics, and its methicillin-resistant strains are a worldwide emergency in clinical medicine. N is reported in the literature as being effective against both *P. aeruginosa* and *S. aureus*, having a MIC (minimal inhibitory concentration) of 2 μg/mL in both cases [44].

Norfloxacin loaded in the scaffolds was characterized by a microbicidal effect slightly higher against *P. aeruginosa* than against *S. aureus* and, moreover, scaffolds loaded with the free drug seem to have an antimicrobial activity higher than those loaded with norfloxacin in the nanocomposite. These could be due to the slower drug release of hybrid scaffolds compared to those loaded with norfloxacin as a free drug. However, the antimicrobial activity was sustained for 48 h.

Although a certain margin of error could be evidenced by the high variability of the results, a significant antimicrobial effect was achieved since all the scaffolds were able to decrease the bioburden by at least 100-fold (a two-log reduction). This suggests that upon implant, the scaffolds were effective for controlling and decreasing bacteria proliferation.

4. Conclusions

Scaffolds entirely based on polysaccharides (pullulan and chitosan plus chondroitin sulfate or hyaluronic acid) were manufactured by means of electrospinning and norfloxacin was loaded as a free drug or as nanocomposite of montmorillonite. The scaffolds were characterized by their homogeneous structures, with fibers of 500 nm diameter when norfloxacin was loaded as a free drug, independent of drug concentration. On the contrary, the presence of nanocomposite caused a certain degree of surface roughness of the fibers with 1000 nm diameters, dramatically influenced by drug concentration. Moreover, this altered entanglement of polymer chains in the scaffolds and caused higher deformability and lower elasticity, compared to the scaffolds loaded with norfloxacin as a free drug, and decreased the mechanical resistance of the systems. The hydration of the scaffolds changed their mechanical properties and the scaffolds were more prone to deformation. This is an advantageous feature, considering their implantation in lesions. Moreover, scaffold degradation occurring via lysozyme secreted during the inflammatory phase of the healing process should ensure scaffold resorption and, simultaneously, drug release. All the scaffolds proved to be degraded via lysozyme and this sustained the drug release (from 50% to 100% in 3 days, depending on system composition), especially when the drug was loaded in the scaffolds as a nanocomposite at 1%. Moreover, the scaffolds were able to decrease the bioburden by at least 100-fold, proving that drug loading in the scaffolds did not impair the antimicrobial activity of norfloxacin. Chondroitin sulfate and montmorillonite in the scaffolds proved to possess a synergic performance in enhancing the fibroblast proliferation without impairing norfloxacin antimicrobial properties. The scaffold based on chondroitin sulfate and containing 1% norfloxacin in nanocomposite was demonstrated to possess adequate stiffness to support fibroblast proliferation and the capability to sustain antimicrobial properties to prevent/treat nonhealing wound infection during the healing process.

5. Patents

Sandri, G., Bonferoni, M.C., Rossi, S., Ferrari, F., electrospun nanofibers and membranes, PCT/IT2017/000160, 2017.

Author Contributions: Conceptualization, G.S.; methodology, G.S.; software, F.F. and M.C.B.; validation, C.V.; investigation, P.G., A.F., M.R.; B.V.; D.M.; data curation, C.A., G.S.; writing—original draft preparation, G.S., M.R., A.F.; writing—review and editing, G.S.; supervision, G.S.; project administration, G.S.; funding acquisition, C.V., G.S., S.R., F.F., M.C.B. All authors have read and agreed to the published version of the manuscript.

Acknowledgments: The authors wish to thank Giusto Faravelli SpA for suppling the polymers.

References

1. Boateng, J.; Matthews, K.; Stevens, H.N.; Eccleston, G.M. Wound Healing Dressings and Drug Delivery Systems: A Review. *J. Pharm. Sci.* **2008**, *97*, 2892–2923. [CrossRef] [PubMed]
2. Velnar, T.; Bailey, T.; Smrkolj, V. The Wound Healing Process: An Overview of the Cellular and Molecular Mechanisms. *J. Int. Med Res.* **2009**, *37*, 1528–1542. [CrossRef] [PubMed]
3. Gupta, A.; Mumtaz, S.; Li, C.-H.; Hussain, I.; Rotello, V.M. Combatting antibiotic-resistant bacteria using nanomaterials. *Chem. Soc. Rev.* **2019**, *48*, 415–427. [CrossRef]
4. Siddiqui, A.R.; Bernstein, J.M. Chronic wound infection: Facts and controversies. *Clin. Dermatol.* **2010**, *28*, 519–526. [CrossRef]
5. Percival, S. Importance of biofilm formation in surgical infection. *BJS* **2017**, *104*, e85–e94. [CrossRef]
6. Van Giau, V.; An, S.S.A.; Hulme, J. Recent advances in the treatment of pathogenic infections using antibiotics and nano-drug delivery vehicles. *Drug Des. Dev. Ther.* **2019**, *13*, 327–343. [CrossRef]
7. Fulaz, S.; Vitale, S.; Quinn, L.; Casey, E. Nanoparticle-Biofilm Interactions: The Role of the EPS Matrix. *Trends Microbiol.* **2019**, *27*, 915–926. [CrossRef]
8. García-Villén, F.; Faccendini, A.; Aguzzi, C.; Cerezo, P.; Bonferoni, M.C.; Rossi, S.; Grisoli, P.; Ruggeri, M.; Ferrari, F.; Sandri, G.; et al. Montmorillonite-norfloxacin nanocomposite intended for healing of infected wounds. *Int. J. Nanomed.* **2019**, *14*, 5051–5060. [CrossRef]
9. Sandri, G.; Rossi, S.; Bonferoni, M.C.; Miele, D.; Faccendini, A.; Del Favero, E.; Di Cola, E.; Cornaglia, A.I.; Boselli, C.; Luxbacher, T.; et al. Chitosan/glycosaminoglycan scaffolds for skin reparation. *Carbohydr. Polym.* **2019**, *220*, 219–227. [CrossRef]
10. Sandri, G.; Miele, D.; Faccendini, A.; Bonferoni, M.C.; Rossi, S.; Grisoli, P.; Taglietti, A.; Ruggeri, M.; Bruni, G.; Vigani, B.; et al. Chitosan/Glycosaminoglycan Scaffolds: The Role of Silver Nanoparticles to Control Microbial Infections in Wound Healing. *Polymers* **2019**, *11*, 1207. [CrossRef]
11. Sahana, T.G.; Rekha, P.D. Biopolymers: Applications in wound healing and skin tissue engineering. *Mol. Boil. Rep.* **2018**, *45*, 2857–2867. [CrossRef] [PubMed]
12. Ajmal, G.; Bonde, G.V.; Thokala, S.; Mittal, P.; Khan, G.; Singh, J.; Pandey, V.K.; Mishra, B. Ciprofloxacin HCl and quercetin functionalized electrospun nanofiber membrane: Fabrication and its evaluation in full thickness wound healing. *Artif. Cells Nanomedicine Biotechnol.* **2019**, *47*, 228–240. [CrossRef] [PubMed]
13. Nejaddehbashi, F.; Hashemitabar, M.; Bayati, V.; Moghimipour, E.; Movaffagh, J.; Orazizadeh, M.; Abbaspour, M. Incorporation of Silver Sulfadiazine into An Electrospun Composite of Polycaprolactone as An Antibacterial Scaffold for Wound Healing in Rats. *Cell J.* **2019**, *21*, 379–390. [PubMed]
14. Grgurić, T.H.; Mijović, B.; Zdraveva, E.; Bajsić, E.G.; Slivac, I.; Ujčić, M.; Dekaris, I.; Trcin, M.T.; Vuković, A.; Kuzmić, S.; et al. Electrospinning of PCL/CEFUROXIM®fibrous scaffolds on 3D printed collectors. *J. Text. Inst.* **2020**, 1–12. [CrossRef]
15. Abdallah, O.; Jalali, F.; Zamani, S.; Isamil, H.I.; Ma, S.; Nasrallah, G.K.; Younes, H.M. Fabrication an Characterization of 3D electrospun biodegradable nanofibers for wound dressing, drug delivery and other tissue engineering applications. *Pharm. Nanotechnol.* **2016**, *4*, 191–201. [CrossRef]
16. Mehta, P.; Zaman, A.; Smith, A.; Rasekh, M.; Haj-Ahmad, R.; Arshad, M.S.; Der Merwe, S.; Chang, M.-W.; Ahmad, Z.; Van Der Merwe, S. Broad Scale and Structure Fabrication of Healthcare Materials for Drug and Emerging Therapies via Electrohydrodynamic Techniques. *Adv. Ther.* **2018**, *2*, 1800024. [CrossRef]
17. Chen, S.; Liu, B.; A Carlson, M.; Gombart, A.F.; A Reilly, D.; Xie, J. Recent advances in electrospun nanofibers for wound healing. *Nanomedicine* **2017**, *12*, 1335–1352. [CrossRef]
18. Kupiec, T.C.; Matthews, P.; Ahmad, R. Dry-heat sterilization of parenteral oil vehicles. *Int. J. Pharm. Compd.* **2013**, *4*, 223–224.
19. Cordenonsi, L.M.; Faccendini, A.; Rossi, S.; Bonferoni, M.C.; Malavasi, L.; Raffin, R.; Schapoval, E.E.S.; Del Fante, C.; Vigani, B.; Miele, D.; et al. Platelet lysate loaded electrospun scaffolds: Effect of nanofiber types on wound healing. *Eur. J. Pharm. Biopharm.* **2019**, *142*, 247–257. [CrossRef]
20. Pharmaceutical Quality/CMC. Transdermal and Topical Delivery Systems—Product Development and Quality Considerations, Guidance for Industry. In *U.S. Department of Health and Human Services*; Food and Drug Administration, Center for Drug Evaluation and Research (CDER), FDA: Rockville, MD, USA, November 2019.

21. Mahmoud, A.A.; Salama, A. Norfloxacin-loaded collagen/chitosan scaffolds for skin reconstruction: Preparation, evaluation and in-vivo wound healing assessment. *Eur. J. Pharm. Sci.* **2016**, *83*, 155–165. [CrossRef]
22. Samanidou, V.F.; Demetriou, C.E.; Papadoyannis, I.N. Direct determination of four fluoroquinolones, enoxacin, norfloxacin, ofloxacin, and ciprofloxacin, in pharmaceuticals and blood serum by HPLC. *Anal. Bioanal. Chem.* **2003**, *375*, 623–629. [CrossRef] [PubMed]
23. Sandri, G.; Bonferoni, M.C.; Ferrari, F.; Rossi, S.; Aguzzi, C.; Mori, M.; Grisoli, P.; Cerezo, P.; Tenci, M.; Viseras, C.; et al. Montmorillonite–chitosan–silver sulfadiazine nanocomposites for topical treatment of chronic skin lesions: In vitro biocompatibility, antibacterial efficacy and gap closure cell motility properties. *Carbohydr. Polym.* **2014**, *102*, 970–977. [CrossRef]
24. Huan, S.; Liu, G.; Han, G.; Cheng, W.; Fu, Z.; Wu, Q.; Wang, Q. Effect of Experimental Parameters on Morphological, Mechanical and Hydrophobic Properties of Electrospun Polystyrene Fibers. *Materials* **2015**, *8*, 2718–2734. [CrossRef]
25. Yu, X.; Zipp, G.L.; Iii, G.W.R.D. The Effect of Temperature and pH on the Solubility of Quinolone Compounds: Estimation of Heat of Fusion. *Pharm. Res.* **1994**, *11*, 522–527. [CrossRef] [PubMed]
26. Irwin, N.; McCoy, C.P.; Carson, L. Effect of pH on the in vitro susceptibility of planktonic and biofilm-grown Proteus mirabilis to the quinolone antimicrobials. *J. Appl. Microbiol.* **2013**, *115*, 382–389. [CrossRef] [PubMed]
27. Sandri, G.; Faccendini, A.; Longo, M.; Ruggeri, M.; Rossi, S.; Bonferoni, M.C.; Miele, D.; Prina-Mello, A.; Aguzzi, C.; Iborra, C.V.; et al. Halloysite- and Montmorillonite-Loaded Scaffolds as Enhancers of Chronic Wound Healing. *pharmaceutics* **2020**, *12*, 179. [CrossRef] [PubMed]
28. Rabbani, M.; Bathaee, H.; Rahimi, R.; Maleki, A. Photocatalytic degradation of p -nitrophenol and methylene blue using Zn-TCPP/Ag doped mesoporous TiO 2 under UV and visible light irradiation. *Desalin. Water Treat.* **2016**, *57*, 1–9. [CrossRef]
29. Tran, T.; Hamid, Z.; Cheong, K. A Review of Mechanical Properties of Scaffold in Tissue Engineering: Aloe Vera Composites. *J. Physics: Conf. Ser.* **2018**, *1082*, 012080. [CrossRef]
30. Pawlaczyk, M.; Lelonkiewicz, M.; Wieczorowski, M. Age-dependent biomechanical properties of the skin. *Adv. Dermatol. Allergol.* **2013**, *30*, 302–306. [CrossRef]
31. Hadjipanayi, E.; Mudera, V.; Brown, R.A. Close dependence of fibroblast proliferation on collagen scaffold matrix stiffness. *J. Tissue Eng. Regen. Med.* **2009**, *3*, 77–84. [CrossRef]
32. Clark, R.A. Biology of Dermal Wound Repair. *Dermatol. Clin.* **1993**, *11*, 647–666. [CrossRef]
33. El-Mohri, H.; Wu, Y.; Mohanty, S.; Ghosh, G. Impact of matrix stiffness on fibroblast function. *Mater. Sci. Eng. C* **2017**, *74*, 146–151. [CrossRef] [PubMed]
34. Saporito, F.; Sandri, G.; Rossi, S.; Bonferoni, M.C.; Riva, F.; Malavasi, L.; Caramella, C.; Ferrari, F. Freeze dried chitosan acetate dressings with glycosaminoglycans and traxenamic acid. *Carbohydr. Polym.* **2018**, *184*, 408–417. [CrossRef] [PubMed]
35. Perez, H.A.; Bustos, A.; Taranto, M.P.; Frias, M.; Ledesma, A.E. Effects of Lysozyme on the Activity of Ionic of Fluoroquinolone Species. *Molecules* **2018**, *23*, 741. [CrossRef] [PubMed]
36. Islam, N.; Wang, H.; Maqbool, F.; Ferro, V. In Vitro Enzymatic Digestibility of Glutaraldehyde-Crosslinked Chitosan Nanoparticles in Lysozyme Solution and Their Applicability in Pulmonary Drug Delivery. *Molecules* **2019**, *24*, 1271. [CrossRef]
37. Dua, K.; Malipeddi, V.R.; Madan, J.R.; Gupta, G.; Chakravarthi, S.; Awasthi, R.; Kikuchi, I.S.; Pinto, T.D.J.A. Norfloxacin and metronidazole topical formulations for effective treatment of bacterial infections and burn wounds. *Interv. Med. Appl. Sci.* **2016**, *8*, 68–76. [CrossRef]
38. Öztürk, E.; Agalar, C.; Öztürk, E. Norfloxacin-loaded Chitosan Sponges as Wound Dressing Material. *J. Biomater. Appl.* **2004**, *18*, 291–303.
39. Sandri, G.; Aguzzi, C.; Rossi, S.; Bonferoni, M.C.; Bruni, G.; Boselli, C.; Cornaglia, A.I.; Riva, F.; Viseras, C.; Caramella, C.; et al. Halloysite and chitosan oligosaccharide nanocomposite for wound healing. *Acta Biomater.* **2017**, *57*, 216–224. [CrossRef]
40. Sandri, G.; Bonferoni, M.C.; Rossi, S.; Ferrari, F.; Aguzzi, C.; Iborra, C.V.; Caramella, C. Clay minerals for tissue regeneration, repair, and engineering. In *Wound Healing Biomaterials*, 2nd ed.; Ågren, S.M., Ed.; Elsevier BV: Sawston, Cambridge, UK, 2016; Volume 2, pp. 385–402.

41. Sandri, G.; Bonferoni, M.C.; Rossi, S.; Ferrari, F.; Mori, M.; Cervio, M.; Riva, F.; Liakos, I.; Athanassiou, A.; Saporito, F.; et al. Platelet lysate embedded scaffolds for skin regeneration. *Expert Opin. Drug Deliv.* **2014**, *12*, 525–545. [CrossRef]
42. Aguzzi, C.; Sandri, G.; Bonferoni, M.C.; Cerezo, P.; Rossi, S.; Ferrari, F.; Caramella, C.; Iborra, C.V. Solid state characterisation of silver sulfadiazine loaded on montmorillonite/chitosan nanocomposite for wound healing. *Colloids Surf. B Biointerfaces* **2014**, *113*, 152–157. [CrossRef]
43. Rossi, S.; Marciello, M.; Sandri, G.; Ferrari, F.; Bonferoni, M.C.; Papetti, A.; Caramella, C.; Dacarro, C.; Grisoli, P. Wound Dressings Based on Chitosans and Hyaluronic Acid for the Release of Chlorhexidine Diacetate in Skin Ulcer Therapy. *Pharm. Dev. Technol.* **2007**, *12*, 415–422. [CrossRef] [PubMed]
44. Norrby, S.R.; Jonsson, M. Antibacterial activity of norfloxacin. *Antimicrob. Agents Chemother.* **1983**, *23*, 15–18. [CrossRef] [PubMed]

11

Correlation between Elemental Composition/Mobility and Skin Cell Proliferation of Fibrous Nanoclay/Spring Water Hydrogels

Fátima García-Villén [1], Rita Sánchez-Espejo [2], Ana Borrego-Sánchez [2], Pilar Cerezo [1], Lucia Cucca [3], Giuseppina Sandri [4] and César Viseras [1,2,*]

1 Department of Pharmacy and Pharmaceutical Technology, Faculty of Pharmacy, University of Granada, Campus of Cartuja, 18071 Granada, Spain; fgarvillen@ugr.es (F.G.-V.); mcerezo@ugr.es (P.C.)

2 Andalusian Institute of Earth Sciences, CSIC-UGR (Consejo Superior de Investigaciones Científicas-Universidad de Granada), Avenida de las Palmeras 4, Armilla, 18100 Granada, Spain; ritase@correo.ugr.es (R.S.-E.); anaborrego@iact.ugr-csic.es (A.B.-S.)

3 Department of Chemistry, University of Pavia, viale Taramelli 12, 27100 Pavia, Italy; lcucca@unipv.it

4 Department of Pharmaceutical Sciences, Faculty of Pharmacy, University of Pavia, viale Taramelli 12, 27100 Pavia, Italy; g.sandri@unipv.it

* Correspondence: cviseras@ugr.es

Abstract: Inorganic hydrogels formulated with spring waters and clay minerals are used to treat musculoskeletal disorders and skin affections. Their underlying mechanism of action for skin disorders is not clear, although it is usually ascribed to the chemical composition of the formulation. The aim of this study was to assess the composition and in vitro release of elements with potential wound healing effects from hydrogels prepared with two nanoclays and natural spring water. In vitro Franz cell studies were used and the element concentration was measured by inductively coupled plasma techniques. Biocompatibility studies were used to evaluate the potential toxicity of the formulation against fibroblasts. The studied hydrogels released elements with known therapeutic interest in wound healing. The released ratios of some elements, such as Mg:Ca or Zn:Ca, played a significant role in the final therapeutic activity of the formulation. In particular, the proliferative activity of fibroblasts was ascribed to the release of Mn and the Zn:Ca ratio. Moreover, the importance of formulative studies is highlighted, since it is the optimal combination of the correct ingredients that makes a formulation effective.

Keywords: sepiolite; palygorksite; spring water; hydrogel; wound healing; proliferation; Franz cell; bioactive elements

---

1. Introduction

Inorganic hydrogels formulated with spring waters and nanoclays are successfully used in the treatment of musculoskeletal disorders and skin affections. There is a general agreement that their therapeutic activity against musculoskeletal disorders is achieved through physical mechanisms such as thermic activity, osmotic pressure and electric conductivity [1–5]. On the other hand, the underlying mechanism of action responsible for the therapeutic skin effects are usually ascribed to the chemical composition of the formulation [1,6–10], although the exact therapeutic activities and mechanisms of action are still unknown.

Several dermatological affections have been successfully treated by formulations that include clay minerals [4,11–14]. Currently, special attention is being paid to wound healing treatments, in which clay minerals have been demonstrated to be very useful [15–18]. During administration of the formulation, elements from the hydrogel could permeate and/or penetrate across the skin barrier. In a previous study, hydrogels prepared with two different fibrous nanoclays were shown to be fully biocompatible and to exert in vitro wound healing activity [17]. More particularly, it was demonstrated that the fibrous nanoclay hydrogels promoted in vitro fibroblast mobility during wound healing processes.

It is well known that adequate concentrations of certain elements, including Ca, Mg, Na and K, in the wound bed are important for enhancing the healing process [19–27]. Transition metals such as Cu, Zn, Mn, Fe, Ag, and Au (among others) have also been demonstrated to play different biological functions in tissue regeneration, as reviewed by Yang et al. [28]. It has also been demonstrated that Zn:Ca ratios reach their maximum during the proliferative stage of wound healing and then decline during the remodeling stage [21]. Moreover, manganese-rich spring waters have been demonstrated to possess wound healing activity [29], and changes in Mg:Ca ratios are essential for a proper wound healing cascade. Consequently, formulations providing adequate bioavailability of elements with wound healing activity will promote the healing process and speed up restoration of the damaged area.

Based on these premises, the aim of this study was to assess the in vitro release and mobility of elements with potential wound healing effects from hydrogels formulated with spring waters and nanoclays that have recently been demonstrated to enhance fibroblast mobility [17]. In vitro Franz cell studies were performed in order to reproduce the topical administration of the formulations and elemental concentration was measured by inductively coupled plasma techniques. The results will be discussed on the basis of both the legal status of elements present in the formulation and their potential therapeutic effects.

2. Materials and Methods

2.1. Materials

Nanoclay/spring water hydrogels were prepared by mixing Alicún thermal station spring water (ALI, Granada, Spain) with two commercial fibrous nanoclays; sepiolite (PS9) and palygorskite (G30). Nanoclays were kindly gifted by the TOLSA group (Madrid, Spain).

Sepiolite hydrogel included in this study was prepared with a concentration of 10% (*w/w*) of PS9 dispersed in ALI spring water (ALIPS9, 250 g in total). Additionally, two palygorskite hydrogels (250 g each), ALIG30@10 and ALIG30@20, were also obtained and their final concentration was 10% *w/w* and 20% *w/w* of G30, respectively. The three formulations were prepared by means of a turbine high-speed agitator (Silverson LT, Chesham, UK) equipped with a high-traction stirrer head of square mesh and working at 8000 rpm for 5 min.

2.2. Methods

2.2.1. Elemental Characterization of Pristine Materials

The elemental composition of ALI, PS9 and G30 was obtained by two Inductively Coupled Plasma techniques: ICP-OES (Optima 8300 ICP–OES Spectrometer, Perkin Elmer, Waltham, MA, USA) and ICP-MS (NexION-300d ICP mass spectrometer, Perkin Elmer), equipped with a triple cone interface and a quadrupole ion deflector using argon for plasma formation. PS9 and G30 were subjected to acid digestion in strong acids (HNO_3 and HF at a 3:5 ratio, Sigma-Aldrich, MO, USA) inside a Teflon reactor, placed in a microwave oven (Millestone ETHOS ONE, Sorisole, Italy). Calibration curves for ICP-OES were obtained by means of standards solution of 1000 ppm for each element. For ICP-MS, single-element standard solutions (Merck, Darmstadt, Germany) were prepared after dilution with 10% HNO_3. Ultrapurified water (milliQ grade) was used in both techniques.

2.2.2. In Vitro Release of Elements

Element mobility from ALIPS9, ALIG30@10 and ALIG30@20 was studied by in vitro release studies performed in Franz diffusion cells system (FDC40020FF, BioScientific Inc., Phoenix, AZ, USA) [30]. This system is purposely designed to reproduce dermal and/or mucosal administration conditions.

The Franz diffusion cells possessed a contact area of 0.64 cm^2 and a total volume of 6.4 mL. Dialysis membranes (cut-off 12–14 kDa, 31.7 mm, Medicall International, London) were used to separate the donor and receptor chambers. The membranes were boiled in ultra-purified water (milli-Q water, ISO 3696) for 10 min in order to hydrate them. Over the membrane, in the donator chamber, known amounts of each hydrogel (approximately 0.025 g) were placed. The receptor chamber was filled with degassed, ultra-purified water. The whole system was maintained at a constant temperature of 32 ± 0.5 °C through thermostatic bath circulation. The experiment lasted for 30 min, which is the typical time of topical nanoclay/spring water hydrogels application. Experiments were performed in sextuplicate. At the end of the experiments, the aqueous content of the receptor chamber was carefully withdrawn and filtered through 0.45 μm single-use, syringe filters (Merck Millipore, Madrid, Spain). Finally, the elemental composition on each sample was assessed by ICP-OES. Element release tests were performed after 48 h and 1 month after hydrogel preparation, in order to study the evolution of the elemental mobility. Hydrogel batches were preserved in static conditions inside closed polyethylene containers, which were placed inside a drawer with an average mean temperature of 20 ± 5 °C. Blanks were also analyzed in order to monitor the elements coming from the materials and the ultra-purified water.

2.2.3. Biocompatibility of ALIG30@20

ALIPS9 and ALIG30@10 hydrogels (both with a solid concentration of 10%) have been demonstrated to be biocompatible against fibroblasts [17]. Moreover, in the very same study, the in vitro scratch assay proved that the hydrogels were able to accelerate wound closure by favoring fibroblast migration. Nonetheless, the ALIG30@10 hydrogel showed insufficient viscosity, as proven in another study that included a full rheological characterization of ALIPS9 and ALIG30@10 hydrogels [30]. The low consistency of a hydrogel could hinder its topical administration due to excessive fluidity of the formulation. Consequently, the ALIG30@20 hydrogel was prepared and its biocompatibility was evaluated. To do so, the methodology described by García-Villén et al. [17] was used. Normal human dermal fibroblasts (NHDFs, PromoCell GmbH, Heidelberg, Germany) were seeded and cultured in Dulbecco's modified Eagle medium (DMEM, Sigma Aldrich®-Merck, Milan, Italy), supplemented with 10% fetal bovine serum (FBS, Euroclone, Milan, Italy), 200 IU/mL penicillin and 0.2 mg/mL streptomycin (PBI International, I). Once cellular confluence was obtained (area 0.34 cm^2/well, density 10^5 cells/cm^2), ALIG30@20 was added to the cell culture in concentrations ranging from 1000 to 5 μg/mL and kept in contact with cells for 24 h. Then, the MTT test (3-(4,5-dimethylthiazol-2-yl)-2,5-diphenyltetrazolium bromide) was performed. DMEM phenol red-free and 50 μL of MTT dissolution were added in each well, the final MTT concentration being 2.5 mg/mL. MTT-NHDF contact was maintained for 3 h before the whole supernatant was withdrawn and substituted by 100 μL of dimethyl sulfoxide solution (DMSO, Sigma-Aldrich®-Merck, Milan, Italy) to dissolve formazan. The absorbance of each well was measured at 570 nm with an ELISA plate reader (Imark Absorbance Reader, Bio-rad, Hercules, CA, USA), with the reference wavelength set at 655 nm. Fibroblast viability was calculated with respect to the viability of the corresponding control (fibroblasts cultured in fresh DMEM, abbreviated as GM). MTT tests over ALIPS9, ALIG30@10 and ALIG30@20 were performed after 1 month of hydrogel preparation.

2.2.4. Selection of Elements Under Study

A wide variety of elements were analyzed in this study. In order to organize and facilitate the interpretation of the results, the discussion will be centered around two main aspects: the potential wound healing activity of the elements and their legal situation regarding cosmetics and medicines regulations. The importance of the latter point lies in the fact that, depending on the final therapeutic activity of the present hydrogels, they could be considered as cosmetics or as medicines [31]. Elements will be classified and addressed according to the European regulations and guidelines summarized in Figure 1. The present study is focused on those elements that are considered "safe" or "non-hazardous".

Additionally, elements without toxicity limits (most of the time not mentioned in the aforementioned regulations) were also included in this study.

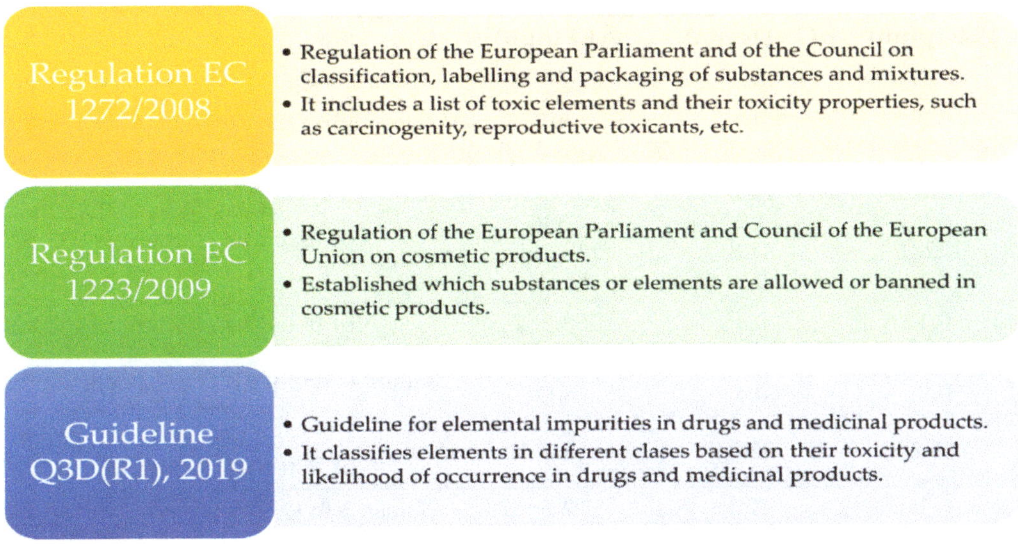

Figure 1. Main regulations [31–33] and guidelines used for the selection of elements, interpretation and discussions of results, ordered by year of publication or latest update.

The guideline for elemental impurities Q3D(R1) [32] of the European Medicines Agency is focused on toxic elements and classifies them in three groups. In view of their limitations and toxicity, all of them with well-defined "permitted daily exposure" (PDE) limits, these elements are not addressed in this manuscript. Nonetheless, there is also a non-defined fourth group that includes elements with low inherent toxicity, without PDE limits. In conclusion, elements in this group should be controlled more for the quality of the final product than for high toxicity and safety considerations. Examples of these elements are Al, B, Ca, Fe, K, Mg, Mn, Na, W and Zn, which are the subject of study of this research. For simplicity throughout the manuscript, these elements are referred to as "class 4". The European Regulation EC 1223/2009 [33] was used to determine those elements whose presence is either allowed or not mentioned in cosmetic products.

2.2.5. Statistical Analysis

Statistical analysis were determined by means of non-parametric Mann–Whitney (Wilcoxon) W test. In all cases, SPSS Statistic software (IBM, version 21, 2012, New York, NY, USA) was used and differences were considered significant at p-values ≤ 0.05.

3. Results and Discussion

3.1. Elemental Characterisation of Pristine Materials

Elemental composition of pristine components (PS9, G30 and ALI) is reported in Table 1. According to the EC 1272/2008, any of the detected elements are not considered as carcinogens.

Major elements in the pristine water (ALI) were Sr, S, Ca, Mg and Na (from higher to lower concentrations). The high presence of S, Ca and Mg are in agreement with the nature of the spring water source [34,35]. Ti, Mn, Mg, Sr, Zn and Al are the major elements present in PS9 and G30. In particular, Zn, Mn, Mg and Al belong to class 4 in the Q3D(R1) guideline [32]. Regarding the cosmetic regulation EC 1223/2009 [33], aluminum is the only one specifically allowed in cosmetics, the rest of them are not mentioned in this regulation. Cu and Ag are elements present in the pristine ingredients that have a "special situation" as far as regulation is concerned, since their presence is allowed in cosmetics (mainly due to their role as colorants) but they are classified as class 3 and 2B by the Q3D(R1).

Table 1. Elemental composition of pristine samples (PS9, G30 and ALI) determined by ICP-OES and ICP-MS. "ND" stands for "Not Detected". For a better understanding, comments about each element are included within the table. Levels of elements marked with * were obtained from [36].

Element	PS9 (ppm)	G30 (ppm)	ALI (ppb)	Comments
Al	15.9	31.9	37	Class 4 Q3D(R1); Allowed in EC 1223/2009
B	0.3	0.3	395	Class 4 in Q3D(R1); Not listed in EC 1223/2009
Ca	2.8	33.3	312,700	Class 4 in Q3D(R1); Not listed as element in EC 1223/2009
Fe	5.2	24.2	58	
K	6.0	1.9	6836	
Mg	122.0	41.8	114,267	
Na	0.1	0.1	49,150	
S	0.1	0.4	388,367	Not listed as element in EC 1223/2009
Mn	177.0	178.5	ND	Class 4 in Q3D(R1); Not listed in EC 1223/2009
W	0.9	0.4	ND	
Zn	81.2	96.1	3.3	Class 4 in Q3D(R1); Not listed as element in EC 1223/2009
Cu *	8.1	11.3	2.5	Class 3 in Q3D(R1); Allowed in EC 1223/2009
Ag *	0.04	0.2	0.1	Class 2B in Q3D(R1); Allowed in EC 1223/2009.
Au *	ND	ND	ND	
Sc	2.7	7.9	1.8	Not listed in EC 1223/2009
Ti	689.6	1820.5	0.2	Not listed as element in EC 1223/2009
Ga	8.2	16.1	0.8	Not listed in EC 1223/2009
Ge	3.2	0.8	0.1	
Tb	43.2	17.9	7.2	
Sr	24.4	106.0	10,049	Not listed as element in EC 1223/2009
Y	6.2	39.9	0.04	Not listed in EC 1223/2009
Nb	3.8	6.1	0.002	
In	ND	0.002	ND	
La	7.7	36.3	ND	
Ce	17.1	48.9	ND	
Pr	2.0	7.5	0.003	
Sm	1.7	5.5	0.001	
Eu	0.2	1.2	0.001	
Gd	1.5	5.6	0.003	
Dy	1.2	4.7	0.002	
Ho	0.2	1.0	0.002	
Er	0.6	2.9	0.002	
Tm	0.1	0.4	0.002	
Yb	0.5	2.4	ND	
Lu	0.1	0.4	0.002	
Hf	44.7	13.9	2.3	
Re	ND	ND	0.01	
Bi	0.1	ND	ND	Not listed as element in EC 1223/2009
Th	4.6	5.6	0.1	Not listed in EC 1223/2009

3.2. *In Vitro Release of Elements*

Elements released from ALIPS9, ALIG30@10 and ALIG30@20 hydrogels are summarized in Table 2. As expected from the nature and composition of the pristine ingredients of both hydrogels, the release of major elements (Ca, K, S, Mg, Na) was not only confirmed but desirable due to their physiologic activities, which will be discussed later. In particular, Ca showed significant release levels in all hydrogels, which is in agreement with the high levels of this element in pristine materials (Table 1).

Moreover, S is the major element present in ALI, which also explains the high release levels of this element from the formulations.

Table 2. Mobility of elements after Franz diffusion cell tests. Major elements are expressed in mg/100 g of hydrogel, while the rest of the elements are expressed as μg/100 g of hydrogel. Mean values ± s.e. ($n = 6$). "ND" stands for "Not Detected". Release levels of elements marked with * were obtained from [36].

Concentration Units	Element	ALIPS9		ALIG30@10		ALIG30@20	
		48 h	1 m	48 h	1 m	48h	1 m
mg/100 g	Ca	11.7 ± 2.91	8.1 ± 1.30	14.9 ± 1.758	30.4 ± 7.379	17.5 ± 3.51	7.0 ± 1.25
	K	1.8 ± 0.843	2.8 ± 0.628	2.7 ± 1.183	1.9 ± 0.491	3.4 ± 1.004	2.6 ± 1.09
	Mg	2.7 ± 0.48	3.7 ± 0.52	2.5 ± 0.237	5.2 ± 1.433	4.9 ± 0.23	3.0 ± 0.48
	Na	5.4 ± 1.40	6.3 ± 1.65	8.8 ± 2.727	10.5 ± 3.185	12.4 ± 1.136	6.43 ± 0.469
	S	14.8 ± 3.80	5.5 ± 2.81	23.3 ± 2.063	11.7 ± 2.162	10.4 ± 2.34	6.7 ± 2.29
	B	0.2 ± 0.016	0.04 ± 0.020	0.1 ± 0.021	ND	0.3 ± 0.062	ND
	Fe	0.06 ± 0.036	0.07 ± 0.028	ND	0.02 ± 0.018	0.1 ± 0.054	0.01 ± 0.009
	Al	ND	0.1 ± 0.056	ND	0.58 ± 0.452	ND	0.67 ± 0.100
μg/100 g	Mn	ND	0.7 ± 0.39	ND	ND	4.9 ± 2.64	7.4 ± 3.69
	W	ND	ND	ND	ND	ND	ND
	Zn	25.9 ± 16.07	165.9 ± 68.51	132.1 ± 38.17	181.4 ± 99.18	164.8 ± 53.09	175.1 ± 80.91
	Cu*	10.8 ± 3.29	3.6 ± 2.17	32.6 ± 11.59	1.5 ± 1.01	20.6 ± 3.725	0.9 ± 0.61
	Ag *, Au *, Sc, Ti, Ge, Tb	ND	ND	ND	ND	ND	ND
	Ga	ND	0.08 ± 0.050	ND	ND	0.2 ± 0.019	0.04 ± 0.001
	Sr	176.5 ± 15.89	148.7 ± 20.37	90.4 ± 18.67	65.9 ± 10.39	82.8 ± 15.64	68.5 ± 7.93
	Y, Nb, In, La, Ce, Pr, Sm, Eu, Gd, Dy, Ho, Er, Tm, Yb, Lu, Hf, Re, Bi, Th	ND	ND	ND	ND	ND	ND

Release levels of Mg were very similar for the three hydrogels. The release of Al increased with time in all cases, not being detected in any of the young hydrogels. On the other hand, the amount of B released after 1 month was lower. The most remarkable release regarding trace elements was shown by Zn and Sr, followed by Cu. Cu release significantly decreased after 1 month in the three hydrogels. As previously reported, the amount of Cu detected in G30 was higher than PS9 (Table 2). This was in agreement with the lower release of both elements in ALIPS9 versus ALIG30@10 and ALIG30@20. Mn release increased with time in ALIPS9 and ALIPS9@20, while it was under the detection limit of the technique for ALIG30@10 experiments. Levels of Mn were the same for both PS9 and G30 (and absent in ALI, Table 1) but ALIG30@20 showed a remarkably higher release of this element.

The rest of the elements were not released or released in very low amounts. Except for Au, Cu and Ag, the rest of the trace elements are not included/mentioned in the EC 1223/2009 regulation [33]. This means that their safety has not been thoroughly assessed or their toxicity is considered non-significant. It is worth mentioning that In and Re were not present in the pristine materials and that they were also not detected during the in vitro release tests. This fact confirmed the absence of contamination with these elements during ALIPS9, ALIG30@10 and ALIG30@20 formulation processes and preservation.

3.3. Biocompatibility of ALIG30@20

Biocompatibility results of ALIPS9@20 are reported in Figure 2. As previously mentioned, G30 and ALIG30@10 results have already been assessed by García-Villén et al. [17]. The reduction in viability produced by the pristine G30 alone at 1 mg/mL was not found in any of the hydrogels. In fact, the viability results of ALIG30@20 demonstrated, once again, that the type of formulation exerts a significant role in the results. That is, despite all tests subjected to the same amount of clay mineral in the culture, the hydrogels increased the biocompatibility. In particular, ALIG30@20 showed cellular viabilities higher than 100% at every concentration ($p > 0.05$ with respect to GM, Figure 2). In view of the experimental results and the statistical analysis, it is possible to state that ALIG30@20 exerts proliferative effects over fibroblasts at the tested concentrations. No other internal statistical differences were found between ALIG30@20 concentrations.

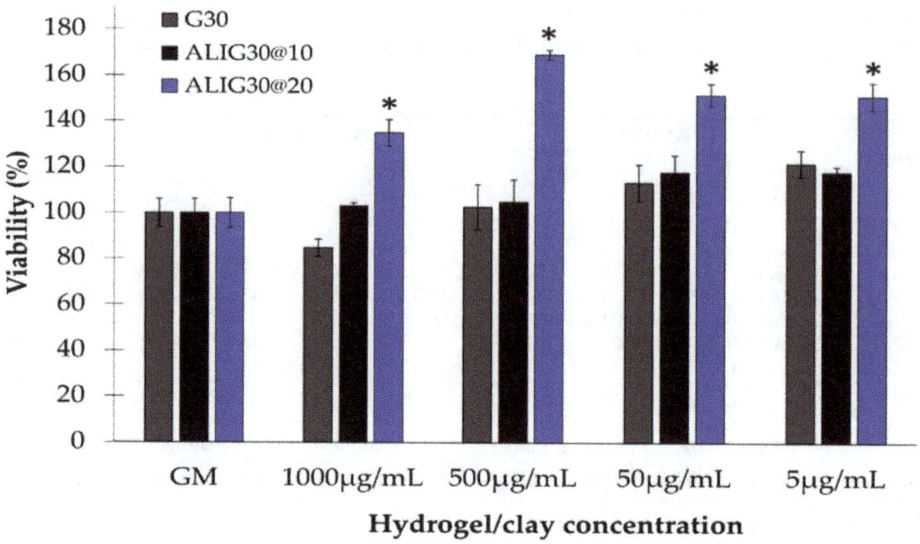

Figure 2. Biocompatibility tests of ALIG30@20 (blue). Viability (%) vs. hydrogel or clay concentration (% w/w). GM (growth medium) indicates the control. G30 and ALIG30@10 results (taken from García-Villén et al. [17]) were included to compare viability results of hydrogels with different concentrations. Mean values ± s.e.; $n = 8$. Significant differences, compared to GM, are marked with (*). Mann–Whitney (Wilcoxon) W tests, p values ≤ 0.05.

4. Discussion

4.1. Release of Elements and Potentially Useful Therapeutic Activities

According to the ICH Q3D(R1) guideline, no PDE limits have been established for class 4 elements [32]. The presence of Al in cosmetics is allowed according to EC 1223/2009 since it specifies that "natural hydrated aluminum silicates ($Al_2O_3{\cdot}2SiO_2{\cdot}2H_2O$) containing calcium, magnesium or iron carbonates, ferric hydroxides, quartz-sand, mica, etc. as impurities" are allowed. Aluminum has shown to be released from 1-month-old hydrogels (Table 2). The WHO has established a tolerable weekly intake of 7 mg/kg of body weight for aluminum [37]. In view of the low bioavailability of aluminum from cosmetic products (≤0.07%) [38–40], applications with more than 213 kg of hydrogel would be necessary to subject patients to potentially dangerous Al doses. Therefore, it is possible to guarantee that ALIPS9, ALIG30@10 and ALIG30@20 are totally safe regarding aluminum release. Additionally, some Al^{3+} "misfolds cell membrane proteins", which gives it antibacterial activity [41].

Ca, Fe, Mn, Zn and S are not listed in this regulation [33], which means that, legally speaking, the presence of these elements does not limit the use of the present hydrogels as cosmetics from a legal point of view. Major elements such Mg, Ca, Na and K are considered as "essential" for both animals and human beings, and their presence in the pristine materials is considered totally safe and, sometimes, even favorable in certain cases. The usefulness of metals during wound healing has also been pointed out by some studies. For instance, it has been demonstrated that wound supplementation of Zn, Cu and Mg would be advisable during the healing process [42].

The amount of K in solids was higher than Na and Ca, though its release from hydrogels was remarkably lower than that of Ca and Na. This result is in agreement with the cation exchange capacity (CEC) of PS9 and G30 reported in previous studies [17], which showed calcium as one of the main exchangeable cations. Additionally, Ca is the second most abundant element in ALI. It has been reported that low concentrations of extracellular potassium may accelerate and favor fibroblast differentiation, thus forming scar tissue [43]. Low intracellular K^+ concentrations favor interleukin-8 expression, which plays an important role in stimulating re-epithelialization, migration and proliferation of dermal cells during wound healing [26]. Therefore, a limited potassium release from both hydrogels would be beneficial during wound healing treatments.

Sodium is the second/third element with higher in vitro release levels (Table 2) and the third/forth element in terms of abundance in the pristine materials (Table 1). Moreover, Na was one of the minor exchanged cations of PS9 and G30. This apparently contradictory result has previously been observed for other clay-based hydrogels subjected to the very same in vitro release methodology [44]. This result could be related to the hydrophilicity of the exchangeable cations of the clay, that follow the order $Ca^{2+} > Na^{+} > K^{+}$ [45]. The higher the hydrophilicity of the element, the higher the ability of water to enter the interlayer space and the higher the exchange capacity. The very same trend has been found for Ca, Na and K release (Table 2) and CEC [17], despite this not being the same exact order of abundance in the pristine materials (Table 1).

Mg release increased with time in ALIPS9 and ALIG30@10, whereas it reduced in ALIG30@20 (Table 2). This element has been shown to easily permeate the skin [46] and possess anti-inflammatory activity, and is thus able to treat skin disorders such as psoriasis and atopic dermatitis [47,48]. The combination of Mg and Ca has been reported to accelerate skin barrier repair, as well as skin hydration by synergic effects [49]. Moreover, apart from the beneficial effects of Mg in the skin, this element, along with Ca, is also essential for good bone and muscle health. Therefore, if any of these elements are able to reach the bloodstream during the hydrogel treatment, they could also help treat other systemic musculoskeletal disorders, such as fibromyalgia [50].

Boron compounds have been demonstrated to be beneficial for wound healing of burned skin and in diabetic wound healing processes, both in vitro and in vivo [51,52]. B has proved useful in several metabolic pathways as well as in the increase of the wound healing rate [53,54]. Release of B decreased with time in the three hydrogels until it reached undetectable levels. Consequently, if any benefit should be obtained from B, those benefits would be at its maximum in young hydrogels.

ALI composition also played an important role in the levels of elements released during the in vitro tests. In fact, the release of S can be totally ascribed to the natural spring water composition (ALI) (Table 1). The release of sulphur reduced with time in all cases (Table 2). Higher S release was reported for ALIG30@10 48 h. For ALIPS9 and ALIG30@20, the release amounts of S were very similar. Differences in ALIG30@10 and ALIG30@20 can be ascribed to the clay mineral concentration. Balneotherapy with sulphurous waters and peloids has been proven to help with several disorders and diseases [55,56]. Specifically, keratolytic, anti-inflammatory, keratoplastic and antipruritic effects have been related to S [57]. Sulphurous mineral waters may be absorbed through the skin causing vasodilation, analgesia, immune response inhibition, and keratolytic effects that reduce skin desquamation [58]. Moreover, S could potentiate angiogenesis (endothelial cell proliferation) and regulate skin immunity. Consequently, the mobility of this element would be positive, since it can ameliorate several skin disorders. In this particular case, to obtain the maximum beneficial effects from sulphur, young hydrogels should be used, when the mobility of this element is maximum.

Mn works as a coenzyme in several biological processes, such as the transition between quiescent and proliferative phases of fibroblasts [59]. Nonetheless, Mn levels contained in healthcare formulations should be controlled due to possible toxic brain accumulation [60–62]. Levels of Mn were the same for pristine PS9 and G30 (while absent in ALI, Table 1). Consequently, it is possible to state that the release of this element is solely due to the clay mineral. Mn release increased with time in ALIG30@20, while it was not measurable in ALIG30@10, probably due to the lower concentration of G30 in this formulation. A study on the bioavailability of manganese from soils revealed that in acid soils, Mn bioavailability grows [63]. Previously it has been shown that G30 and PS9 hydrogels prepared with ALI water suffer from a reduction in pH values during the first 6 months [64]. This modification of the pH could be the explanation for a higher release of Mn after 1 month in ALIPS9 and ALIG30@20. In terms of safety, ALIG30@10 would be the safest formulation, since Mn release was not detectable during Franz cells study.

Zinc is a class 4 element, but it is not listed in EC 1223/2009. The ALIPS9 hydrogel showed an increase in Zn release with time, while ALIG30@20 showed stable levels (Table 2). The increase in Zn release in ALIPS9 and ALIG30@10 could also be related to pH changes in the formulation with time, although the literature results are contradictory [63]. Regarding safety and regulations, Zn did possess a defined PDE level in the Q3D(R1) [32] (13,000 μg/day for both oral and parenteral routes). Moreover, the WHO defined a provisional maximum tolerable daily intake amount of 18–60 mg/day for an adult of 60 kg. As previously mentioned, it has been reported that this element could compromise renal and hepatic functions when high doses reach the bloodstream. Nonetheless, Zn has also been demonstrated to be essential for keratinocyte and fibroblast proliferation, differentiation and survival. Its deficiency has been related to different disorders such as acquired acrodermatitis enteropathica, biotic deficiency, alopecia and delayed wound healing. Moreover, Zn concentration is usually higher in the epidermis than in the dermis [65,66]. Consequently, the mobility of Zn from the studied hydrogels is seen as a positive and potentially useful feature for wound healing. Moreover, the released amount of Zn in Franz cells can be considered safe, since it was below the WHO and PDE limits previously mentioned and they are intended to be topically administered.

Together with Zn, Cu is a useful element in terms of wound healing [67] and its presence is allowed in cosmetics by EC 1223/2009. This element has been demonstrated to increase the expression of TGF-β1 in ex vivo skin models, thus leading to higher pro-collagen 1 and elastin production by fibroblasts [67]. Moreover, Cu has been demonstrated to enhance skin cell migration (keratinocytes and fibroblasts), which is crucial for wound healing [68,69]. ALIPS9 and ALIG30@10 were shown to favor fibroblast migration in a previous study [17], which could be related to copper release. Additionally, copper possesses an antimicrobial effect and has been proposed as an ingredient for wound dressings [70]. In fact, some clay minerals with Cu were demonstrated to be the most effective against *Escherichia coli* and *Staphylococcus aureus*. Release levels of Cu revealed that, to obtain the aforementioned effects, extemporaneous hydrogels should be used (Table 2).

Ga showed minimum mobility in both hydrogels (Table 2) and significantly reduced mobility in ALIG30@20 after 1 month. Higher release levels in ALIG30@20 versus ALIPS9 can be ascribed to a higher concentration of this element in G30 pristine material (Table 1). This element is not addressed in any of the aforementioned regulations [32,33,71,72] since it is currently considered a relatively non-toxic element for humans. Antimicrobial activity of Ga has been reported [73,74], which could be of use for the treatment of infected wounds. A biocompatible, gallium-loaded, antimicrobial, artificial dermal scaffold has been recently proposed [75]. Other biomedical uses of Ga have also been previously reported due to its low toxicity [76–81]. In view of the existing bibliography and the present results, extemporaneous ALIG30@20 hydrogels would be a proper choice to obtain antimicrobial activity.

Strontium mobility was one of the most remarkable among the trace elements, mainly because of its presence in ALI. The presence of this element in cosmetics is not considered determinant in terms of safety, maybe because symptoms of Sr overdose are not yet clear in humans. What is more, despite the in vivo studies performed in animals, no Sr limits have been established for humans (since dietary intake variations did not induced acute toxicity symptoms) [82,83]. Wound healing effects of strontium chloride hexahydrate has been evaluated in vivo. This strontium salt was shown to reduce TNF-α expression in the wound site and, therefore, reduce inflammation [84], which is of special use in chronic inflammatory disorders. The antioxidant effect is also related to Sr, according to previous studies [85] that used strontium-substituted bioglass for tissue engineering purposes. Strontium has also been included in wound dressings as a wound healing promoter [86] and has been demonstrated to exert useful systemic effects when it reaches the bloodstream [87–90]. In conclusion, the release of Sr release is desirable, ALIPS9 being the formulation providing the highest levels of this element.

4.2. Mobility of Elements

The sole presence of an element or chemical compound in a formulation does not mean that it would exert its therapeutic effect: it also needs to be released and be able to reach the active site.

Moreover, the release process can be determined by different factors, one of them being its location in the formulation (clay structure or the spring water) or the age of the system [36,91]. Element mobility is a normalized parameter that allows comparisons between released levels of different elements. It can be calculated as the ratio between total concentration in the formulation and the released concentration. Mobility values of elements in ALIPS9 and ALIG30@20 hydrogels are plotted in Figure 3. In this figure, the delimited areas within the graphic were defined in a speculative manner. As can be seen from the dispersion (Figure 3), the majority of the elements showed a mobility lower than 2%.

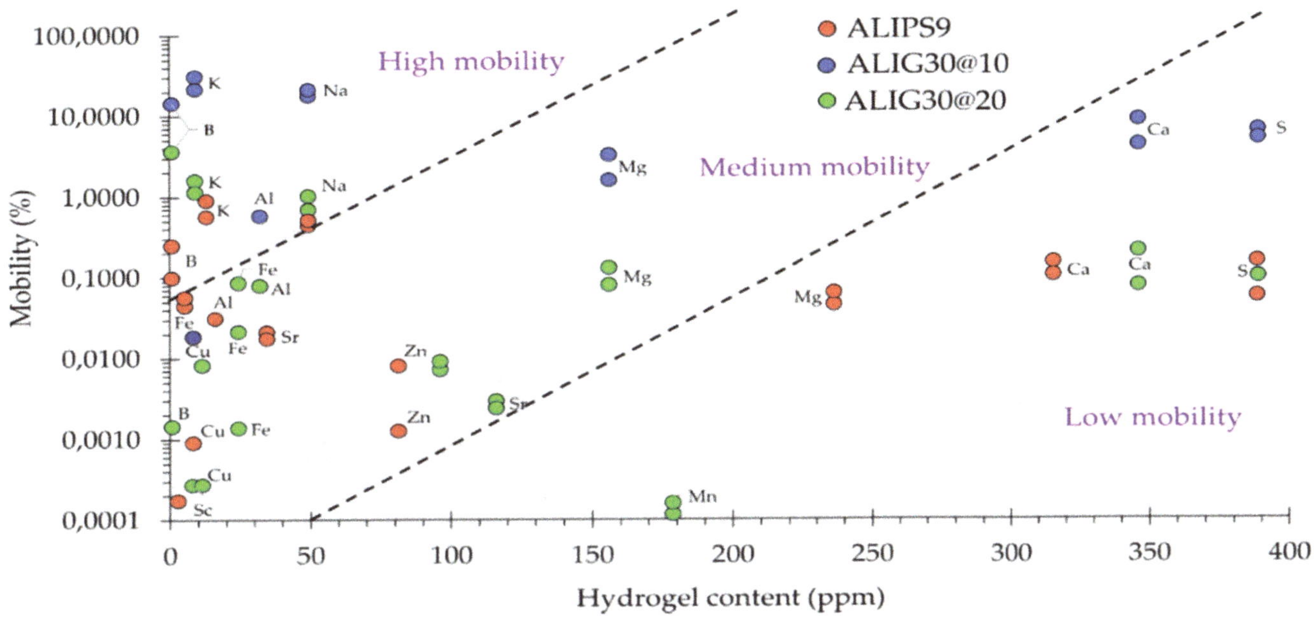

Figure 3. Percentage of mobility (logarithmic scale) versus total content of the element in ALIPS9, ALIG30@10 and ALIG30@20 hydrogels (ppm). "High", "Medium" and "Low mobility" areas are hypothetical. Non-detected elements (mobility = 0%) do not appear in the logarithmic scale.

Even if Ca, S and Mg were present in remarkable amounts in the studied formulations, their released levels were very low in proportion, thus giving rise to low element mobility. This result demonstrates that, despite the spring water having remarkable amounts of these elements, their mobility is probably limited by the presence of the solid phase. Consequently, the solid and the liquid phases of the formulations establish a very close interaction that affects the final performance of the system, something that highlights the necessity to fully characterize this kind of formulation. Another visible result is the higher mobility of elements in ALIG30@10 with respect to ALIG30@20 and ALIPS9, which also demonstrates that the type and the concentration of the clay mineral exert a remarkable influence. Elements in the "medium mobility" area (Figure 3) were located in this section since they have low mobility (<1%) together with low concentration (<150 ppm) in the final formulation.

In view of the mobility results, K, Na, B and Al are the elements with the highest mobility. They showed relatively low amounts in the hydrogels but their mobility was clearly significantly higher with respect to the rest of the elements. We hypothesized that the high mobility of the aforementioned elements could be related to both the hydrophilicity of cations (previously mentioned in Section 4.1) and to a small/absent interaction between the pristine ingredients and, therefore, the released levels ascribed to the influence of the liquid phase (ALI) more than to the solid phase. That is, even if K, Na and B were not the main major elements in the pristine ingredients, the low interaction between K, Na and B (coming from ALI) with fibrous clay structure let these elements be relatively "free" within the system and, therefore, more prone to move. This hypothesis is confirmed by the fact that the mobility of elements in ALIG30@10 is higher than in ALIG30@20, due to the lower amount of G30 in the former. In this formulation, the reduced amount of clay mineral implies less retention of the elements and, therefore, higher mobility.

Spider diagrams represent more clearly the different mobility of elements between the same hydrogels at 48 h and 1 month (Figure 4). This comparison reveals that nanoclay/spring water hydrogels are "living formulations" since their ingredients constantly interact with each other, changing the final properties of the system. The area of ALIG30@10 (48 h and 1 month) is higher than the area of ALIPS9 and ALIG30@20, which is in agreement with the previous mobility results (Figure 4). The "liveliness" of the hydrogels can be ascribed to the different elemental equilibriums established between the solid and liquid phases in the formulation (adsorption and desorption equilibriums). Upholding this hypothesis, the solid phase mainly influenced the time-mobility of Cu, Mn, Ga, Al, B, and Fe, either increasing or reducing the corresponding mobility, depending on each particular case.

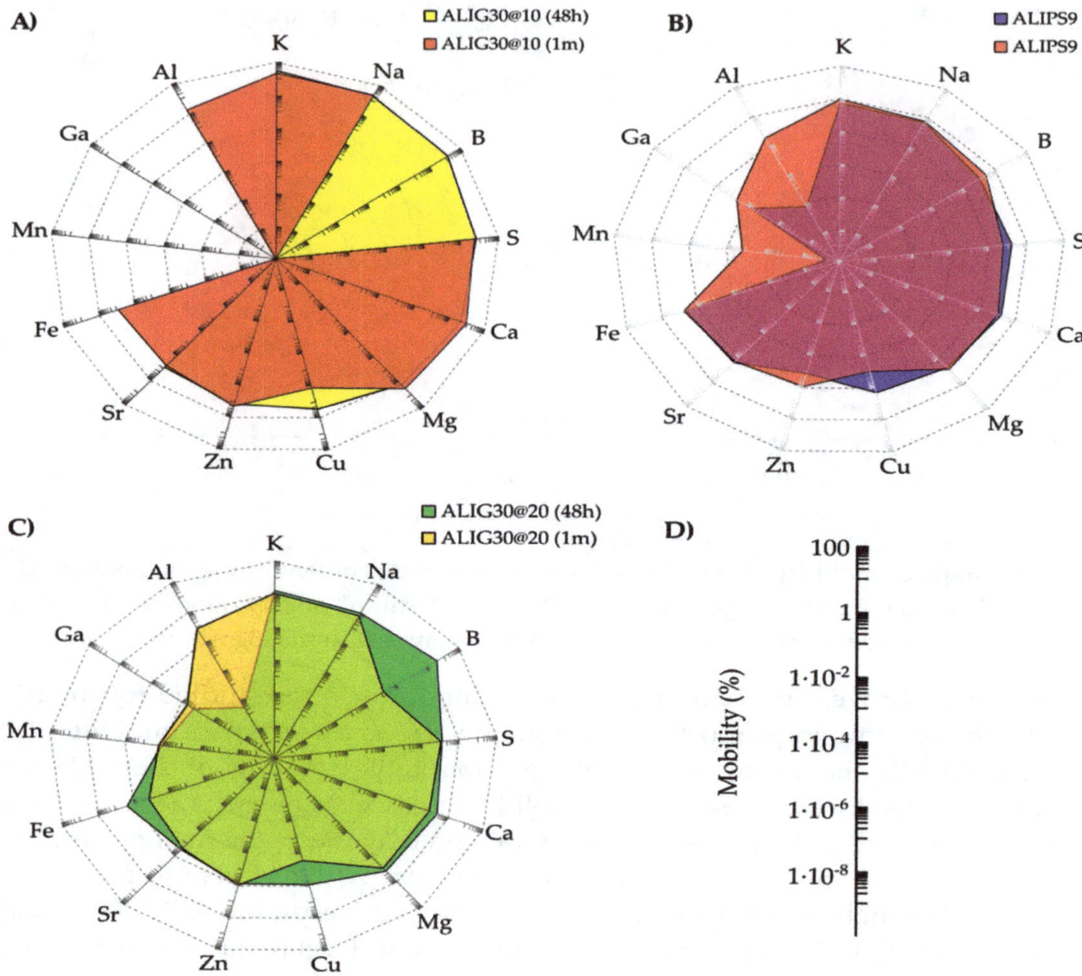

Figure 4. Spider diagrams of element mobility. (**A**) ALIG30@10; (**B**) ALIPS9 (**C**) ALIG30@20. For simplicity, the scale of the diagrams has been represented independently in (**D**).

The reduction of some elements' mobility with time (for instance B, Mg, Al, Zn, Mn, and Na) could also be explained by the stabilization of the system, and the clay better adsorbing/retaining these elements as time passes. In fact, clay minerals have been widely used for decontamination purposes due to their remarkable adsorptive properties [92–95]. Moreover, rheological changes have also been detected is these samples. A different structure of the system network could modify the mobility of certain elements and vice versa [91]. As can be seen in Appendix A (Figure A1), both ALIG30@20 and ALIPS9 suffered rheological changes within one month. Moreover, it is also possible from these results to hypothesize that the rheological performance of the system could also be influencing the element mobility. ALIPS9 and ALIG30@20, having a much more structured internal network (Figure A1), could hinder the mobility of elements that will find a more intricate path to travel towards the exterior. On the other hand, ALIG30@10 was shown to have a less structured gel network (see García-Villén et al. [64] for information on the rheology of ALIG30@10).

4.3. Biocompatibility of ALIG30@20

In vitro biocompatibility of clay minerals has been widely studied [15,96–99]. Some clay minerals have already been shown to have proliferating activity in cellular cultures, such as montmorillonite and halloysite [100,101]. Nonetheless, the induction of cellular proliferation by palygorskite clay mineral is a rare result [102]. This result leads us to hypothesize that if ALIG30@10 was biocompatible and able to induce fibroblast motility during in vitro wound healing [17], ALIG30@20, with proliferative activity, is also a promising formulation for wound healing treatments, especially during the proliferative stage. The different performance between these two hydrogels could be due to physicochemical differences of the systems. That is, different rheological behaviors as well as different chemical performances of both hydrogels could be the factors governing the biocompatibility results. Moreover, the present results could also be due to the combination of both physical and chemical performances of the formulations. Table A1 shows the theoretical amount of mobile element released in the fibroblast culture during MTT tests. These calculations have been made in order to correlate Franz cells results with those of MTT.

Mn has been reported as an active ingredient of spring waters with wound healing activity [29] This, together with the Mn released results in ALIG30@10 and ALIG30@20 (Table 2), leads us to propose manganese as one of the possible factors explaining the proliferative effect of ALIG30@20 versus ALIG30@10 (Figure 2).

Calcium and zinc have been demonstrated to actively participate in cellular growth, in particular the Zn:Ca ratio, which was demonstrated to increase Zn:Ca during cell proliferation and the decline Zn:Ca during the remodeling phase [20,21,103]. This is due to a redistribution of calcium within dermal cells during the wound healing cascade [104], which is dependent on certain trace elements such as zinc. In fact, extracellular calcium has been shown to stimulate DNA synthesis in cultured fibroblasts in the presence of Zn [105]. This has been mainly ascribed to the cofactor role of Zn in different enzymes involved in fibroblast growth. Moreover, Zn also plays an important role as a structural component of essential proteins. Some in vitro studies demonstrated that, even if proper growth factors and nutrients are present in the fibroblast culture medium, deficiencies of Zn translate to insufficient intracellular calcium and, ultimately, to impaired fibroblast proliferation [106,107]. From the release values of these elements, the Zn:Ca ratio of ALIG30@10 was 0.00465 and 0.01060 for ALIG30@20 (obtained from Table A1), which could be a significant factor inducing the proliferation of fibroblasts in ALIG30@20. It is also worth pointing out the fact that G30 showed a remarkable amount of Zn, thus being the ingredient providing this element. On the other hand, the major amount of Ca is provided by ALI. Any of the formulation ingredients on their own have been shown to induce cellular proliferation (see MTT results in García-Villén et al. [17] and Figure 2). This indicates that both ALI and G30, properly combined in a certain concentration, are necessary to induce fibroblast proliferation. Consequently, the proliferative effect is ascribed to the formulation itself, proving once again the major importance of formulative studies. By the same token, the Ca:Mg ratio also changes along the wound healing cascade. In fact, an increase in Mg levels is observed to favor cellular migration. Grzesiak and Pierschbacher stated that the Mg:Ca ratio was close to 1 during the migratory phase, and it reversed during the rest of the process [108]. ALIPS9 and ALIG30@10 hydrogels (aged for 1 month) showed Mg:Ca ratios (Table 2) closest to 1, which is in agreement with the induction of fibroblast migration already demonstrated for these formulations [17]. Nonetheless, the ALIG30@20 Mg:Ca ratio was significantly distant from this value, which happens during the proliferative phase.

The present results ultimately lead us to think that, apart from the amount of elements released from each hydrogel, their ratio and specific identity highly influence the final therapeutic performance of the formulation. Notwithstanding the fact that further studies are needed, it is noteworthy that the present formulations have the potential to be combined and administered at different times of the wound treatment by virtue of their chemical performance

5. Conclusions

The present study deals with the in vitro release and mobility of potentially bioactive elements present in semisolid gel-like formulations obtained by mixing sepiolite and palygorskite with a natural spring water. Hydrogels were subjected to in vitro Franz cell tests and the elements released were analyzed by inductively coupled plasma techniques. Then, the element release and mobility were compared with in vitro biocompatibility tests of the very same formulation. The results demonstrated that, unlike other formulations, the potential therapeutic activity of nanoclay/spring water hydrogels should be studied in depth and characterized.

Clay/spring water hydrogels are "living formulations" since their ingredients constantly interact with each other, changing the properties of the system. For instance, the presence of an element in high concentration does not mean it would be released in high amounts. Moreover, the high release of bioactive elements is not a *sine qua non* to obtain maximum therapeutic effect. In fact, the ALIG30@20 hydrogel, with lower elemental mobility, not only proved to be biocompatible, but to exert potential proliferative effects over fibroblast cultures. According to the present in vitro release studies, it is possible to state that the ratios of the elements released play a significant role in the final therapeutic activity of the formulation. Moreover, the importance of formulative studies is again highlighted, since it is the optimal combination of the correct ingredients that makes a formulation effective.

As a general conclusion, the present study demonstrates that synergistic effects can be achieved from the formulation of the liquid phase in a semisolid system, in which elemental composition of the solid phase and structure of the system will determine elements' mobility and, ultimately, the therapeutic effects.

Author Contributions: Data curation, F.G.-V.; Funding acquisition, P.C., G.S. and C.V.; Methodology, F.G.-V., R.S.-E. and G.S.; Supervision, C.V.; Writing—original draft, F.G.-V.; Writing—review & editing, A.B.-S., P.C., L.C. and C.V All authors have read and agreed to the published version of the manuscript.

Acknowledgments: This project was supported by the Spanish research group CTS-946. Technical support was provided by the CIC (Centro de Instrumentación Científica, University of Granada) and the IACT (Instituto Andaluz de Ciencias de la Tierra, CSIS-UGR). Special thanks to TOLSA group (Madrid), who kindly gifted clay minerals samples, and Alicún de las Torres thermal station, who provided spring water samples for the study.

Appendix A

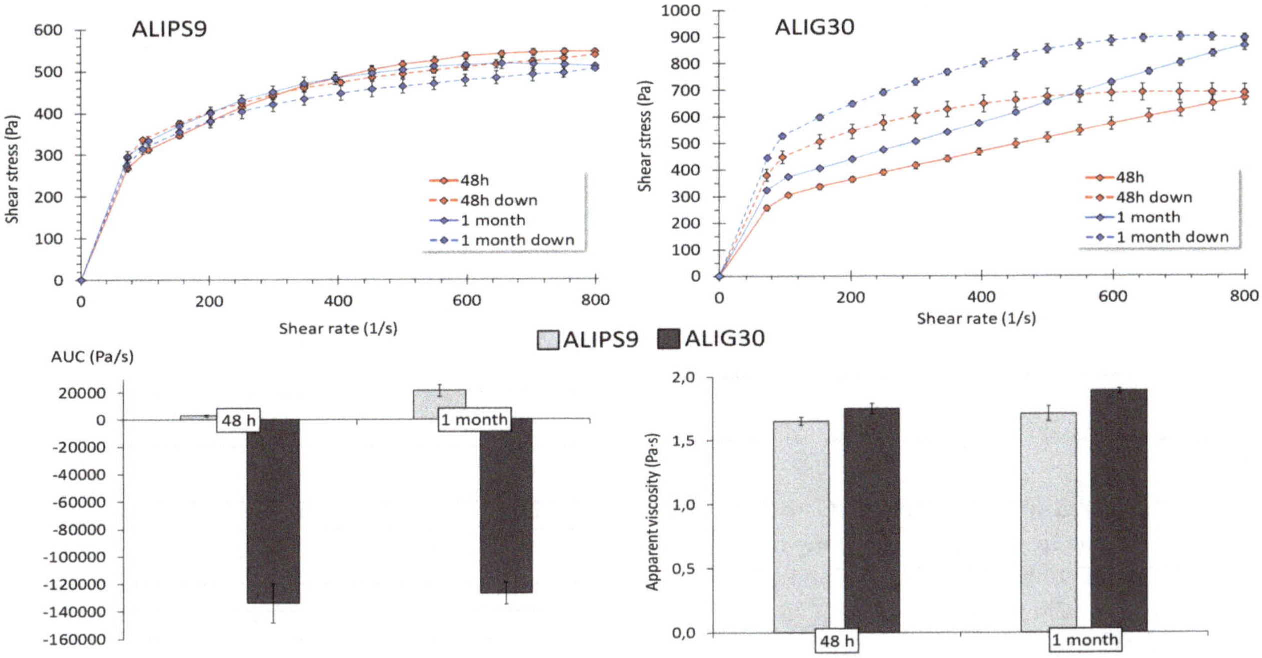

Figure A1. Rheological characterization of ALIPS9 and ALIG30@20 hydrogels after 48 h and 1 month. Up: flow curves (from 70 to 800 s^{-1}, mean values ± s.d., $n = 6$). Down: hysteresis areas (mean values ± s.d., $n = 6$) and apparent viscosities (250 s^{-1}, mean values ± s.d., $n = 6$). Positive *AUC* values indicates thixotropic behavior, while negative ones correspond to anti-thixotropic profile.

Table A1. Amount of mobile elements released from the corresponding hydrogels into fibroblast cultures (MTT well-plate). Results were calculated from Franz experiments at 1 month and expressed in nanograms. NM stands for "Not Released".

Hydrogel	Element (ng)	Amount of Hydrogel in Cell Wells During MTT Test			
		1000 μg/mL	500 μg/mL	50 μg/mL	5 μg/mL
ALIPS9	Al	2.25	1.13	0.11	0.01
	B	0.79	0.39	0.04	0.004
	Ca	161.5	80.7	8.08	0.81
	K	55.3	27.6	2.76	0.28
	Mg	73.8	36.9	3.69	0.37
	Na	125.7	62.8	6.28	0.63
	S	109.4	54.7	5.47	0.55
	Fe	1.46	0.73	0.07	0.01
	Sr	2.97	1.49	0.15	0.01
	Zn	3.32	1.66	0.17	0.02
	Mn	0.01	0.01	0.0007	0.0001
	Cu	0.07	0.04	0.0036	0.0004
ALIG30@10	Al	11.6	5.78	0.58	0.06
	B	NR	NR	NR	NR
	Ca	608.3	304.1	30.41	3.04
	K	38.3	19.1	1.91	0.19
	Mg	103.1	51.6	5.16	0.52
	Na	210.7	105.3	10.53	1.05
	S	234.0	117.0	11.70	1.17
	Fe	0.42	0.21	0.02	0.002
	Sr	1.32	0.66	0.07	0.01
	Zn	2.83	1.41	0.14	0.01
	Mn	NR	NR	NR	NR
	Cu	0.036	0.018	0.002	0.0002

Table A1. *Cont.*

Hydrogel	Element (ng)	Amount of Hydrogel in Cell Wells During MTT Test			
		1000 μg/mL	500 μg/mL	50 μg/mL	5 μg/mL
ALIG30@20	Al	6.72	3.36	0.34	0.03
	B	0.001	$5{\cdot}10^{4}$	$5{\cdot}10^{-5}$	$5{\cdot}10^{-6}$
	Ca	165.2	82.6	8.26	0.83
	K	25.9	12.9	1.29	0.13
	Mg	29.7	14.8	1.48	0.15
	Na	84.8	42.4	4.24	0.42
	S	79.4	39.7	3.97	0.4
	Fe	0.09	0.04	$4.4{\cdot}10^{-3}$	$4.4{\cdot}10^{-4}$
	Sr	0.69	0.34	0.03	0.003
	Zn	1.75	0.88	0.09	0.01
	Mn	0.07	0.04	0.0004	$3.7{\cdot}10^{-4}$
	Cu	0.01	0.005	$4.6{\cdot}10^{-4}$	$4.6{\cdot}10^{-5}$

References

1. Tateo, F.; Ravaglioli, A.; Andreoli, C.; Bonina, F.; Coiro, V.; Degetto, S.; Giaretta, A.; Orsini, A.M.; Puglia, C.; Summa, V. The in-vitro percutaneous migration of chemical elements from a thermal mud for healing use. *Appl. Clay Sci.* **2009**, *44*, 83–94. [CrossRef]
2. Fioravanti, A.; Cantarini, L.; Guidelli, G.M.; Galeazzi, M. Mechanisms of action of spa therapies in rheumatic diseases: What scientific evidence is there? *Rheumatol. Int.* **2011**, *31*, 1–8. [CrossRef] [PubMed]
3. Fioravanti, A.; Perpignano, G.; Tirri, G.; Cardinale, G.; Gianniti, C.; Lanza, C.E.; Loi, A.; Tirri, E.; Sfriso, P.; Cozzi, F. Effects of mud-bath treatment on fibromyalgia patients: A randomized clinical trial. *Rheumatol. Int.* **2007**, *27*, 1157–1161. [CrossRef]
4. Cozzi, F.; Raffeiner, B.; Beltrame, V.; Ciprian, L.; Coran, A.; Botsios, C.; Perissinotto, E.; Grisan, E.; Ramonda, R.; Oliviero, F.; et al. Effects of mud-bath therapy in psoriatic arthritis patients treated with TNF inhibitors. Clinical evaluation and assessment of synovial inflammation by contrast-enhanced ultrasound (CEUS). *Jt. Bone Spine* **2015**, *82*, 104–108. [CrossRef] [PubMed]
5. Fioravanti, A.; Karagulle, M.; Bender, T.; Karagülle, M.Z. Balneotherapy in osteoarthritis: Facts, fiction and gaps in knowledge. *Eur. J. Integr. Med.* **2017**, *9*, 148–150. [CrossRef]
6. Sukenik, S.; Flusser, D.; Codish, S.; Abu-Shakra, M. Balneotherapy at the Dead Sea area for knee osteoarthritis. *Isr. Med. Assoc. J.* **1999**, *1*, 83–85.
7. Andreoli, C.; Rascio, N. The algal flora in the Thermal Baths of Montegrotto Terme (Padua). Its distribution over one-year period. *Int. Rev. Hydrobiol.* **1975**, *60*, 857–871. [CrossRef]
8. Quintela, A.; Terroso, D.; Almeida, S.; Reis, A. Geochemical and microbiological characterization of some Azorean volcanic muds after maturation. *Res. J. Chem. Environ.* **2010**, *14*, 66–74.
9. Pesciaroli, C.; Viseras, C.; Aguzzi, C.; Rodelas, B.; González-López, J. Study of bacterial community structure and diversity during the maturation process of a therapeutic peloid. *Appl. Clay Sci.* **2016**, *132*, 59–67. [CrossRef]
10. Drobnik, J.; Stebel, A. Central European ethnomedical and officinal uses of peat, with special emphasis on the Tołpa peat preparation (TPP): An historical review. *J. Ethnopharmacol.* **2019**, *246*, 112248. [CrossRef]
11. Elkayam, O.; Ophir, J.; Brener, S.; Paran, D.; Wigler, I.; Efron, D.; Even-Paz, Z.; Politi, Y.; Yaron, M. Immediate and delayed effects of treatment at the Dead Sea in patients with psoriatic arthritis. *Rheumatol. Int.* **2000**, *19*, 77–82. [CrossRef] [PubMed]
12. Delfino, M.; Russo, N.; Migliaccio, G.; Carraturo, N. Experimental study on efficacy of thermal muds of Ischia Island combined with balneotherapy in the treatment of psoriasis vulgaris with plaques. *La Clin. Ter.* **2003**, *154*, 167–171.
13. Harari, M. Beauty is not only skin deep: The Dead Sea features and cosmetics. In *Anales de Hidrología Médica*; Universidad Complutense de Madrid: Madrid, Spain, 2012; Volume 5, pp. 75–88.
14. Argenziano, G.; Delfino, M.; Russo, N. Mud and baththerapy in the acne cure. *La Clin. Ter.* **2004**, *155*, 125.

15. Sandri, G.; Bonferoni, M.C.; Rossi, S.; Ferrari, F.; Aguzzi, C.; Viseras, C.; Caramella, C. Clay minerals for tissue regeneration, repair, and engineering. In *Wound Healing Biomaterials*; Agren, M.S., Ed.; Elsevier: Amsterdam, The Netherlands, 2016; pp. 385–402.
16. García-Villén, F.; Faccendini, A.; Aguzzi, C.; Cerezo, P.; Bonferoni, M.C.; Rossi, S.; Grisoli, P.; Ruggeri, M.; Ferrari, F.; Sandri, G.; et al. Montmorillonite-norfloxacin nanocomposite intended for healing of infected wounds. *Int. J. Nanomed.* **2019**, *14*, 5051–5060. [CrossRef] [PubMed]
17. García-Villén, F.; Faccendini, A.; Miele, D.; Ruggeri, M.; Sánchez-Espejo, R.; Borrego-Sánchez, A.; Cerezo, P.; Rossi, S.; Viseras, C.; Sandri, G. Wound Healing Activity of Nanoclay/Spring Water Hydrogels. *Pharmaceutics* **2020**, *12*, 467. [CrossRef]
18. García-Villén, F.; Souza, I.M.; Barbosa, R.D.M.; Borrego-Sánchez, A.; Sánchez-Espejo, R.; Ojeda-Riascos, S.; Iborra, C.V.; Viseras, C. Natural Inorganic Ingredients in Wound Healing. *Curr. Pharm. Des.* **2020**, *26*, 621–641. [CrossRef]
19. Sasaki, Y.; Sathi, G.A.; Yamamoto, O. Wound healing effect of bioactive ion released from Mg-smectite. *Mater. Sci. Eng. C* **2017**, *77*, 52–57. [CrossRef]
20. Lansdown, A.B.G.; Sampson, B.; Rowe, A. Sequential changes in trace metal, metallothionein and calmodulin concentrations in healing skin wounds. *J. Anat.* **1999**, *195*, 375–386. [CrossRef]
21. Lansdown, A.B.G. Calcium: A potential central regulator in wound healing in the skin. *Wound Repair Regen.* **2002**, *10*, 271–285. [CrossRef]
22. Dubé, J.; Rochette-Drouin, O.; Lévesque, P.; Gauvin, R.; Roberge, C.J.; Auger, F.A.; Goulet, D.; Bourdages, M.; Plante, M.; Germain, L.; et al. Restoration of the Transepithelial Potential Within Tissue-Engineered Human Skin In Vitro and During the Wound Healing Process In Vivo. *Tissue Eng. Part A* **2010**, *16*, 3055–3063. [CrossRef]
23. Fairley, J.A.; Marcelo, C.L.; Hogan, V.A.; Voorhees, J.J. Increased Calmodulin Levels in Psoriasis and Low Ca++ Regulated Mouse Epidermal Keratinocyte Cultures. *J. Investig. Dermatol.* **1985**, *84*, 195–198. [CrossRef] [PubMed]
24. Karvonen, S.-L.; Korkiamäki, T.; Ylä-Outinen, H.; Nissinen, M.; Teerikangas, H.; Pummi, K.; Karvonen, J.; Peltonen, J. Psoriasis and Altered Calcium Metabolism: Downregulated Capacitative Calcium Influx and Defective Calcium-Mediated Cell Signaling in Cultured Psoriatic Keratinocytes. *J. Investig. Dermatol.* **2000**, *114*, 693–700. [CrossRef] [PubMed]
25. Gao, Y.; Jin, X. Needle-punched three-dimensional nonwoven wound dressings with density gradient from biocompatible calcium alginate fiber. *Text. Res. J.* **2019**, *89*, 2776–2788. [CrossRef]
26. Hotta, E.; Hara, H.; Kamiya, T.; Adachi, T. Non-thermal atmospheric pressure plasma-induced IL-8 expression is regulated via intracellular K + loss and subsequent ERK activation in human keratinocyte HaCaT cells. *Arch. Biochem. Biophys.* **2018**, *644*, 64–71. [CrossRef] [PubMed]
27. Shim, J.H.; Lim, J.W.; Kim, B.K.; Park, S.J.; Kim, S.W.; Choi, T.H. KCl Mediates K+Channel-Activated Mitogen-Activated Protein Kinases Signaling in Wound Healing. *Arch. Plast. Surg.* **2015**, *42*, 11–19. [CrossRef]
28. Yang, G.; Zhang, M.; Qi, B.; Zhu, Z.; Yao, J.; Yuan, X.; Sun, D. Nanoparticle-Based Strategies and Approaches for the Treatment of Chronic Wounds. *J. Biomater. Tissue Eng.* **2018**, *8*, 455–464. [CrossRef]
29. Chebassier, N.; Ouijja, E.H.; Viegas, I.; Dreno, B. Stimulatory effect of boron and manganese salts on keratinocyte migration. *Acta Derm. Venereol.* **2004**, *84*, 191–194. [CrossRef] [PubMed]
30. COLIPA. *Guidelines for Percutaneous Absorption/Penetration*; COLIPA: Brussels, Belgium, 1997; pp. 1–36.
31. EU. *Manual of the Working Group on Cosmetic Products (Sub-Group on Borderline Products) on the Scope of Application of the Cosmetics Regulation*; EU: Brussels, Belgium, 2017; pp. 1–33.
32. ICH. *Guideline for Elemental Impurities Q3D (R1)*; ICH: Geneva, Switzerland, 2019.
33. EU. *Regulation (EC) No 1223/2009 on Cosmetic Products*; EU: Brussels, Belgium, 2009; pp. 1–151.
34. Prado, A.J.P. Sistema termal de Alicún de las Torres (Granada) como análogo natural de escape de CO_2 en forma de DIC: Implicaciones paleoclimáticas y como sumidero de CO_2. Ph.D. Thesis, Universidad Complutense de Madrid, Madrid, Spain, 2011.
35. Prado-Pérez, A.J.; Del Villar, L.P. Dedolomitization as an analogue process for assessing the long-term behaviour of a CO_2 deep geological storage: The Alicún de las Torres thermal system (Betic Cordillera, Spain). *Chem. Geol.* **2011**, *289*, 98–113. [CrossRef]

36. García-Villén, F.; Sánchez-Espejo, R.; Borrego-Sánchez, A.; Cerezo, P.; Perioli, L.; Iborra, C.A.V. Safety of Nanoclay/Spring Water Hydrogels: Assessment and Mobility of Hazardous Elements. *Pharmaceutics* **2020**, *12*, 764. [CrossRef]
37. WHO. *Trace Elements in Human Nutrition and Health*; World Health Organization: Geneva, Switzerland, 1996; pp. 1–360.
38. Flarend, R.; Bin, T.; Elmore, D.; Hem, S.L. A preliminary study of the dermal absorption of aluminium from antiperspirants using aluminium-26. *Food Chem. Toxicol.* **2001**, *39*, 163–168. [CrossRef]
39. De Ligt, R.; Van Duijn, E.; Grossouw, D.; Bosgra, S.; Burggraaf, J.; Windhorst, A.; Peeters, P.A.; Van Der Luijt, G.A.; Alexander-White, C.; Vaes, W.H. Assessment of Dermal Absorption of Aluminum from a Representative Antiperspirant Formulation Using a 26Al Microtracer Approach. *Clin. Transl. Sci.* **2018**, *11*, 573–581. [CrossRef] [PubMed]
40. Pineau, A.; Guillard, O.; Fauconneau, B.; Favreau, F.; Marty, M.H.; Gaudin, A.; Vincent, C.M.; Marrauld, A.; Marty, J.P. In vitro study of percutaneous absorption of aluminum from antiperspirants through human skin in the FranzTM diffusion cell. *J. Inorg. Biochem.* **2012**, *110*, 21–26. [CrossRef] [PubMed]
41. Morrison, K.D.; Misra, R.; Williams, L.B. Unearthing the Antibacterial Mechanism of Medicinal Clay: A Geochemical Approach to Combating Antibiotic Resistance. *Sci. Rep.* **2016**, *6*, 19043. [CrossRef] [PubMed]
42. Wlaschek, M.; Singh, K.; Sindrilaru, A.; Crisan, D.; Scharffetter-Kochanek, K. Iron and iron-dependent reactive oxygen species in the regulation of macrophages and fibroblasts in non-healing chronic wounds. *Free Radic. Biol. Med.* **2019**, *133*, 262–275. [CrossRef]
43. Grasman, J.; Williams, M.D.; Razis, C.G.; Bonzanni, M.; Golding, A.S.; Cairns, D.M.; Levin, M.; Kaplan, D. Hyperosmolar Potassium Inhibits Myofibroblast Conversion and Reduces Scar Tissue Formation. *ACS Biomater. Sci. Eng.* **2019**, *5*, 5327–5336. [CrossRef]
44. Khiari, I.; Sánchez-Espejo, R.; García-Villén, F.; Cerezo, P.; Aguzzi, C.; López-Galindo, A.; Jamoussi, F.; Viseras, C. Rheology and cation release of tunisian medina mud-packs intended for topical applications. *Appl. Clay Sci.* **2019**, *171*, 110–117. [CrossRef]
45. Bish, D. Parallels and Distinctions between Clay Minerals and Zeolites. In *Developments in Clay Science*; Elsevier Ltd.: Amsterdam, The Netherlands, 2006; pp. 1097–1112.
46. Kass, L.; Rosanoff, A.; Tanner, A.; Sullivan, K.; McAuley, W.; Plesset, M. Effect of transdermal magnesium cream on serum and urinary magnesium levels in humans: A pilot study. *PLoS ONE* **2017**, *12*, e0174817. [CrossRef]
47. Schempp, C.M.; Dittmar, H.C.; Hummler, D.; Simon-Haarhaus, B.; Schöpf, E.; Simon, J.C.; Schulte-Mönting, J.; Christoph, M. Magnesium ions inhibit the antigen-presenting function of human epidermal Langerhans cells in vivo and in vitro. Involvement of ATPase, HLA-DR, B7 molecules, and cytokines. *J. Investig. Dermatol.* **2000**, *115*, 680–686. [CrossRef]
48. Chandrasekaran, N.C.; Sanchez, W.Y.; Mohammed, Y.H.; Grice, J.E.; Roberts, M.S.; Barnard, R.T. Permeation of topically applied Magnesium ions through human skin is facilitated by hair follicles. *Magnes. Res.* **2016**, *29*, 35–42. [CrossRef]
49. Denda, M.; Katagiri, C.; Hirao, T.; Maruyama, N.; Takahashi, M. Some magnesium salts and a mixture of magnesium and calcium salts accelerate skin barrier recovery. *Arch. Dermatol. Res.* **1999**, *291*, 560–563. [CrossRef]
50. Engen, D.J.; McAllister, S.J.; Whipple, M.O.; Cha, S.; Dion, L.J.; Vincent, A.; Bauer, B.A.; Wahner-Roedler, D.L. Effects of transdermal magnesium chloride on quality of life for patients with fibromyalgia: A feasibility study. *J. Integr. Med.* **2015**, *13*, 306–313. [CrossRef]
51. Demirci, S.; Doğan, A.; Karakus, E.; Halici, Z.; Topçu, A.; Demirci, E.; Şahin, F.; Halıcı, Z. Boron and Poloxamer (F68 and F127) Containing Hydrogel Formulation for Burn Wound Healing. *Biol. Trace Elem. Res.* **2015**, *168*, 169–180. [CrossRef] [PubMed]
52. Demirci, S.; Doğan, A.; Aydın, S.; Dülger, E.Ç.; Şahin, F. Boron promotes streptozotocin-induced diabetic wound healing: Roles in cell proliferation and migration, growth factor expression, and inflammation. *Mol. Cell. Biochem.* **2016**, *417*, 119–133. [CrossRef] [PubMed]
53. Benderdour, M.; Van Bui, T.; Hess, K.; Dicko, A.; Belleville, F.; Dousset, B. Effects of boron derivatives on extracellular matrix formation. *J. Trace Elem. Med. Boil.* **2000**, *14*, 168–173. [CrossRef]

54. Chebassier, N.; El Houssein, O.; Viegas, I.; Dreno, B. In vitro induction of matrix metalloproteinase-2 and matrix metalloproteinase-9 expression in keratinocytes by boron and manganese. *Exp. Dermatol.* **2004**, *13*, 484–490. [CrossRef]
55. Sieghart, D.; Liszt, M.; Wanivenhaus, A.; Bröll, H.; Kiener, H.; Klösch, B.; Steiner, G. Hydrogen sulphide decreases IL-1β-induced activation of fibroblast-like synoviocytes from patients with osteoarthritis. *J. Cell. Mol. Med.* **2015**, *19*, 187–197. [CrossRef]
56. Carbajo, J.M.; Maraver, F. Sulphurous Mineral Waters: New Applications for Health. *Evid. Based Complement. Altern. Med.* **2017**, *2017*, 8034084. [CrossRef]
57. Rodrigues, L.; Valentim, E.E.; Florenzano, J.; Cerqueira, A.; Soares, A.; Schmidt, T.; Santos, K.; Teixeira, S.; Ribela, M.; Rodrigues, S.F.; et al. Protective effects of exogenous and endogenous hydrogen sulfide in mast cell-mediated pruritus and cutaneous acute inflammation in mice. *Pharmacol. Res.* **2017**, *115*, 255–266. [CrossRef]
58. Nasermoaddel, A.; Kagamimori, S. Balneotherapy in medicine: A review. *Environ. Health Prev. Med.* **2005**, *10*, 171–179. [CrossRef]
59. Sarsour, E.H.; Venkataraman, S.; Kalen, A.L.; Oberley, L.W.; Goswami, P. Manganese superoxide dismutase activity regulates transitions between quiescent and proliferative growth. *Aging Cell* **2008**, *7*, 405–417. [CrossRef]
60. Erikson, K.M.; Aschner, M. Manganese: Its Role in Disease and Health. *Essent. Met. Med.* **2019**, *19*, 253–266.
61. Lucchini, R.G.; Aschner, M.; Landrigan, P.J.; Cranmer, J.M. Neurotoxicity of manganese: Indications for future research and public health intervention from the Manganese 2016 conference. *Neurotoxicology* **2018**, *64*, 1–4. [CrossRef] [PubMed]
62. Horning, K.J.; Caito, S.W.; Tipps, K.G.; Bowman, A.B.; Aschner, M. Manganese Is Essential for Neuronal Health. *Annu. Rev. Nutr.* **2015**, *35*, 71–108. [CrossRef] [PubMed]
63. Dinic, Z.; Maksimović, J.; Stanojković-Sebić, A.; Pivić, R. Prediction Models for Bioavailability of Mn, Cu, Zn, Ni and Pb in Soils of Republic of Serbia. *Agronomy* **2019**, *9*, 856. [CrossRef]
64. García-Villén, F.; Sánchez-Espejo, R.; López-Galindo, A.; Cerezo, P.; Viseras, C. Design and characterization of spring water hydrogels with natural inorganic excipients. *Appl. Clay Sci.* **2020**, *197*, 105772. [CrossRef]
65. Ogawa, Y.; Kinoshita, M.; Shimada, S.; Kawamura, T. Zinc and Skin Disorders. *Nutrients* **2018**, *10*, 199. [CrossRef]
66. Ogawa, Y.; Kawamura, T.; Shimada, S. Zinc and skin biology. *Arch. Biochem. Biophys.* **2016**, *611*, 113–119. [CrossRef]
67. Ogen-Shtern, N.; Chumin, K.; Cohen, G.; Borkow, G. Increased pro-collagen 1, elastin, and TGF-β1 expression by copper ions in an ex-vivo human skin model. *J. Cosmet. Dermatol.* **2019**, *19*, 1522–1527. [CrossRef]
68. Tenaud, I.; Leroy, S.; Chebassier, N.; Dreno, B. Zinc, copper and manganese enhanced keratinocyte migration through a functional modulation of keratinocyte integrins. *Exp. Dermatol.* **2000**, *9*, 407–416. [CrossRef]
69. Qiao, Y.; Ping, Y.; Zhang, H.; Zhou, B.; Liu, F.; Yu, Y.; Xie, T.; Li, W.; Zhong, D.; Zhang, Y.; et al. Laser-Activatable CuS Nanodots to Treat Multidrug-Resistant Bacteria and Release Copper Ion to Accelerate Healing of Infected Chronic Nonhealing Wounds. *ACS Appl. Mater. Interfaces* **2019**, *11*, 3809–3822. [CrossRef]
70. Ul-Islam, M.; Khan, T.; Khattak, W.A.; Park, J.K. Bacterial cellulose-MMTs nanoreinforced composite films: Novel wound dressing material with antibacterial properties. *Cellulose* **2013**, *20*, 589–596. [CrossRef]
71. Health Canada. Natural Health Products Ingredients Database. Available online: http://webprod.hc-sc.gc.ca/nhpid-bdipsn/search-rechercheReq.do (accessed on 18 December 2019).
72. Health Canada. *Quality of Natural Health Products Guide—Natural and Non-Prescription Health Products Directorate*; Health Canada: Ottawa, ON, Canada, 2015; Available online: https://www.canada.ca/en/health-canada/services/consumer-product-safety/reports-publications/industry-professionals.html (accessed on 18 December 2019).
73. Goss, C.; Kaneko, Y.; Khuu, L.; Anderson, G.D.; Ravishankar, S.; Aitken, M.L.; Lechtzin, N.; Zhou, G.; Czyz, D.M.; McLean, K.; et al. Gallium disrupts bacterial iron metabolism and has therapeutic effects in mice and humans with lung infections. *Sci. Transl. Med.* **2018**, *10*, eaat7520. [CrossRef] [PubMed]
74. Young, M.; Ozcan, A.; Lee, B.; Maxwell, T.; Andl, T.; Rajasekaran, P.; Beazley, M.J.; Tetard, L.; Santra, S. N-acetyl Cysteine Coated Gallium Particles Demonstrate High Potency against Pseudomonas aeruginosa PAO1. *Pathogens* **2019**, *8*, 120. [CrossRef] [PubMed]

75. Xu, Z.; Chen, X.; Tan, R.; She, Z.; Chen, Z.-H.; Xia, Z. Preparation and characterization of a gallium-loaded antimicrobial artificial dermal scaffold. *Mater. Sci. Eng. C* **2019**, *105*, 110063. [CrossRef] [PubMed]
76. Song, H.; Kim, T.; Kang, S.; Jin, H.; Lee, K.; Yoon, H.J. Ga-Based Liquid Metal Micro/Nanoparticles: Recent Advances and Applications. *Small* **2020**, *16*, e1903391. [CrossRef] [PubMed]
77. Nguyen, P.; Knapp-Wachsner, A.; Hsieh, C.G.; Kamangar, N. Pulmonary Kaposi Sarcoma without Mucocutaneous Involvement: The Role of Sequential Thallium and Gallium Scintigraphy. *J. Clin. Imaging Sci.* **2019**, *9*, 12–15. [CrossRef] [PubMed]
78. Kimura, Y.; Seguchi, O.; Mochizuki, H.; Iwasaki, K.; Toda, K.; Kumai, Y.; Kuroda, K.; Nakajima, S.; Tateishi, E.; Watanabe, T.; et al. Role of Gallium-SPECT-CT in the Management of Patients With Ventricular Assist Device-Specific Percutaneous Driveline Infection. *J. Card. Fail.* **2019**, *25*, 795–802. [CrossRef]
79. Jalali, A.; Zahmatkesh, M.H.; Jalilian, A.R.; Borujeni, A.T.; Alirezapour, B. Preparation and Biological Evaluation of 67Gallium- Labeled Iranian Hemiscorpius Lepturus Scorpion Venom. *Curr. Radiopharm.* **2020**, *13*, 99–106. [CrossRef]
80. Chitambar, C.R. Medical Applications and Toxicities of Gallium Compounds. *Int. J. Environ. Res. Public Health* **2010**, *7*, 2337–2361. [CrossRef]
81. Melnikov, P.; Matos, M.D.F.C.; Malzac, A.; Teixeira, A.R.; De Albuquerque, D.M. Evaluation of in vitro toxicity of hydroxyapatite doped with gallium. *Mater. Lett.* **2019**, *253*, 343–345. [CrossRef]
82. Bartley, J.C.; Reber, E.F. Toxic Effects of Stable Strontium in Young Pigs. *J. Nutr.* **1961**, *75*, 21–28. [CrossRef] [PubMed]
83. Kirrane, B.M.; Nelson, L.S.; Hoffman, R.S. Massive Strontium Ferrite Ingestion without Acute Toxicity. *Basic Clin. Pharmacol. Toxicol.* **2006**, *99*, 358–359. [CrossRef] [PubMed]
84. Hayta, S.B.; Durmuş, K.; Altuntaş, E.E.; Yildiz, E.; Hisarciklıo, M.; Akyol, M.; Durmuş, K.; Yıldız, E.; Hisarcıklıo, M. The reduction in inflammation and impairment in wound healing by using strontium chloride hexahydrate. *Cutan. Ocul. Toxicol.* **2018**, *37*, 24–28. [CrossRef] [PubMed]
85. Jebahi, S.; Oudadesse, H.; Jardak, N.; Khayat, I.; Keskes, H.; Khabir, A.; Rebai, T.; El Feki, H.; El Feki, A. Biological therapy of strontium-substituted bioglass for soft tissue wound-healing: Responses to oxidative stress in ovariectomised rats. *Ann. Pharm. Fr.* **2013**, *71*, 234–242. [CrossRef] [PubMed]
86. Li, S.; Li, L.; Guo, C.; Qin, H.; Yu, X. A promising wound dressing material with excellent cytocompatibility and proangiogenesis action for wound healing: Strontium loaded Silk fibroin/Sodium alginate (SF/SA) blend films. *Int. J. Biol. Macromol.* **2017**, *104*, 969–978. [CrossRef]
87. Gunawardana, D.H.; Lichtenstein, M.; Better, N.; Rosenthal, M. Results of Strontium-89 Therapy in Patients with Prostate Cancer Resistant to Chemotherapy. *Clin. Nucl. Med.* **2004**, *29*, 81–85. [CrossRef]
88. Nielsen, S.P. The biological role of strontium. *Bone* **2004**, *35*, 583–588. [CrossRef]
89. Cabrera, W.E.; Schrooten, I.; De Broe, M.E.; D'Haese, P.C. Strontium and Bone. *J. Bone Miner. Res.* **1999**, *14*, 661–668. [CrossRef]
90. Buehler, J.; Chappuis, P.; Saffar, J.-L.; Tsouderos, Y.; Vignery, A. Strontium ranelate inhibits bone resorption while maintaining bone formation in alveolar bone in monkeys (*Macaca fascicularis*). *Bone* **2001**, *29*, 176–179. [CrossRef]
91. Sánchez-Espejo, R.; Cerezo, P.; Aguzzi, C.; Galindo, A.L.; Machado, J.; Viseras, C. Physicochemical and in vitro cation release relevance of therapeutic muds "maturation". *Appl. Clay Sci.* **2015**, *116*, 1–7. [CrossRef]
92. Adeleye, S.A.; Clay, P.G.; Oladipo, M.O.A. Sorption of caesium, strontium and europium ions on clay minerals. *J. Mater. Sci.* **1994**, *29*, 954–958. [CrossRef]
93. Missana, T.; Garcia-Gutierrez, M.; Alonso, U. Sorption of strontium onto illite/smectite mixed clays. *Phys. Chem. Earth Parts A B C* **2008**, *33*, S156–S162. [CrossRef]
94. Vengris, T.; Binkien, R.; Sveikauskait, A. Nickel, copper and zinc removal from waste water by a modified clay sorbent. *Appl. Clay Sci.* **2001**, *18*, 183–190. [CrossRef]
95. Sun, W.; Selim, H.M. Kinetics of Molybdenum Adsorption and Desorption in Soils. *J. Environ. Qual.* **2018**, *47*, 504–512. [CrossRef] [PubMed]
96. Mousa, M.; Evans, N.D.; Oreffo, R.O.C.; Dawson, J.I. Clay nanoparticles for regenerative medicine and biomaterial design: A review of clay bioactivity. *Biomaterials* **2018**, *159*, 204–214. [CrossRef] [PubMed]
97. Salcedo-Bellido, I.; Sandri, G.; Aguzzi, C.; Bonferoni, C.; Cerezo, P.; Sánchez-Espejo, R.; Viseras, C.; Bonferoni, M.C. Intestinal permeability of oxytetracycline from chitosan-montmorillonite nanocomposites. *Colloids Surf. B Biointerfaces* **2014**, *117*, 441–448. [CrossRef] [PubMed]

98. Salcedo, I.; Aguzzi, C.; Sandri, G.; Bonferoni, M.C.; Mori, M.; Cerezo, P.; Sánchez, R.; Viseras, C.; Caramella, C. In vitro biocompatibility and mucoadhesion of montmorillonite chitosan nanocomposite: A new drug delivery. *Appl. Clay Sci.* **2012**, *55*, 131–137. [CrossRef]
99. Tenci, M.; Rossi, S.; Aguzzi, C.; Carazo, E.; Sandri, G.; Bonferoni, M.C.; Grisoli, P.; Viseras, C.; Caramella, C.; Ferrari, F. Carvacrol/clay hybrids loaded into in situ gelling films. *Int. J. Pharm.* **2017**, *531*, 676–688. [CrossRef]
100. Carazo, E.; Sandri, G.; Cerezo, P.; Lanni, C.; Ferrari, F.; Bonferoni, C.; Viseras, C.; Aguzzi, C.; Ianni, C. Halloysite nanotubes as tools to improve the actual challenge of fixed doses combinations in tuberculosis treatment. *J. Biomed. Mater. Res. Part A* **2019**, *107*, 1513–1521. [CrossRef]
101. Cervini-Silva, J.; Ramírez-Apan, M.T.; Kaufhold, S.; Ufer, K.; Palacios, E.; Montoya, A. Role of bentonite clays on cell growth. *Chemosphere* **2016**, *149*, 57–61. [CrossRef]
102. Wang, S.; Zhao, Y.; Luo, Y.; Wang, S.; Shen, M.; Tomás, H.; Zhu, M.; Shi, X. Attapulgite-doped electrospun poly (lactic-co-glycolic acid) nanofibers enable enhanced osteogenic differentiation of human mesenchymal stem cells. *RSC Adv.* **2015**, *5*, 2383–2391. [CrossRef]
103. Zhang, L.-L.; Du, J.; Tang, C.-S.; Jin, H.; Huang, Y. Inhibitory Effects of Sulfur Dioxide on Rat Myocardial Fibroblast Proliferation and Migration. *Chin. Med. J.* **2018**, *131*, 1715–1723. [CrossRef] [PubMed]
104. Lansdown, A.B.G. Physiological and Toxicological Changes in the Skin Resulting from the Action and Interaction of Metal Ions. *Crit. Rev. Toxicol.* **1995**, *25*, 397–462. [CrossRef]
105. Huang, J.-S.; Mukherjee, J.J.; Chung, T.; Crilly, K.S.; Kiss, Z. Extracellular calcium stimulates DNA synthesis in synergism with zinc, insulin and insulin-like growth factor I in fibroblasts. *Eur. J. Biochem.* **1999**, *266*, 943–951. [CrossRef]
106. O'Dell, B.L.; Browning, J.D. Zinc Deprivation Impairs Growth Factor-Stimulated Calcium Influx into Murine 3T3 cells Associated with Decreased Cell Proliferation. *J. Nutr.* **2011**, *141*, 1036–1040. [CrossRef] [PubMed]
107. O'Dell, B.L.; Browning, J.D. Impaired Calcium Entry into Cells Is Associated with Pathological Signs of Zinc Deficiency. *Adv. Nutr.* **2013**, *4*, 287–293. [CrossRef]
108. Grzesiak, J.J.; Pierschbacher, M.D. Shifts in the concentrations of magnesium and calcium in early porcine and rat wound fluids activate the cell migratory response. *J. Clin. Investig.* **1995**, *95*, 227–233. [CrossRef]

12

Influence of Chitin Source and Polymorphism on Powder Compression and Compaction: Application in Drug Delivery

Linda Al-Hmoud [1], Deeb Abu Fara [1,*], Iyad Rashid [2], Babur Z. Chowdhry [3] and Adnan A. Badwan [2]

1. Chemical Engineering Department, School of Engineering, University of Jordan, Amman 11942, Jordan; l.alhmoud@ju.edu.jo
2. Research and Innovation Centre, The Jordanian Pharmaceutical Manufacturing Company (JPM), P.O. Box 94, Naor 11710, Jordan; irashid@jpm.com.jo (I.R.); adnanbadwan@gmail.com (A.A.B.)
3. School of Science, Faculty of Engineering & Science, University of Greenwich, Medway Campus, Chatham Maritime, Kent ME4 4TB, UK; b.z.chowdhry@greenwich.ac.uk

* Correspondence: abufara@ju.edu.jo

Academic Editor: Leonard Ionut Atanase

Abstract: The objective of the research reported herein is to compare the compaction properties of three different chitin extracts from the organisms most used in the seafood industry; namely crabs, shrimps and squids. The foregoing is examined in relation to their polymorphic forms as well as compression and compaction behavior. Chitin extracted from crabs and shrimps exhibits the α-polymorphic form whilst chitin extracted from squid pins displays a β-polymorphic form. These polymorphs were characterized using FTIR, X-ray powder diffraction and scanning electron microscopy. Pore diameter and volume differ between the two polymorphic powder forms. The β form is smaller in pore diameter and volume. Scanning electron microscopy of the two polymorphic forms shows clear variation in the arrangement of chitin layers such that the α form appears more condensed due to the anti-parallel arrangement of the polymer chains. True, bulk and tapped densities of these polymorphs and their mixtures indicated poor flowability. Nevertheless, compression and compaction properties obtained by applying Heckle and Kawakita analyses indicated that both polymorphs are able to be compacted with differences in the extent of compaction. Chitin compacts, regardless of their origin, showed a very high crushing strength with very fast dissolution which makes them suitable for use as fast mouth dissolving tablets. Moreover, when different chitin powders are granulated with two model drugs, i.e., metronidazole and spiramycin they yielded high crushing strength and their dissolution profiles were in accordance with compendial requirements. It is concluded that the source of chitin extraction is as important as the polymorphic form when compression and compaction of chitin powders is carried out.

Keywords: chitin; polymorphs; chitin sources; chitin characterization; disintegration; dissolution; crushing strength; compression analysis

---

1. Introduction

Chitin (CH; poly-β-(1,4)-*N*-acetyl glucosamine) occurs in the exoskeletons of crustaceans, insects and the cell walls of algae and fungi. CH has a protective and supporting function; it is responsible for the rigidity of the exoskeletons of insects and crustacean, and its presence in the cell walls of fungi and algae facilitates movement [1]. Currently, there are no synthetic methods for preparing CH. As a result, methods to obtain CH are dependent on extraction from crustaceans and algae. Usually, these methods are carried out in the following sequence: deproteinization, demineralization and discoloration [2]. The methods of preparation, as well as physical and chemical characterization of CH, are the subject of an extensive review by Daraghmah et al. [1].

Usually, CH exists in different organisms in its "complexed" forms with proteins, carbohydrates, or lipids. This means that CH, in order to interact with other chemical functional groups in the tissues of organisms, must have free functional binding groups. This is clear evidence that CH must have some deacetylated domains which means it cannot be isolated in pure form. Consequently, purification of CH involves freeing this insoluble material from various debris and other active matter such as deacetylated derivatives; namely, chitosan (CHS) and glucosamine. It seems that there is no clear demarcation between extraction and purification of CH which is therefore obtained with different molecular weights ranging from hundreds to thousands of kDa. Regardless of variations in molecular weight, CH can occur in three distinct existing polymorphic forms: α, β and γ. CH polymer chains in the α polymorph are aligned in an anti-parallel fashion, whilst in β polymorphs the alignment occurs in parallel. In the γ form the CH polymer chains are arranged in a pattern whereby two parallel chains are in one direction whilst the third is in the opposite direction [1]. Whether or not the anatomical variation of CH in a particular organism affects the mechanical properties of extracted CH is still the subject of active research.

CH is a polymer which is insoluble in water and other conventional solvents. It has a structure deprived of active functional groups. This leaves the CH surface without any reactive functional groups with no ability to react with any chemical moieties; thus, it is chemically inert. In addition, its lack of absorption in the human body allows it to be considered as a pharmacologically inert material. This means it is an ideal material to be used as a pharmaceutical excipient from both a chemical and pharmacological perspective [3,4]. Furthermore, CH is classified as grass in the FDA classification for materials safety usage [5]. This unique characteristic keeps the door open for future use as a pharmaceutical excipient particularly in liquid and solid dosage forms. The challenge in utilizing CH in solid pharmaceutical preparations is its powder flow and mechanical characteristics, including compaction and compression [6].

It may be advantageous to highlight the similarity of CH with the most popular excipient in pharmaceutical solid dosage form preparations, i.e., cellulose and its derivatives such as micro crystalline cellulose (MCC) [7]. MCC shares with CH its β-(1,4) glycosidic bond, and its relative chemical and pharmacological inertness. Researchers in the CH field are attempting to emulate and test if the same techniques which have been successfully used to modify MCC can be applied in the field of CH research, particularly in solid pharmaceutical dosage form preparations [8,9].

It is well known that, like MCC, CH and CHS powder flow properties suffer from low bulk density. This causes unsmooth flow which is attributed to the fibrous nature of these natural polymers [6,10]. Attempts to alleviate this drawback have been tested by adding silicon dioxide to CH and CHS powders [11,12]. The addition of silicon dioxide facilitates smooth flow in tableting machines. Furthermore, combining CH/CHS with Avicel PH201, starch 1500, calcium carbonate or gelatin have been tested and were found to dramatically improve the flow behavior of the composite powders [13–15]. The improvement in flow properties has encouraged novel applications of these composites in producing pharmaceutical solid dosage forms excipients, especially as direct compression excipients. It is worth mentioning that various attempts to utilize CH as a novel solid drug delivery system were carried out by Daraghmeh et.al. [16], whereby CH was co-processed with mannitol to produce orodispersible tablets able to disintegrate in the mouth within a few seconds. Furthermore, CH was formulated, by Gana et.al. [17], with cephalosporins and metal silicates in order to obtain an insight into the effect of pH on the CH surface and its influence on drug stability. Abu Fara et al. [8] used roller compaction to improve CH powder flow qualities and to make its compression and compaction characteristics compatible for use in industrial pharmaceutical machines. Additionally, there are some on-going trials to extend the use of CH and CHS as excipients in a similar method followed in improving MCC powder flow using spray drying [6,18]. Such studies, show that

CH is a suitable solid pharmaceutical excipient. As a result, it can be concluded that CH powder modification is essential in order to commercialize this novel excipient.

Natural polymers usually contain crystalline and amorphous domains in their structure. The balance between these two components controls the powder flow behavior. It has been reported that during the compaction of MCC, its crystalline domains are responsible for fragmentation while its amorphous domains are responsible for polymer plasticity, which induces bonding [7]. This is confirmed in the case of lactose, whereby amorphous lactose offers better compactibility than the crystalline form [19,20]. Accordingly, it seems that an amorphous powder is more compactable but the bulk density is usually lower than the crystalline material. Consequently, studying the impact of the crystalline-amorphous balance on powder flow is a pre-requisite to its industrial use. However, a review of the scientific literature does not show if CH polymorphs differ in their response towards compression and compaction.

CH has diverse functions in different tissues in an organism; e.g., the CH in the lining of the gastrointestinal tract in some organisms is more flexible to suite its functional role and has more elasticity than exoskeleton CH, which is a harder material. Such functionality raises the question whether CH polymorphs behave in a similar manner when compressed, or does the functional use dictate their mechanical strength, as expressed in different tissues of organism? As sea food remains from industrial packaging contain a mixture of CH with various origins, it would be interesting to compare extracted CH from the most utilized CH sources, namely shrimp, crab and squid. These organisms are known to have α (shrimp and crab) and β (squid) CH polymorphs. Such polymorphs can be differentiated by their powder X-ray diffraction patterns. It would be interesting to test each polymorph individually and discern the differences in their compaction and compression behavior.

The present work focuses on pharmaceutical powder compression and compaction properties of CH extracted from the most widely used sea food organisms namely crabs, shrimps, and squids. The influence of variation in α and β CH polymorphic forms due to CH extraction source on compression and compaction is explored. Hence it may be possible to ascertain whether CH sources must be processed separately or collectively prior to their extraction.

2. Results

2.1. Bulk, Tapped Density and True Density

The bulk, tapped, and true densities of CH from different sources, as well as of their mixtures (Sh9Sq1, Sh7Sq3, and Sh5Sq5) are presented in Table 1. Crab (CH-Cr) and shrimp (CH-Sh) CHs have much higher bulk and tapped densities than squid CH (CH-Sq).

Table 1. True, bulk and tapped densities, HR, and CI of CHs from different sources and their mixtures.

Sample *	Bulk Density (kg/m^3)	Tapped Density (kg/m^3)	True Density (kg/m^3)	HR	CI
CH-Cr	332 ± 9	531 ± 9	1400 ± 30	1.60 ± 0.04	60 ± 4
CH-Sh	280 ± 6	401 ± 6	1700 ± 40	1.43 ± 0.02	43 ± 2
CH-Sq	190 ± 4	338 ± 4	1200 ± 20	1.78 ± 0.03	78 ± 3
CH-Sh9Sq1	255 ± 6	402 ± 6	1650 ± 35	1.58 ± 0.03	58 ± 3
CH-Sh7Sq3	252 ± 6	403 ± 6	1550 ± 30	1.60 ± 0.03	60 ± 3
CH-Sh5Sq5	242 ± 5	403 ± 5	1450 ± 25	1.67 ± 0.02	67 ± 2

* CH-Cr = crab CH, CH-Sh = shrimp CH, CH-Sq = squid CH, CH-Sh9Sq1 = mixture of 90 wt% shrimp CH and 10 wt% squidCH, CH-Sh7Sq3 = mixture of 70 wt% shrimpCH and 30 wt% squid CH, CH-Sh9Sq1 = mixture of 50 wt% shrimp CH and 50 wt% squid CH.

To study the effect of mixing CH from different sources, CH-Sh was chosen as representative of α-CH, and mixed with CH-Sq (β-CH) in different compositions, as shown in Table 1. With respect to bulk and tapped densities, such mixtures manifested intermediate values between the low (CH-Sq) and high (CH-Sh) bulk and tapped densities.

In comparing the powder flowability of CH from different sources, the Carr index (CI) and Hausner ratio (HR) were determined [21]. Flowability results, as illustrated in Table 1, indicate that CH from different sources, as well as their mixtures, exhibit extremely poor flowability. Flow interpretation criteria based on HR and CI is given in the literature [21]. As for densities, the mixtures manifested intermediate HR and CI values between the low and high values presented by CH-Sh and CH-Sq, respectively.

2.2. Water Content

The water content of CH from different sources are presented in Table 2. The water content of CH-Cr and CH-Sh is almost half that of CH-Sq.

Table 2. Water content of CH extracted from different sources.

Sample	CH-Cr	CH-Sh	CH-Sq
Water content (wt %)	5.44 ± 0.06	4.84 ± 0.05	8.65 ± 0.06

2.3. Porosity of Powders

The porosity parameters of the three CH powder samples are shown in Table 3. The pore volume of crab and shrimp CHs are of similar values, whereas that of squid CH is ~20% less. On the other hand, crab CH has the largest pore diameter and squid CH has the smallest.

Table 3. Porosity parameters for CH-Cr, CH-Sh, and CH-Sq.

Sample	Pore Volume (cm^3/g)	Average Pore Diameter (nm)
CH-Cr	$(7.308 \pm 0.003) \times 10^{-3}$	5.68 ± 0.01
CH-Sh	$(6.977 \pm 0.003) \times 10^{-3}$	4.32 ± 0.01
CH-Sq	$(5.353 \pm 0.002) \times 10^{-3}$	3.70 ± 0.01

2.4. FTIR

The Fourier-transform infrared (FT-IR) spectra of α-CH (CH-Cr and CH-Sh) and β-CH (CH-Sq) are shown in Figure 1. For α-CH, the amide I band is split at about 1650 and 1620 cm^{-1} (Figure 1a,b), whereas it is a single sharp band at about 1657 cm^{-1} for β-CH (Figure 1c). The amide II band appears at about 1555 and 1559 cm^{-1} for α- and β-CH, respectively. Both polymorphs show strong absorption bands in the 3100–3285 cm^{-1} region which correspond to the N–H group. Bands in the 2840–2960 cm^{-1} region are due to CH, CH_2, and CH_3 in both CH polymorphs [1].

2.5. X-ray Powder Diffraction (XRPD) Analysis

The XRPD profiles of CH from different sources are presented in Figure 2. The XRPD patterns of crab (CH-Cr) and shrimp CH (CH-Sh) show four sharp crystalline reflections indicative of α-CH at $2\theta = 9.3, 19.1, 20.6$, and 23.2°.

The XRPD pattern of squid CH (CH-Sq) shows two broad crystalline peaks at 8.7 and 19.8° which indicates that squid CH is of the β-CH type. The crystal size of CH-Cr and CH-Sh is almost the same. Squid CH has a smaller crystal size than crab and shrimp as its pattern peaks at 9° and 19° are much wider for CH-Sq than the corresponding ones for CH-Cr and CH-Sh. Table 4 shows the crystalline index (I_{CR}) of the three CH samples. These results indicate that α-CH has a more crystalline structure because of its inter-sheet and intra-sheet structure [22,23]. Crystalline index (I_{CR}) is used to estimate the degree of deacetylation (DDA) of CH using a method reported by Zhang et al. [24]. DDA results presented in Table 4 shows that α-CHs (CH-Cr and CH-Sh) is less deacetylated than β-CH (CH-Sq), which conforms with findings reported in the literature [1,2,22].

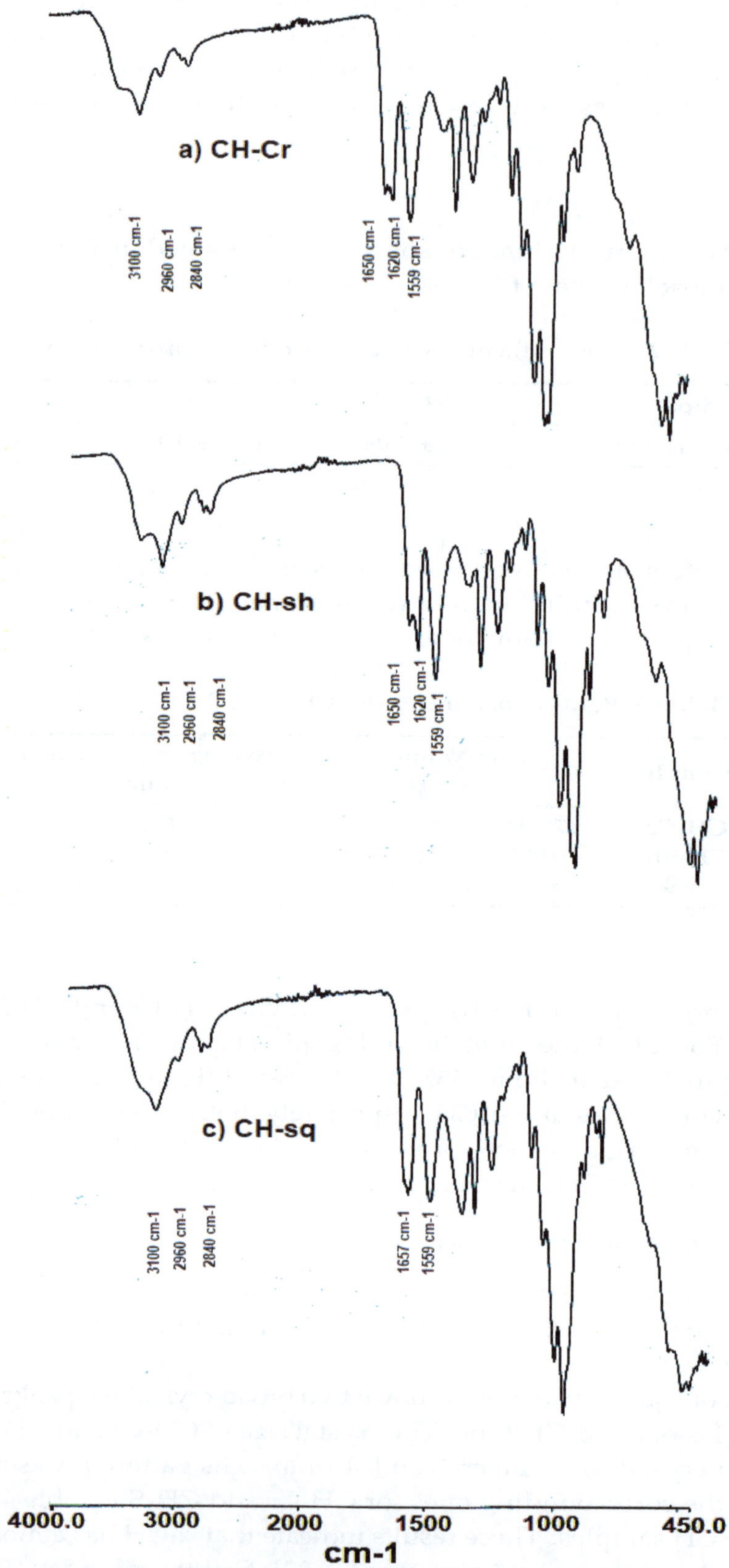

Figure 1. FTIR spectra of (**a**) CH-Cr, (**b**) CH-Sh (**b**), and (**c**) CH-Sq.

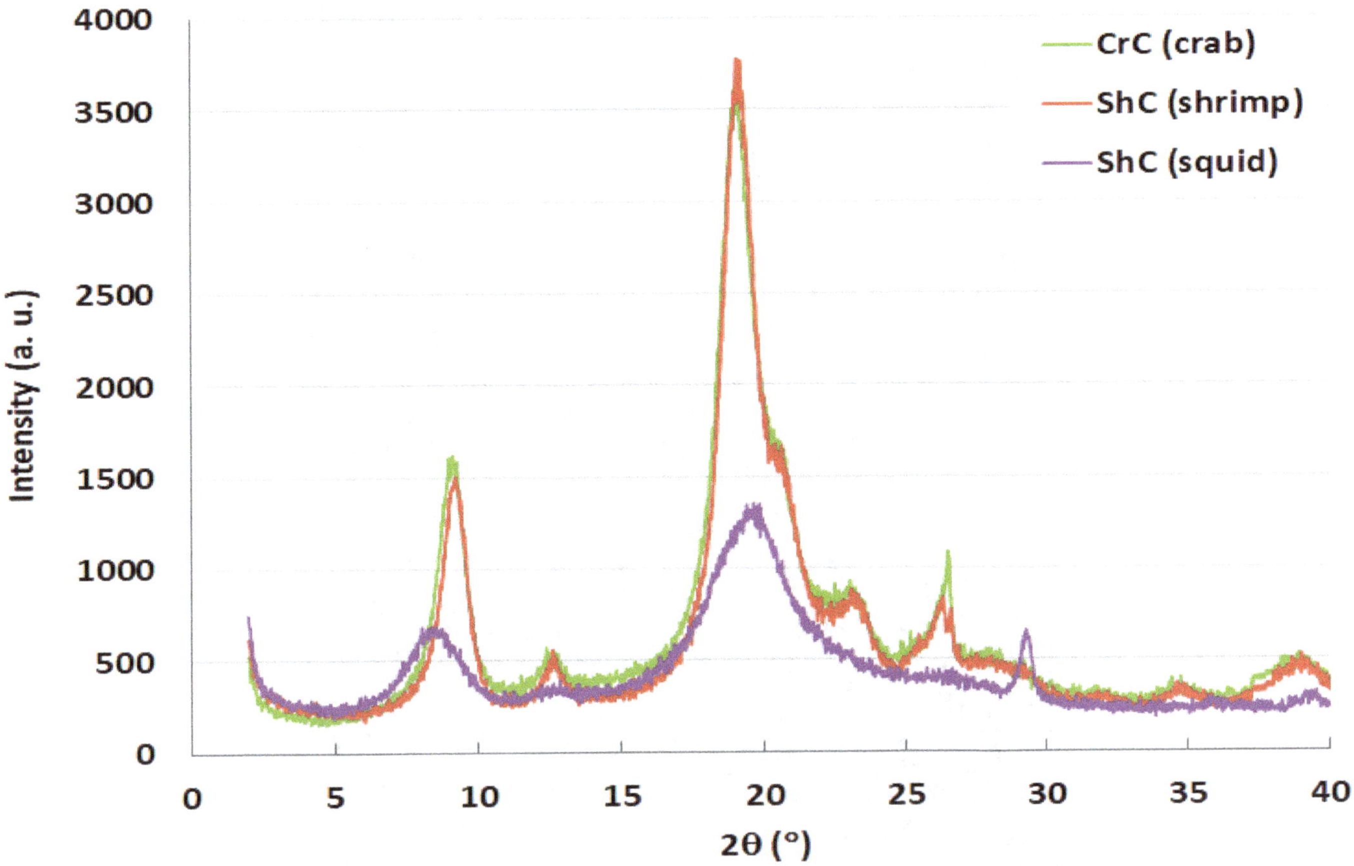

Figure 2. X-ray powder diffraction (XRPD) patterns of CH-Cr, CH-Sh, and CH-Sq CH.

Table 4. Crystalline index (I_{CR}) and degree of deacetylation (DDA) of CH extracted from different sources.

Sample	CH-Cr	CH-Sh	CH-Sq
I_{CR} (%)	84.3 ± 0.1	85.2 ± 0.1	72.1 ± 0.2
DDA (%)	26.1 ± 0.6	24.9 ± 0.5	42.3 ± 0.7

2.6. Scanning Electron Microscope (SEM)

SEM was used to highlight the contribution of micro-irregularities to powder physical properties by visualizing the surface of CH particles from different sources. Figures 3–5 present SEM images of crab (CH-Cr), shrimp (CH-Sh), and squid (CH-Sq) CHs at a magnification of 8000×, 16,000×, and 30,000×, respectively. Figure 6 presents SEM images with measurement of fibers thicknesses of shrimp (CH-Sh) CH at 16,000× and 60,000× magnifications, and of squid (CH-Sq) CH at 5000× magnification.

At 8000× magnification (Figure 3) it is difficult to see any significant difference amongst the different CH samples. At 16,000× magnification (Figure 4) it can be noticed that squid chitin fibers are more organized than crab and shrimp CH samples. At 30,000× magnification (Figure 5) shrimp CH showed two types of fibers; one forming the layers, and the other connecting the layers. Squid CH layers have no connecting fibers.

The data in Figure 6 shows that the fibers forming shrimp CH layers have a thickness of ~200 nm (Figure 6a), where the layers are about 1 µm apart, and the fibers connecting them have a thickness of 35–45 nm (Figure 6b). On the other hand, squid chitin layers are around 60 nm apart and no connecting fibers can be observed at ×50,000 magnification (Figure 6c).

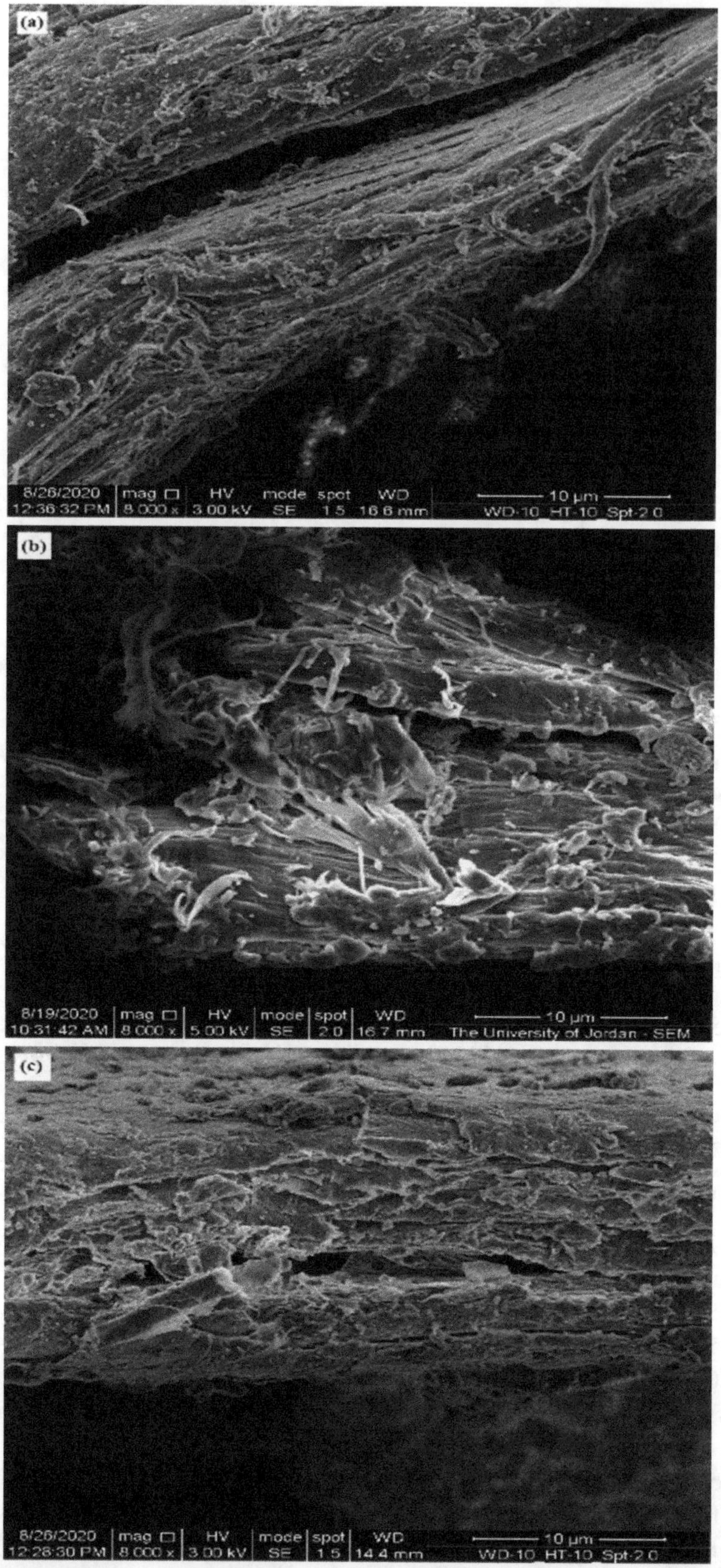

Figure 3. SEM image of (**a**) crab (CH-Cr), (**b**) shrimp (CH-Sh), and (**c**) squid (CH-Sq) CHs at 8000× magnification.

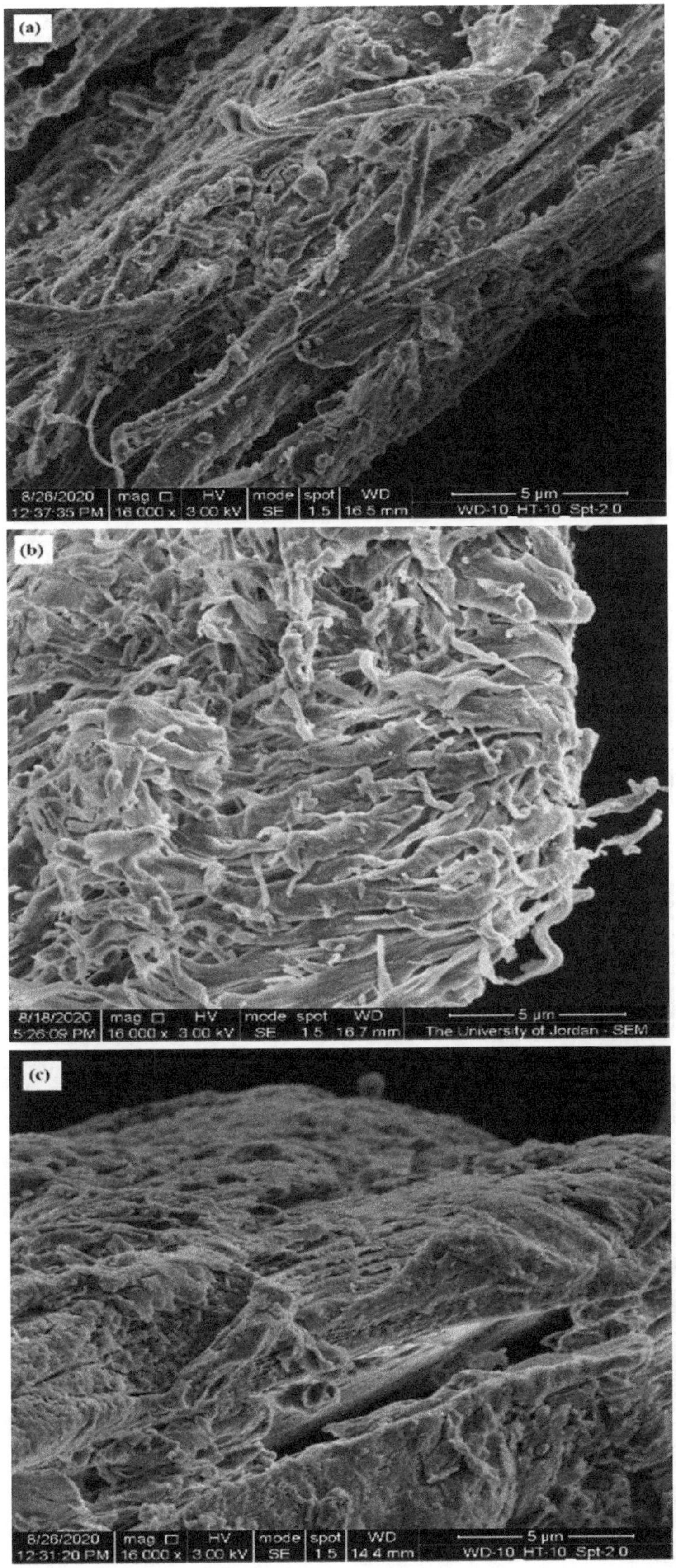

Figure 4. SEM image of (**a**) crab (CH-Cr), (**b**) shrimp (CH-Sh), and (**c**) squid (CH-Sq) CHs at 16,000× magnification.

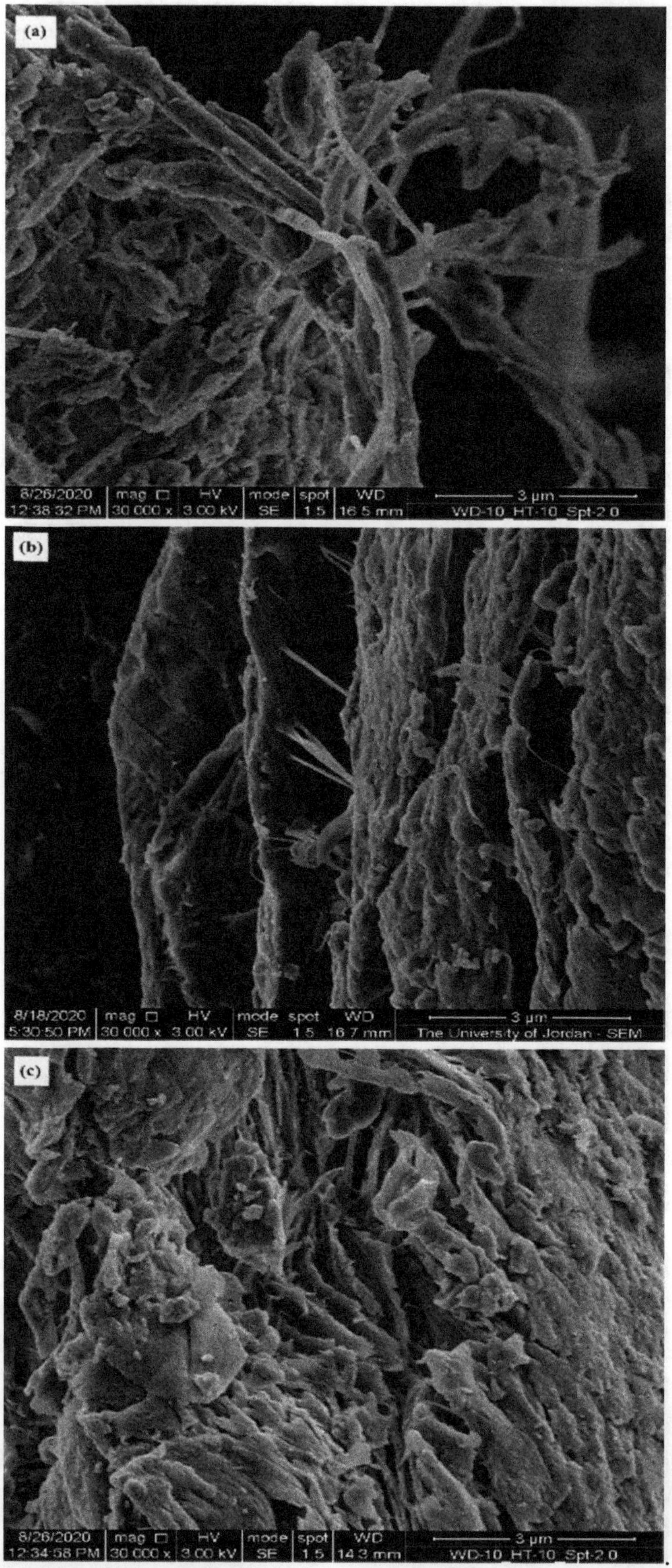

Figure 5. SEM image of (**a**) crab (CH-Cr), (**b**) shrimp (CH-Sh), and (**c**) squid (CH-Sq) CHs at 30,000× magnification.

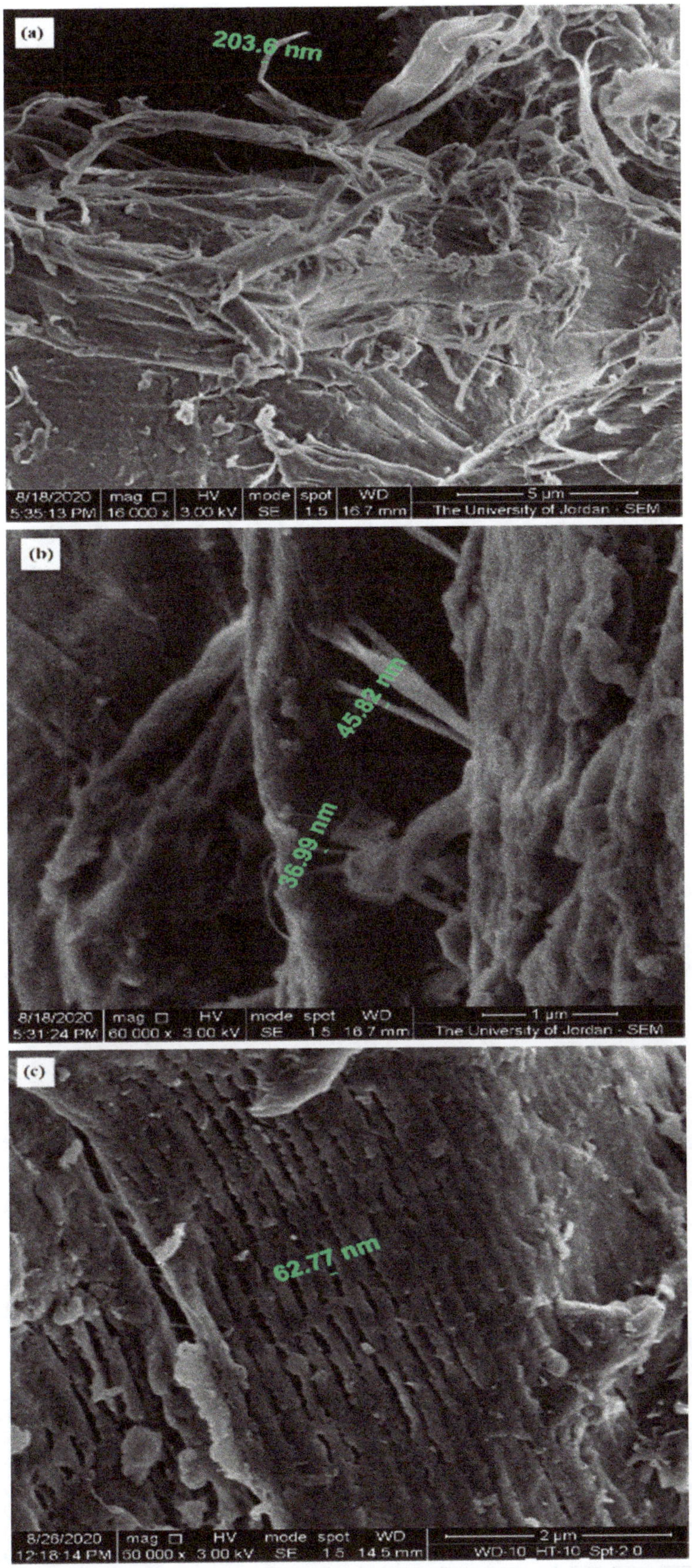

Figure 6. SEM image with measurement of fiber thickness of (**a**) shrimp (CH-Sh) CH at 16,000× magnification, (**b**) shrimp (CH-Sh) CH at 60,000× magnification, and (**c**) squid (CH-Sq) CH at 50,000× magnification.

2.7. Compression Analysis

The three main parameters (a, P_k and ab) obtained via Kawakita analysis (as illustrated in Section 4.2.7. Compression Analysis) were analyzed in an attempt to interpret the compression behavior of the three samples of CH and their mixtures. The data in Figure 7 shows the Kawakita plots of CH-Cr, CH-Sh, and CH-Sq CHs, and Figure 8 shows the Kawakita plots of shrimp/squid CH mixtures; CH-Sh9Sq1, CH-Sh7Sq3, and CH-Sh5Sq5. Table 5 presents the values of Kawakita parameters for the different chitin types and their mixtures.

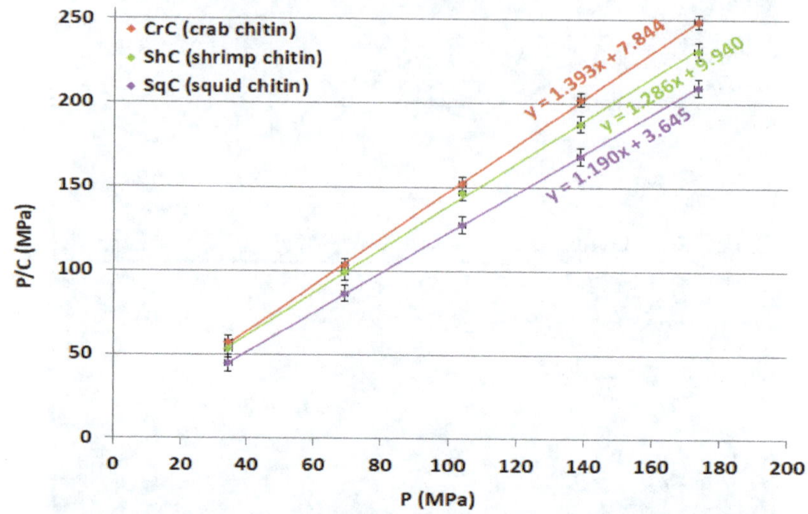

Figure 7. Kawakita plots of crab (CH-Cr), shrimp (CH-Sh), and squid (CH-Sq) CHs.

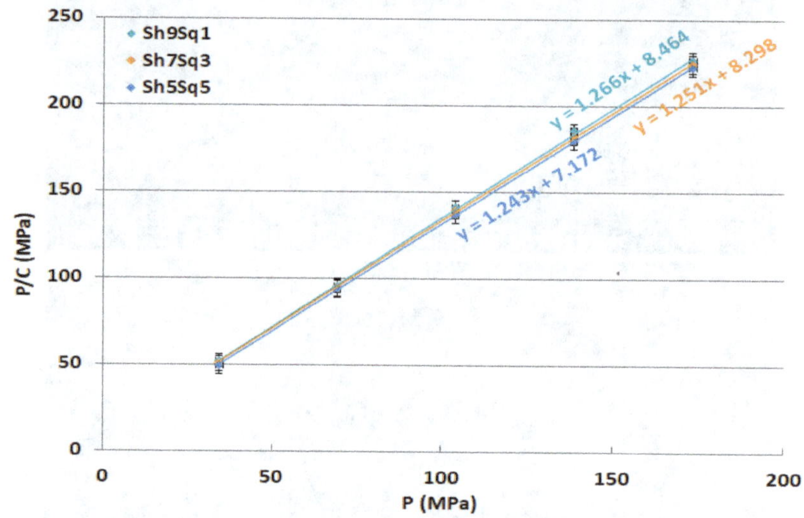

Figure 8. Kawakita plots of CH-Sh9Sq1, CH-Sh7Sq3, and CH-Sh5Sq5 CH mixtures.

Table 5. Kawakita parameters of CH-Cr, CH-Sh, and CH-Sq and their mixtures.

Sample	Slope	Intercept (MPa)	a = 1/Slope	b = Slope/Intercept (1/MPa)	ab (1/MPa)	P_K = 1/b (MPa)
CH-Cr	1.393 ± 0.066	7.84 ± 0.36	0.7179	0.178	0.127	5.63
CH-Sh	1.286 ± 0.061	9.94 ± 0.46	0.7778	0.129	0.101	7.73
CH-Sq	1.190 ± 0.056	3.65 ± 0.17	0.8406	0.326	0.274	3.06
CH-Sh9Sq1	1.266 ± 0.060	8.46 ± 0.39	0.7899	0.150	0.118	6.68
CH-Sh7Sq3	1.251 ± 0.059	8.30 ± 0.38	0.7997	0.151	0.121	6.64
CH-Sh5Sq5	1.243 ± 0.059	7.17 ± 0.33	0.8046	0.173	0.139	5.77

The maximum volume reduction that can be attained (a) illustrates that CH-Cr has the lowest a value with CH-Sq having the highest volume reduction when a compression force is applied.

In addition, the results of the three mixtures show that the volume reduction value increases with increasing percentage of squid CH in the mixture.

P_K, which represents the pressure needed to reduce the value of (a) to half its initial value, is the most important Kawakita parameter to be tested. This is because it represents how hard the CH granules are, and therefore their ability to be used in direct compression applications. Table 5 shows that the P_K value of shrimp CH (CH-Sh) is the highest among the three types of CH. P_K value of mixture containing shrimp and squid CHs at different fractional content; CH-Sh9Sq1, CH-Sh7Sq3, and CH-Sh5Sq5, decreases with increasing squid CH fraction.

The last Kawakita parameter used in this work to describe the compression behavior is ab. This parameter gives an indication of the degree of rearrangement of powder particles. As Table 6 shows, squid CH (CH-Sq) has the highest the extent of particle rearrangement (ab) upon compression. The value of ab is the lowest for shrimp CH (CH-Sh). The data in Table 6 also indicates that mixtures containing shrimp and squid CHs in different fractions; CH-Sh9Sq1, CH-Sh7Sq3, and CH-Sh5Sq5, show ab values that increase with increasing squid fraction of CH.

Table 6. Heckel parameters of CH-Cr, CH-Sh, and CH-Sq and their mixtures.

Sample	Slope (K)	Intercept (A)	P_Y(MPa)=1/K
CH-Cr	6.71×10^{-3}	0.7336	149
CH-Sh	2.69×10^{-3}	0.5739	372
CH-Sq	1.08×10^{-2}	0.8627	93
CH-Sh9Sq1	3.20×10^{-3}	0.5782	306
CH-Sh7Sq3	4.40×10^{-3}	0.6051	227
CH-Sh5Sq5	4.94×10^{-3}	0.6868	202

Compression analysis was further examined using the empirical Heckel model of compression analysis. In this model, the yield pressure (P_Y) represents a critical outcome whereby it reflects the type and extent of deformation, i.e., plastic/elastic or brittle-fracture. The data in Table 6 and Figure 9 illustrates the yield pressure values for all tested powders. Results show that P_Y ranking of pure CHs follows the order: shrimp chitin > crab chitin > squid CH. Adding squid CH to shrimp CH reduced the P_Y value, and the more squid CH content in the mixture, the lower its P_Y value: CH-Sh9Sq1 > CH-Sh7Sq3 > CH-Sh5Sq5.

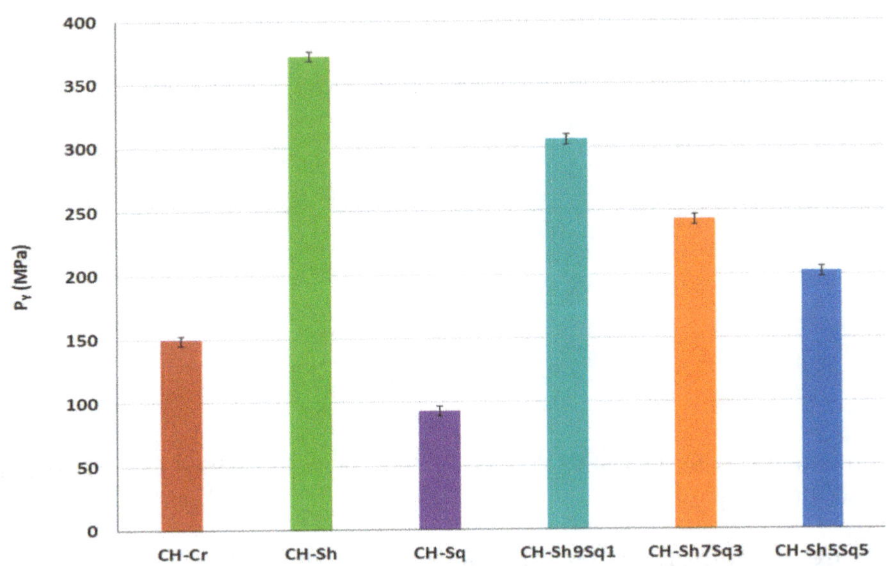

Figure 9. Heckel parameter (P_Y) for CH-Cr, CH-Sh, and CH-Sq and their mixtures.

2.8. *Work of Compression*

When powders of different types are compressed using the GTP, the instrument displays the force displacement curve during the descending/compression and decompression of the powders. The work of compression (W_C), which is the area under the compression curves of the of the F-D profiles, is shown in Figures 10 and 11. W_C values were calculated at each compression force used. The results shown in Figure 10 indicate that at all loads, the W_C of shrimp CH (CH-Sh) > W_C of crab CH (CH-Cr) > W_C of squid CH (CH-Sq).

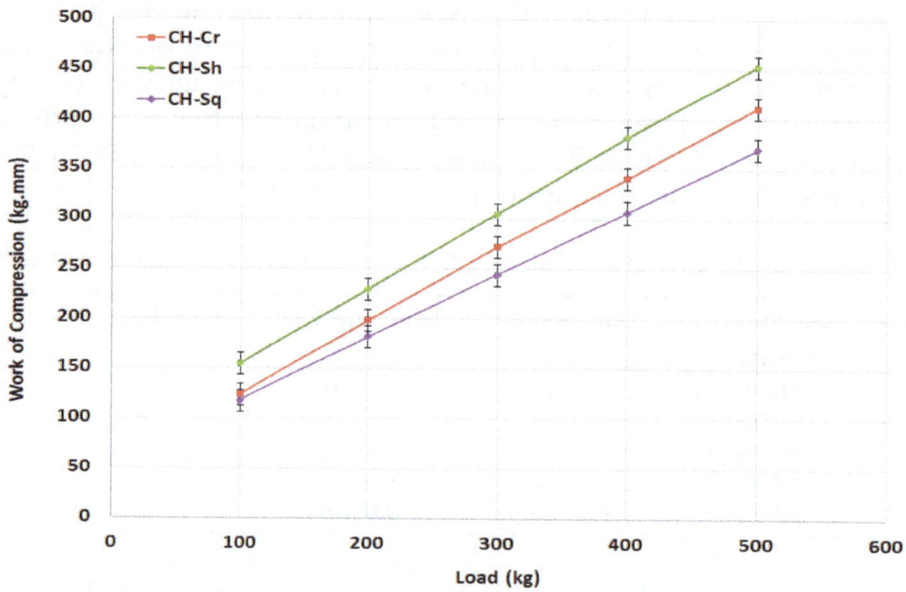

Figure 10. Compression work for CH-Cr, CH-Sh, and CH-Sq CHs.

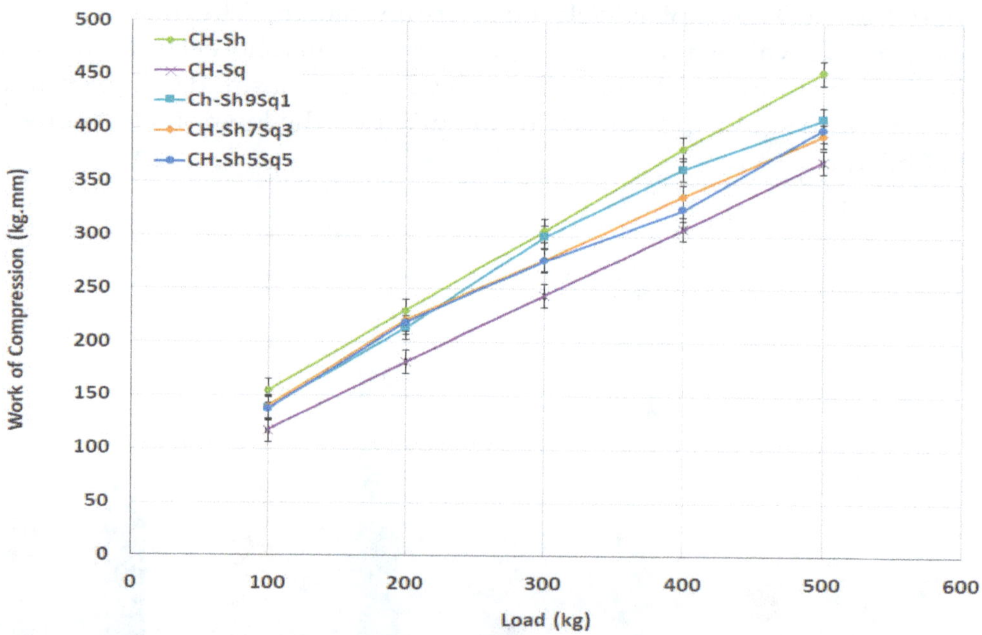

Figure 11. Compression work for CH-Sh9Sq1, CH-Sh7Sq3, and CH-Sh5Sq5 CH mixtures in comparison with pure CH-Sh and CH-Sq.

The data in Figure 11 demonstrates the effect of adding β-CH (CH-Sq) to α-CH (CH-Sh) in different fractional contents. Mixtures containing different amounts of β-CH have W_C values close to each other at low compression loads (100 and 200 kg), while at higher loads W_C decreases with increasing the amount of added CH-Sq.

2.9. Tablet Crushing Strength

Tablet crushing strength for CH from different sources are presented in Table 7. CH-Cr and CH-Sh tablet crushing strength is almost half that of CH-Sq tablet crushing strength. The crushing strength of the mixture is closer in value to that of CH-Sq.

Table 7. Tablet crushing strength.

Sample	CH-Cr	CH-Sh	CH-Sq	CH-Sh9Sq1	CH-Sh7Sq3	CH-Sh5Sq5
Crushing Strength (*N*)	54 ± 2	115 ± 3	310 ± 5	121 ± 3	155 ± 4	195 ± 4

2.10. Tablet Disintegration

All tablets have recorded disintegration times of less than 10 s irrespective of CS source or mixtures comprised thereof.

2.11. Characterization of Metronidazole/Spiramycin Tablets Comprising Drug/CH

Tablet dissolution data are illustrated in Table 8 and in Figures 12 and 13. Figure 12 demonstrates that full drug release of metronidazole/α-CH (crab and shrimp) matrix is achieved within 15 min of dissolution time. This is faster than tablets comprising metronidazole/β-CH (squid) matrix which achieved full drug release within 30 min of dissolution time. Tablets comprising metronidazole/CH mixture (50 wt% shrimp and 50 wt% squid) as well as Rodogyl® tablets also achieved full drug release within 30 min of dissolution time.

Table 8. Time for full drug release for metronidazole® (125 mg) and spiramycin® (0.75 M UI) tablets comprising compacted pure CHs from different sources, and CH mixture (CH-Sh5Sq5) compared to Rodogyl® tablets.

Excipient Used in Tablet Preparation	Metronidazole® Complete Dissolution Time (min)	Spiramycin® Complete Dissolution Time (min)
CH-Cr	15	45
CH-Sh	15	30
CH-Sq	30	45
CH-Sh5Sq5	30	45
Rodogyl®	30	60

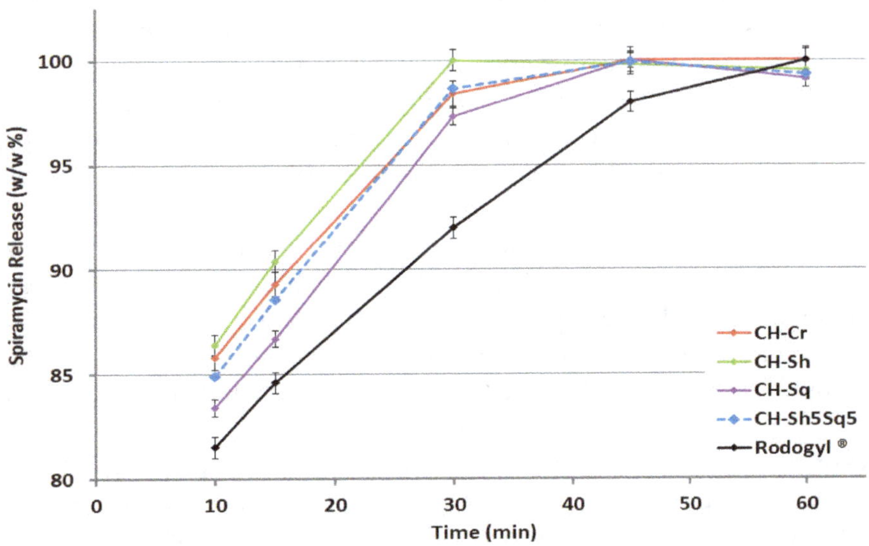

Figure 12. Dissolution profile for metronidazole (200 mg) tablets comprising compacted CHs or CH mixture (CH-Sh5Sq5) compared to Rodogyl® tablets.

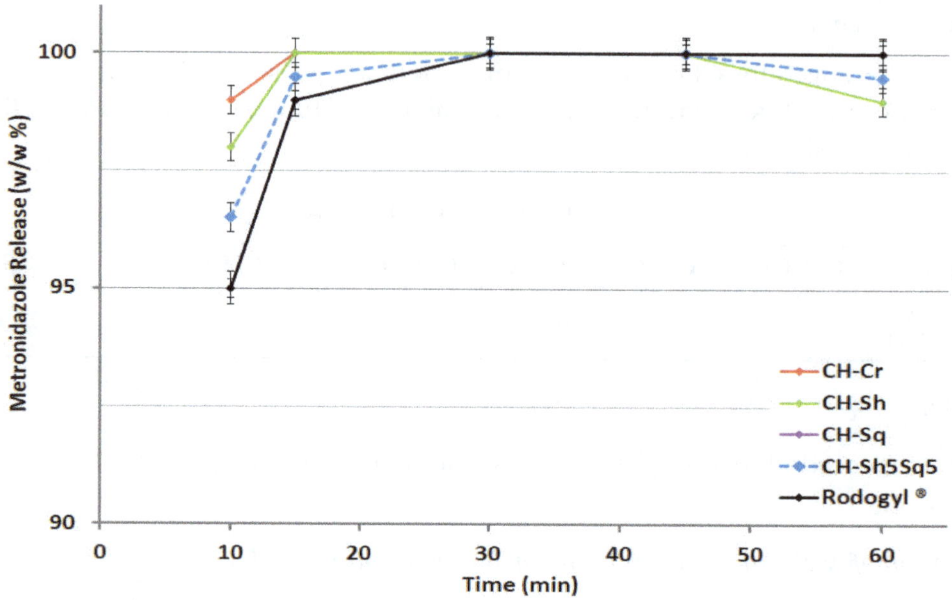

Figure 13. Dissolution profile of spiramycin (0.75 M UI) tablets comprising compacted CHs or CH mixture (CH-Sh5Sq5) compared to Rodogyl® tablets.

Results presented in Figure 13 demonstrates that full drug release of spiramycin/shrimp CH matrix was achieved within 30 min of dissolution time, and within 45 min of dissolution time for the other types of CH, as well as for CH mixtures. This was faster than Rodogyl® tablets which achieved full drug release within 60 min of dissolution time.

3. Discussion

The prime objective of the present investigation was to test CHs extracted from different sources to assess their similarity and suitability for use as a future excipient in pharmaceutical solid dosage form preparations. The final goal is to reach a conclusion whether remains from the sea food packaging industry need to be classified according to their source prior to CH extraction process. This concern becomes evident when one screens the different scientific literature on CH, where there are indications that CH from different sources are chemically similar, but their mechanical properties vary [25].

The strategy followed in this work was to compare CH from crabs and shrimps, both of which belong to α polymorph, in order to find out if the variation in CH source has any influence on the extracted polymer compression and compaction properties. Furthermore, a comparison between α and β-CH polymorphs extracted from squid pins, regarding their compression and compaction behavior, was also conducted. Mixtures of the two polymorphs were also prepared, and their physical and mechanical properties were studied. Whether or not these polymorphic forms could facilitate compaction of two model drugs, namely metronidazole and spiramycin, which are difficult to compress on their own, was tested.

It is well known that shrimps, crabs and squids are the most used organisms in the sea food packaging industry [26]. These organisms differ in their species and their extracted CH is confined to the three well characterized and known polymorphs; α, β and γ. It is essential to first confirm this primary information. The Fourier-transform infrared (FT-IR) spectra of CH-Cr, CH-Sh, and CH-Sq are shown in Figure 1. Distinct vibrational bands appear at a wavelength of 1620–1660 with a distinct split in the band for α-chitin (Figure 1a,b), while there is a single sharp band for β-CH (Figure 1c). This confirms different previous reports on CH of α and β polymorphs [23,27]. Further confirmation of the polymorphic type was carried out using X-ray powder diffraction, Figure 2. The γ polymorph is scarce due to its limited occurrence in the lining of the digestive system of different organisms such as squid. Consequently, the present investigation was limited to a comparison of the compression and compaction behavior of the most commercially available two polymorphs, α and β. Such a comparison helps to clarify if the source of CH extraction causes variation in their related mechanical properties when compacted.

In addition to identifying polymorphic forms of molecules, XRPD has been used as a tool to shed light on the crystallinity and arrangement of CH in different polymer fibers. Figure 2 confirms α polymorph in CH-Cr and CH-Sh, and β polymorph in CH-Sq. The crystalline index, Table 5, shows that the α polymorph is more crystalline than the β polymorph; 84–85% in CH-Cr and CH-Sh, and 73% in CH-Sq. SEM images, Figures 3–6 show the parallel arrangements of β-CH sheets with clear spacing. This is indicative of their ability to hydrate and gel much more than α polymorph [23,27]. Interestingly, the β polymorph shows a smaller pore size and pore volume which may indicate that the value of the parameter a (the capillary water effect) may contribute to its functional strength and flexibility in squid pins. Indeed, the water content determination of CH-Sq shows almost double the value of Ch-Cr and CH-Sh (Table 3). This dramatic variation in water content is an important difference which can be beneficial in the use of CH as excipients for pharmaceutical solid dosage forms. Water content results are consistent with the fact that β-CH (CH-Sq) is more susceptible to intra-crystalline hydration than α-CH (CH-Cr and CH-Sh) due to its lack of intra-sheet hydrogen bonds [23].

Bulk densities of the three types of CH (Table 2) are different although shrimp and crab are similar in polymorphic form. The difference between shrimp and crab CH measured bulk densities may be due to a difference in material arrangements in nature in those living organisms depending on their functional use. Such variation has been previously reported, where extracted CHs from male and female grasshoppers show some differences in CH content and surface morphology [27]. Accordingly, one would expect to observe some variations in CH extracted even from the same species. The higher crab and shrimp chitin bulk densities indicate that these powder samples comprise denser aggregated particles. Such aggregation could be a result of particle-particle adherence which may be attributed to the highly fibrous structure of CH-Cr and CH-Sh, whereas CH-Sq displays a structure which is much less fibrous (Figures 5 and 6). The plain surface of CH-Sq with no fibrous extensions is responsible for the absence of an interlocking structural network, which consequently leads to the formation of aggregated particles in CH-Cr and CH-Sh.

As expected, all types of CH did not provide good flowability as indicated by their HR and CI values (Table 2), which is attributed to their low bulk densities. The foregoing has led, various workers, to suggestion that these powders be treated by roller compaction or slugging before using them as excipients [8]. Thus CH-Sh would be more favorable for tablet compression than CH-Cr and CH-Sq since it has the lowest HR and CI values.

Parameters from Heckle and Kawakita equations indicate that shrimp powder is more resistance to compression than the other two sources. This is reflected in the force required for compression (P_K) which is significantly higher in value than for the other two CH samples (Table 6). Such variation makes the work required for compression higher, as emphasized in the data in Figure 10. Indeed, this is a real indication that differences in CH properties, such as bulk and tapped densities, are reflected in the compression forces required to convert the powders into compacts. The mechanical properties of CH are similar to cellulose derivatives e.g., micro crystalline cellulose (MCC), where reports have shown that various cellulose polymorphs behave differently in response to compaction forces. MCC requires a disintegration agent when used in tablet manufacturing whilst CH powders are self-disintegrating. This is advantageous in terms of the use of CH for pharmaceutical dosage forms which need to be dissolved in the buccal cavity.

The three parameters extracted from the Kawakita equation, namely a, ab, and P_K, are interesting. CH from different sources, which show differences in particle morphology and crystallography, has concurrently shown differences in powder compression behavior. Among the three types, CH-Sq (β-CH) displays the highest volume reduction (a), particle rearrangement (ab), and the lowest compression force (P_K) to reduce the powder bed volume (Table 6). In other words, in order to produce a compact, CH-Sq requires the smallest force to yield the highest volume reduction in comparison with CH-Cr and CH-Sh (α-CHs). This may be attributed to the anti-parallel and parallel arrangement of α-

and β-polymorphs, respectively. As a matter of fact, CH-Cr and CH-Sh responses to compression vary although they belong to the same polymorph. This may be due to variation in the mechanical strength of the extracted materials. Concurrently, examining the results from Heckel analysis (Table 7) CH-Sq is the highest plastically deforming material, it can be stated that compression of the less fibrous and less aggregated material, i.e., CH-Sq, is more mechanically engaged in the deformation of the highly plastic material than the more fibrous one, i.e., CH-Cr and CH-Sh. Such a high extent of deformation shown by CH-Sq contributes to the high reduction of its powder bed volume upon compression compared to CH-Cr and CH-Sh. Moreover, the high extent of deformation of CH-Sq enables the appearance of fresh new surfaces for surface-to-surface contact and bridging [28,29]. Thus, compacts made of CH-Sq have a higher crushing strength than compacts made of CH-Cr and CH-Sh (Table 8).

Although the α-polymorph is more resistant to reduction in size compared to the β-polymorph, such behavior does not hinder both polymorphs from possessing an excellent crushing strength and very short disintegration time. This means direct compression of these individual powders can be utilized in preparing tablets or films which can dissolve in the mouth within seconds liberating the active content. This property can be highly advantageous and utilized in oral dissolving tablets, which are required to dissolve fast but at the same time be composed of a hard compact. The extracted CH polymorphs fit very well for such a function and future research potentially bodes well in this direction. However, due to its fast dissolving characteristics, CH can be used as a disintegrating agent; indeed, this has been previously reported [1,11]. Both polymorphs can be used as direct compression excipients in pharmaceutical formulations, either as whole or partially, and their need for a driving force for compaction is low, allowing ease of use in tableting machines.

Bearing in mind that the work/energy of compression is the product of force and displacement, CH-Sq manifested the lowest energy needed for compression (Figure 10), since it manifested the lowest compression force (or lowest P_K) needed to produce the hardest compacts (Tables 6 and 8). Irrespective of the fact that hard compacts can be made using CH-Sq, a disintegration time of less than one minute, like other CH sources, makes the super-disintegration power of CH independent of tablet hardness.

The dissolution performance of formulations containing CH from different sources was studied and compared with Rodogyl® formulation, which contains a superdisintegrant and a filler with disintegrant action [29] in addition to two drugs: spiramycin and metronidazole. The drug release profile for the two drugs formulated with CH-Cr, CH-Sh, and CH-Sq and the mixture CH-Sh5Sq5 showed that 8.3% CH was sufficient to attain faster and complete drug release compared to Rodogyl®, for both spiramycin and metronidazole (Figures 12 and 13). However, the release of the two drugs in formulations containing CH-Sq was slightly slower than that in formulations containing CH-Cr and CH-Sh. Nevertheless, the mixture containing CH-Sh5Sq5 speeded up the drug release from CH-Sq formulations for both drugs. This makes it necessary to use more than one source of CH in the drug formulations. Thus, a combination of CH sources is recommended to attain optimized tablet physical properties and optimum drug release profile.

Mixtures of CH polymorphs demonstrate an optimized action when compacted. This results in a satisfactory mixture suitable to be compressed and compacted. At first glance, this may suggest to gather remains from sea food packaging industry without classification, but such process shall yield CH with different characteristics depending on the percentage of squid remains involved in extraction process. Such operational procedure will result in lack of consistency in the extracted CH in each produced batch, which would in turn influence the manufactured dosage forms. Consequently, separating the organisms before CH extraction would yield a homogeneous CH powder, enabling pharmaceutical formulator to take advantage when formulating dosage forms by adding the required polymorph in the formulation stage depending on required properties. Alpha polymorph CH is reasonably less expensive than beta polymorph which reserve this polymorph for certain required formulation functions. Indeed, this polymorph can be used to form tablets or films with excellent hardness capable of withstanding mechanical vibrations encountered throughout manufacturing, packaging and transferring steps. The main advantage of CH as an excipient is its ability to form hard compacts with a very short disintegration time. This gives this excipient an advantage compared to excipients based on cellulose derivatives, without any need to add a disintegrating agent to formulations containing CH. Thus, CH is a suitable future excipient. Differences in sources or polymorphic form extend its usage particularly as a solid dosage form excipient suitable for drugs required to be released in a very-short time. CH must be extracted using a single species process, whereby the extracted CH has a well-defined function.

As a general remark, these raw excipients must be exposed to a process of compaction; for example, by using roller compaction, as has been previously reported by our group [8]. The variation in compaction properties between different sources of CH and their mixtures suggest that separation of sources yielding different polymorphs has an advantage in producing excipients with functional properties e.g., as a disintegrant or as filler. CH is chemically and pharmacologically inert and can be considered as a future pharmaceutical excipient.

4. Materials and Methods

4.1. Materials

CH powder from shrimp (CH-Sh) was obtained from G.T.C. Bio Corporation (Qingdao, China). The powder was sieved and the portion of particle size less than 90 μm was used for further analysis, characterization and testing. CH samples from crab (CH-Cr) and squid (CH-Sq) were also obtained from G.T.C. Bio Corporation in the form of flakes and fibers, respectively. They were ground using a ring mill, the powder was sieved and the portion of particle size less than 90 μm was used for further analysis, characterization, and testing. To study the effect of mixing chitin from different sources, CH-Sh was chosen as representative of α-chitin, and mixed with CH-Sq (β-chitin) using the compositions shown in Table 9; these mixtures were characterized and analyzed.

Table 9. Composition of CH mixtures (weight %).

Mixture	CH-Sh	CH-Sq
CH-Sh9Sq1	90	10
CH-Sh7Sq3	70	30
CH-Sh5Sq5	50	50

4.2. Methods

4.2.1. True, Bulk, and Tapped Density Measurement, and Flow Determination

The bulk density of chitin powder samples (shrimp, crab and squid) in g/mL was measured by pouring the powder into a 25 mL volumetric cylinder. The bulk density of all samples was calculated as the ratio of the mass over the volume it occupies. Tapped density measurements were carried out by physical tapping of the cylinder for 100 mechanical taps then dividing the mass over the tapped volume. The cylinder was tapped again for 200 mechanical taps. If the decrease in volume (V_{100}–V_{200}) was less than 2 mL then the V_{200} was considered. If the difference was greater than 2 mL, the increments are repeated, such as the 200 taps, until the difference between succeeding measurements was less than or equal to 2 mL.

The reduction in powder bulk volume due to tapping is considered to be an indication of powder flowability which was evaluated by the Hausner ratio (HR) and Carr Index (CI). As HR and CI increase in value, the flowability is reduced.

HR is calculated using Equation (1), and CI is calculated using Equation (2):

$$HR = \frac{\rho_{tapped}}{\rho_{bulk}} \quad (1)$$

$$CI = 100 \times \left(\frac{\rho_{tapped} - \rho_{bulk}}{\rho_{bulk}} \right) \tag{2}$$

Flow interpretation criteria based on HR and CI is given in the literature [21]. True density was determined by fitting compaction data, i.e., compaction pressure versus tablet density, according to the method reported by Sun [30].

4.2.2. Water Content Determination

CH samples were analyzed for water content by placing the samples in a porcelain crucible and drying them in a conventional oven at 105 °C to constant weight.

4.2.3. Determination of the Porosity of Powders

Brunauer-Emmett-Teller (BET) pore volume, and pore diameter were determined by physical adsorption of nitrogen gas using a Nova 2200 multi-speed high gas sorption analyzer (version 6.11, Quantachrome Co., Syosset, NY, USA). Samples were subjected to nitrogen gas for adsorption under isothermal conditions at 77 K. The samples were initially placed in a vacuum oven at 60 °C for 24 h. An empty reference cell (Sartorius, analytic, A120s, Göttingen, Germany) and the sample (~500 mg) were placed in the chambers.

4.2.4. FTIR Spectrophotometry

IR spectrophotometry was carried out using Perkin Elmer Spectrum Two UATR FTIR spectrometer (Akron, OH, USA) with a resolution of 4 cm^{-1}, data interval of 2 cm^{-1} and a scan speed of 0.2 cm/s operating in the range of 450–4000 cm^{-1}. The ATR sample base plate was equipped with a Diamond ZnSe crystal; an infrared background was collected for all FTIR measurements. Samples (2–5 mg) were placed on the ATR crystal and a pressure was applied to compress the sample in order to obtain the spectra. The IR spectra of CH samples (raw, ball milled, and roller compacted) were examined.

4.2.5. X-ray Powder Diffraction (XRPD), Crystalline Index (ICR) and Degree of Deacetalyion (DDA)

XRPD test was carried out using an X-ray powder diffractometer (Bruker, Karlsruhe, Germany) in 2-theta range of 2–40° 2θ in reflection mode. The X-ray compartment is a D2 Phaser comprising a copper tube, using Kα X-rays of 300 watts of power at 1.54184 Å wavelength. DIFFRAC.SUITE™ computer software was used to analyze the data obtained.

The crystalline index (I_{CR}) was calculated from the normalized diffractograms. The intensities of the peaks at 110 lattices (I_{110}, at $2\theta \cong 20°$ corresponding to maximum intensity) and at $2\theta \cong 16°$ (amorphous diffraction) were used to calculate I_{CR} using Equation (3) according to Al Sagheer et al. [22]:

$$I_{CR} = 100 \times \left(\frac{I_{110} - I_{am}}{I_{110}} \right) \tag{3}$$

Chitin degree of deacetylation (DDA) is estimated using a method reported Zhang et al. [24], which reported the linear correlation between the crystalline index (I_{CR}) and the degree of chitin deacetylation (DDA) shown in Equation (4):

$$I_{CR}(\%) = 103.97 - 0.7529\ DDA(\%) \tag{4}$$

4.2.6. Scanning Electron Microscopy (SEM)

The morphology of samples was determined using a Inspect F50 SEM (FEI Company, Eindhoven, The Netherlands), operated at an accelerating voltage from 1–30 kV. Samples (≈0.5 mg) were mounted on graphite tape to an aluminum stub. The powder was then sputter-coated with platinum (Emitech K550X, Qourum Technology, Lewes, UK).

4.2.7. Compression Analysis

CH powder samples (crab, shrimp, squid, and their mixtures) were compressed into tablets using an instrumental single punch bench top tablet press (GTP-1, Gamlen Tablet Press Ltd., Nottingham, UK). Compression was carried out at a punch speed of 60 mm/min by applying five different loads: 100, 200, 300, 400, 500 kg. The samples poured into the die of the GTP had a common weight of 100 ± 1 mg. The diameter of the die was 6 mm. The machine was run by software to display the force-displacement (F-D) curve. Kawakita and Heckel models (Equations (5) and (7), respectively) were utilized to describe the compression analysis of the powders [31,32].

Kawakita analysis describes a linear relationship between the ratio P/C and P, Equation (5), where P is the pressure in MPa, and C is the volume reduction. From the slope and intercept of this relationship, constants 'a' and 'b' can be deduced; 'a' represents the maximum volume reduction that can be attained by the powder. '$1/b$' or 'P_K' is another parameter that represents the force required to reduce the powder bed volume to half its maximum value:

$$\frac{P}{C} = \frac{P}{a} + \frac{1}{ab} \tag{5}$$

Volume reduction (C) is calculated using Equation (6):

$$C = 1 - \frac{\rho_b}{\rho_c} \tag{6}$$

where ρ_b and ρ_c are bulk and compact densities (kg/m^3), respectively.

Heckel analysis describes a relationship between the logarithm of the inverse of compact porosity (ε) and the pressure applied, as shown in Equation (7):

$$\ln \frac{1}{\varepsilon} = KP + A \tag{7}$$

Porosity is calculated using the Equation (8):

$$\varepsilon = 1 - \rho_r \tag{8}$$

where ρ_r is the relative density of the compact, and is calculated using the Equation (9):

$$\rho_r = \frac{\rho_c}{\rho_T} \tag{9}$$

where ρ_c and ρ_T are compact and true densities (kg/m^3), respectively.

The inverse of the Heckel equation slope or '$1/K$' is an important parameter which assigns Sh5Sq5the type of deformation of materials; whether plastic/elastic or brittle-fracture. This parameter is called the yield pressure and is signified by the symbol 'P_Y'.

4.2.8. Application of Chitin Excipient Using Metronidazole/Spiramycin as Model Drugs

For dissolution analysis, a sample (100 g) comprising 56.3 g of spiramycin, 30.1 g of metronidazole, 1.9 g of sorbitol powder (solubilizer), and 8.7 g of CH (either CH-Cr, CH-Sh, CH-Sq, or the mixture CH-Sh5Sq5) were granulated with 100 mL of 3% *w/w* povidone K30 aqueous solution. The granules were dried at 60 °C for 3 h, then sieved at mesh #18 (particle size = 1 mm). A sample of 415 mg was compressed using a Manesty single punch tablet machine (Manesty F3 single stroke tablet press; West Pharma Services Ltd., Dorset, UK) at an applied force of 35 kN using a 10 mm circular shallow biconvex punch. Rodogyl® tablets were used as a reference.

Apparatus II (USP) dissolution tests were performed using an Erweka DT6 system (Langen, Germany) with paddles running at 50 rpm. 900 mL of 0.1 N HCl was used as the dissolution medium. The amount of drug released was analyzed by measuring the absorbance using a UV spectrophotometer (LABINDIA UV/VIS, UV 3000, Maharashtra, India) at a wavelength of 320 nm for metronidazole, and of 230 nm for spiramycin.

For crushing force and disintegration tests, 415 mg of chitin powder (either CH-Cr, CH-Sh, CH-Sq, or the mixtures CH-Sh9Sq1, CH-Sh7Sq3, and CH-Sh5Sq5) was compressed using the Manesty single punch tablets machine at an applied force of 35 kN using a 10 mm circular shallow biconvex punch. The average crushing force and disintegration time of 10 chitin tablets produced were measured using crushing force tester (Pharma Test PTB 311E. Hainburg, Germany) and disintegration tester (CALEVA, Dorest, UK), respectively.

5. Conclusions

Chitin is chemically and pharmacologically inert and can be considered as a future pharmaceutical excipient especially for immediate release tablets, as it can form hard compacts with a very short disintegration time. Depending on the source, CH varies marginally in compression properties. Consequently, CH must be extracted using a single species process. Variations in polymorphic form would not hinder the use of chitin as a pharmaceutical excipient. In order for an excipient comprising chitin to perform ideally in compression and compaction properties, α- and β- polymorphic types would be mixed. In this perspective, α-CH will provide the high bulk density, good flowability, and low water absorption aspects, whereas the β-polymorph will provide the mechanical strength. These aspects were attributed to the difference in crystallinity, fibrous nature, pore size and pore volume of α- and β-CHs.

Author Contributions: Conceptualization, D.A.F. and A.A.B.; data curation, L.A.-H. and I.R.; formal analysis, L.A.-H. and D.A.F.; investigation, L.A.-H., D.A.F. and A.A.B.; methodology, L.A.-H. and D.A.F.; project administration, A.A.B.; software, L.A.-H.; supervision, D.A.F.; writing—original draft, L.A.-H., D.A.F., I.R. and A.A.B.; writing—review & editing, B.Z.C. and A.A.B. All authors have read and agreed to the published version of the manuscript.

Acknowledgments: The authors would like to thank The University of Jordan and University of Greenwich for their ongoing support. The authors also wish to thank the Jordanian Pharmaceutical Manufacturing Co. (JPM) for providing materials, laboratory and testing facilities. The authors would like also to thank Hatim Al-Khatib from the School of Pharmacy, University of Jordan for providing lab facilities for some sample analysis.

References

1. Daraghmeh, N.H.; Chowdhry, B.Z.; Leharne, S.A.; Al Omari, M.M.; Badwan, A.A. Chitin. *Profiles Drug Subst. Excip. Relat. Methodol.* **2011**, *36*, 35–102. [CrossRef]
2. Roberts, G.A.F. *Chitin Chemistry*; Palgrave Macmillan Press Ltd.: London, UK, 1992; pp. 54–115.
3. Budavari, S. (Ed.) *The Merck Index*, 13th ed.; Merck and Co.: Kenilworth, NJ, USA, 2001.
4. Uragami, T.; Tokura, S. *Material Science of Chitin and Chitosan*; Springer: Berlin, Germany; Kodansha: Tokyo, Japan, 2006.
5. Bellich, B.; D'Agostino, I.; Semeraro, S.; Gamini, A.; Cesàro, A. "The Good, the Bad and the Ugly" of Chitosans. *Mar. Drugs* **2016**, *14*, 99. [CrossRef]
6. Badwan, A.A.; Rashid, I.; Al Omari, M.M.; Darras, F.H. Chitin and Chitosan as Direct Compression Excipients in Pharmaceutical Applications. *Mar. Drugs* **2015**, *13*, 1519–1547. [CrossRef]
7. Abu Fara, D.; Rashid, I.; Al-Hmoud, L.; Chowdhry, B.Z.; Badwan, A.A. A New Perspective of Multiple Roller Compaction of Microcrystalline Cellulose for Overcoming Re-Compression Drawbacks in Tableting Processing. *Appl. Sci.* **2020**, *10*, 4787. [CrossRef]
8. Abu Fara, D.; Al-Hmoud, L.; Rashid, I.; Chowdhry, B.Z.; Badwan, A.A. Understanding the Performance of a Novel Direct Compression Excipient Comprising Roller Compacted Chitin. *Mar. Drugs* **2020**, *18*, 115. [CrossRef] [PubMed]

9. Patole, R.K.; Sav, A.K.; Amin, P.D. A Novel Directly Compressible Co-Processed Excipient for Sustained Release Formulation. *J. Appl. Pharm. Sci.* **2013**, *3*, 89–97.
10. El-hefian, E.A.; Yahaya, A.H. Rheological study of chitosan and its blends: An overview. *Maejo Int. J. Sci. Technol.* **2010**, *4*, 210–220.
11. Rashid, I.; Eftaiha, A.F.; Badwan, A.; Al-Remawi, M. Chitin–Silicon dioxide coprecipitate as a novel superdisintegrant. *J. Pharm. Sci.* **2008**, *97*, 4955–4969. [CrossRef] [PubMed]
12. Alonso, B.; Belamie, E. Chitin–Silica Nanocomposites by Self-Assembly. *Angew. Chem. Int. Ed.* **2010**, *49*, 8201–8204. [CrossRef]
13. Rojas, J.; Buckner, I.; Kumar, V. Co-proccessed excipients with enhanced direct compression functionality for improved tableting performance. *Drug Dev. Ind. Pharm.* **2012**, *38*, 1159–1170. [CrossRef]
14. Chaheen, M.; Sanchez-Ballester, N.M.; Bataille, B.; Yassine, A.; Belamie, E.; Sharkawi, T. Development of co-processed chitin-calcium carbonate as multifunctional tablet excipient for direct compression. *J. Pharm. Sci.* **2018**, *107*, 2152–2159. [CrossRef] [PubMed]
15. Chaheen, M.; Bataille, B.; Yassine, A.; Belamie, E. Development of Co-processed Chitin-Calcium Carbonate as Multifunctional Tablet Excipient for Direct Compression, Part 2: Tableting Properties. *J. Pharm. Sci.* **2019**, *108*, 3319–3328. [CrossRef] [PubMed]
16. Daraghmeh, N.; Chowdhry, B.Z.; Leharne, S.A.; Al Omari, M.M.H.; Badwan, A.A. Co-Processed Chitin-Mannitol as a New Excipient for Oro-Dispersible Tablets. *Mar. Drugs* **2015**, *13*, 1739–1764. [CrossRef]
17. Gana, F.Z.; Rashid, I.; Badwan, A.; Alkhamis, K.A. Determination of Solid-State Acidity of Chitin–Metal Silicates and their Effect on the Degradation of Cephalosporin Antibiotics. *J. Pharm. Sci.* **2012**, *101*, 2398–2407. [CrossRef] [PubMed]
18. Wei, Y.; Huang, Y.H.; Cheng, K.; Song, C. Investigations of the Infuences of Processing Conditions on the Properties of Spray Dried Chitosan Tripolyphosphate Particles loaded with Theophylline. *Sci. Rep.* **2020**, *10*, 1155. [CrossRef]
19. Abu Fara, D.; Rashid, I.; Alkhamis, K.; Al-Omari, M.; Chowdhry, B.Z.; Badwan, A.A. Modification of a-lactose monohydrate as a direct compression excipient using roller compaction. *Drug Dev. Ind. Pharm.* **2018**, *44*, 2038–2047. [CrossRef]
20. Abu Fara, D. A comparison of industrial lactose obtained by roller compaction with spray dried lactose and α-lactose monohydrate using compression analysis techniques. *J. Excip. Food Chem.* **2019**, *10*, 41–54.
21. The United States Pharmacopeia. Powder Flow, Page 618 of PF 28(2) [March–April 2002]. 9D. Available online: https://www.usp.org/sites/default/files/usp/ducument/harmonization/gen-chapter/g05_pf_30_6_2004.pdf (accessed on 15 October 2020).
22. Al Sagheer, F.; Al-Sughayer, M.; Muslim, S.; Elsabee, M. Extraction and characterization of chitin and chitosan from marine sources in Arabian Gulf. *Carbohydr. Polym.* **2009**, *77*, 410–419. [CrossRef]
23. Jang, M.K.; Kong, B.G.; Jeong, Y.I.; Lee, C.H.; Nah, J.W. Physicochemical characterization of α-chitin, β-chitin, and γ-chitin separated from natural resources. *J. Polym. Sci. A Polym. Chem.* **2004**, *42*, 3423–3432. [CrossRef]
24. Zhang, Y.; Xue, C.; Xue, Y.; Gao, R.; Zhang, X. Determination of the degree of deacetylation of chitin and chitosan by X-ray powder diffraction. *Carbohydr. Res.* **2005**, *340*, 1914–1917. [CrossRef]
25. Hepburn, H.R.; Chandler, H.D. Tensile Mechanical Properties and Transconformational Changes of Chitins. In Proceedings of the First International Conference on Chitin/Chitosan, MIT Sea Grant Program, Cambridge, MA, USA, 11–13 April 1977; pp. 124–143.
26. National Marine Fisheries Service. Fisheries of the United States, 2018. U.S. Department of Commerce, NOAA Current Fishery Statistics No. 2018; 2020. Available online: https://www.fisheries.noaa.gov/national/commercial-fishing/fisheries-united-states-2018 (accessed on 15 October 2020).
27. Kaya, M.; Lelešius, E.; Nagrockaitė, R.; Sargin, I.; Arslan, G.; Mol, A.; Baran, T.; Can, E.; Bitim, B. Differentiations of Chitin Content and Surface Morphologies of Chitins Extracted from Male and Female Grasshopper Species. *PLoS ONE* **2015**, *10*, e0115531. [CrossRef] [PubMed]
28. Alakayleh, F.; Rashid, I.; Al Omari, M.M.; Al-Sou'Od, K.; Chowdhry, B.Z.; Badwan, A.A. Compression profiles of different molecular weight chitosans. *Powder Technol.* **2016**, *299*, 107–118. [CrossRef]
29. Abrégée, F. Spiramycine/Metronidazole Biogaran 1,5 MUI/250 Mg Cp Pellic. Available online: https://www.vidal.fr/Medicament/spiramycine_metronidazole_biogaran-68905.htm (accessed on 15 October 2020).
30. Sun, C.C. A Novel Method for Deriving True Density of Pharmaceutical Solids Including Hydrates and Water-Containing Powders. *J. Pharm. Sci.* **2004**, *93*, 646–653. [CrossRef] [PubMed]

Permissions

All chapters in this book were first published by MDPI; hereby published with permission under the Creative Commons Attribution License or equivalent. Every chapter published in this book has been scrutinized by our experts. Their significance has been extensively debated. The topics covered herein carry significant findings which will fuel the growth of the discipline. They may even be implemented as practical applications or may be referred to as a beginning point for another development.

The contributors of this book come from diverse backgrounds, making this book a truly international effort. This book will bring forth new frontiers with its revolutionizing research information and detailed analysis of the nascent developments around the world.

We would like to thank all the contributing authors for lending their expertise to make the book truly unique. They have played a crucial role in the development of this book. Without their invaluable contributions this book wouldn't have been possible. They have made vital efforts to compile up to date information on the varied aspects of this subject to make this book a valuable addition to the collection of many professionals and students.

This book was conceptualized with the vision of imparting up-to-date information and advanced data in this field. To ensure the same, a matchless editorial board was set up. Every individual on the board went through rigorous rounds of assessment to prove their worth. After which they invested a large part of their time researching and compiling the most relevant data for our readers.

The editorial board has been involved in producing this book since its inception. They have spent rigorous hours researching and exploring the diverse topics which have resulted in the successful publishing of this book. They have passed on their knowledge of decades through this book. To expedite this challenging task, the publisher supported the team at every step. A small team of assistant editors was also appointed to further simplify the editing procedure and attain best results for the readers.

Apart from the editorial board, the designing team has also invested a significant amount of their time in understanding the subject and creating the most relevant covers. They scrutinized every image to scout for the most suitable representation of the subject and create an appropriate cover for the book.

The publishing team has been an ardent support to the editorial, designing and production team. Their endless efforts to recruit the best for this project, has resulted in the accomplishment of this book. They are a veteran in the field of academics and their pool of knowledge is as vast as their experience in printing. Their expertise and guidance has proved useful at every step. Their uncompromising quality standards have made this book an exceptional effort. Their encouragement from time to time has been an inspiration for everyone.

The publisher and the editorial board hope that this book will prove to be a valuable piece of knowledge for researchers, students, practitioners and scholars across the globe.

List of Contributors

Fátima García-Villén, Rita Sánchez-Espejo, Ana Borrego-Sánchez, Pilar Cerezo and César Viseras
Department of Pharmacy and Pharmaceutical Technology, Faculty of Pharmacy, University of Granada, Campus of Cartuja, 18071 Granada, Spain
Andalusian Institute of Earth Sciences, CSIC-UGR, Avenida de las Palmeras 4, 18100 Armilla, Granada, Spain

Luana Perioli
Department of Pharmaceutical Sciences, University of Perugia, 06123 Perugia, Italy

Giuseppina Sandri
Department of Pharmaceutical Sciences, Faculty of Pharmacy, University of Pavia, viale Taramelli 12, 27100 Pavia, Italy
Department of Drug Sciences, Faculty of Pharmacy, University of Pavia, Taramelli Street 12, 27100 Pavia, Italy

Angela Faccendini, Marco Ruggeri, Silvia Rossi, Maria Cristina Bonferoni, Dalila Miele, Pietro Grisoli, Barbara Vigani and Franca Ferrari
Department of Drug Sciences, Faculty of Pharmacy, University of Pavia, Taramelli Street 12, 27100 Pavia, Italy

Marysol Longo
Department of Drug Sciences, University of Pavia, Viale Taramelli 12, 27100 Pavia, Italy
Trinity Translational Medicine Institute, Trinity College Dublin, Dublin 8, Dublin, Ireland

Adriele Prina-Mello
Trinity Translational Medicine Institute, Trinity College Dublin, Dublin 8, Dublin, Ireland

Cesar Viseras and Carola Aguzzi
Department of Pharmacy and Pharmaceutical Technology, Faculty of Pharmacy, University of Granada, Campus of Cartuja s/n, 18071 Granada, Spain

Cinzia Pagano and Maurizio Ricci
Department of Pharmaceutical Sciences, University of Perugia, 06123 Perugia Italy

Loredana Latterini
Department of Chemistry, Biology and Biotechnology, University of Perugia, 06123 Perugia, Italy

Alessandro Di Michele
Department of Physics and Geology, University of Perugia, 06123 Perugia, Italy

Francesca Luzi and Debora Puglia
Civil and Environmental Engineering Department, University of Perugia, UdR INSTM, 05100 Terni, Italy

César Antonio Viseras Iborra
Department of Pharmacy and Pharmaceutical Technology, Faculty of Pharmacy, University of Granada, Campus of Cartuja, 18071 Granada, Spain

Stefania Racovita, Ana Maria Macsim and Silvia Vasiliu
"Petru Poni" Institute of Macromolecular Chemistry, Grigore Ghica Voda Alley, No. 41A, 700487 Iasi, Romania

Nicolae Baranov
Department of Natural and Synthetic Polymers, Faculty of Chemical Engienering and Environmental Protection, "Gheorghe Asachi" Technical University of Iasi, Prof. Dr. Docent Dimitrie Mangeron Street, No. 73, 700050 Iasi, Romania
Faculty of Chemistry, "Al. I. Cuza" University, Carol 1 Bvd., No. 11, 700506 Iasi, Romania

Catalina Lionte
Faculty of Medicine, "Gr. T. Popa" University of Medicine and Pharmacy, Universitatii Street, No.16, 700115 Iasi, Romania

Corina Cheptea
Department of Biomedical Sciences, Faculty of Biomedical Bioengineering, "Gr. T. Popa" University of Medicine and Pharmacy, Kogalniceanu Street No. 9-13, 700454 Iasi, Romania

Valeriu Sunel
Faculty of Chemistry, "Al. I. Cuza" University, Carol 1 Bvd., No. 11, 700506 Iasi, Romania

Marcel Popa
Department of Natural and Synthetic Polymers, Faculty of Chemical Engienering and Environmental Protection, "Gheorghe Asachi" Technical University of Iasi, Prof. Dr. Docent Dimitrie Mangeron Street, No. 73, 700050 Iasi, Romania
Academy of Romanian Scientists, Splaiul Independentei Street No. 54, 050085 Bucuresti, Romania

Jacques Desbrieres
Institut des Sciences Analytiques et de Physico-Chimie Pour l'Environnement et les Materiaux (IPREM), Pau and Pays de l'Adour University (UPPA), UMR CNRS 5254, Helioparc Pau Pyrenees, 2, av. President Angot, 64053 Pau CEDEX 09, France

Francesca Maestrelli, Marzia Cirri, Paola Mura and Letizia Brunetti
Department of Chemistry, University of Florence, via Schiff 6, Sesto Fiorentino, 50019 Florence, Italy

César Viseras Iborra
Department of Pharmacy and Pharmaceutical Technology, University of Granada, Campus de Cartuja, s/n 18071 Granada, Spain
Andalusian Institute of Earth Sciences, CSIC-University of Granada, Avda. de Las Palmeras 4, 18100 Armilla (Granada), Spain

C. Ignacio Sainz-Díaz
Instituto Andaluz de Ciencias de la Tierra, CSIC-University of Granada, Av. de las Palmeras 4, 18100 Granada, Spain

Yangyang Luo, Ahmed Humayun, Teresa A. Murray, Benjamin S. Kemp, Antwine McFarland and Xuan Liu
Molecular Sciences & Nanotechnology, Louisiana Tech University, Ruston, LA 71272, USA

David K. Mills
School of Biological Sciences and the Center for Biomedical Engineering, Louisiana Tech University, Ruston, LA 71272, USA

Maurizio Valleri
Menarini Manufacturing Logistics and Services, s.r.l. (AMMLS), 50019 Florence, Italy

Lucia Cucca
Department of Chemistry, University of Pavia, viale Taramelli 12, 27100 Pavia, Italy

Linda Al-Hmoud and Deeb Abu Fara
Chemical Engineering Department, School of Engineering, University of Jordan, Amman 11942, Jordan

Babur Z. Chowdhry
School of Science, Faculty of Engineering & Science, University of Greenwich, Medway Campus, Chatham Maritime, Kent ME4 4TB, UK

Iyad Rashid and Adnan A. Badwan
Research and Innovation Centre, The Jordanian Pharmaceutical Manufacturing Company (JPM), Naor 11710, Jordan

Index

www.ingramcontent.com/pod-product-compliance
Lightning Source LLC
LaVergne TN
LVHW082209200926
848484LV00008B/2235